REPRODUCTIVE MEDICINE

A Millennium Review

The Proceedings of the 10th World Congress
on Human Reproduction

Edited by

Elsimar M. Coutinho
and
Paulo Spinola

Federal University of Bahia, School of Medicine
Salvador, Bahia, Brazil

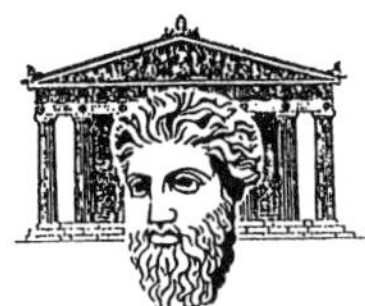

The Parthenon Publishing Group

International Publishers in Medicine, Science & Technology

NEW YORK   LONDON

Library of Congress Cataloging-in-Publication Data

Data available on application

British Library Cataloguing in Publication Data

Reproductive medicine : a millennium review
  1. Human reproduction
  I. Coutinho, Elsimar M.   II. Spinola, P.
  616.6
ISBN 1-85070-088-5

Published in the USA by
The Parthenon Publishing Group Inc.
One Blue Hill Plaza
PO Box 1564, Pearl River
New York 10965, USA

Published in the UK and Europe by
The Parthenon Publishing Group Limited
Casterton Hall, Carnforth
Lancs. LA6 2LA, UK

Copyright © 1999 Parthenon Publishing Group

First published 1999

Typeset by AMA DataSet Ltd., Preston, UK
Printed and bound in Brazil

REPRODUCTIVE MEDICINE

A Millennium Review

Contents

List of principal contributors

R. Abdelmassih
Rua Maestro Elias Lobo, 805
Jardim Paulista
01433-000 São Paulo
Brazil

C. Athayde
Maternidade Climério de Oliveira
Rua do Limoeiro, No. 1
Salvador
40055-150 Bahia
Brazil

G. Benagiano
Ministerio della Sanita
Istituto Superiore di Sanita
Viale Regina Elena, 299
00161 Rome
Italy

Z. Ben-Rafael
Department of Obstetrics and Gynecology
Rabin Medical Center
Beilinson Campus
49372 Petah-Tikva
Israel

M. Busacca
Second Department of Obstetrics &
    Gynecology
University of Milan
Via Commenda 12
20122 Milan
Italy

J. Cohen
Centre de Stérilité de L'Hôpital de Sevres
8, rue de Marignan
75008 Paris
France

E. M. Coutinho
CEPARH
Rua Caetano Moura, 35
Salvador
40055-150 Bahia
Brazil

P. G. Crosignani
First Department of Obstetrics and
    Gynecology
University of Milan
Via Commenda 12
20122 Milan
Italy

S. Daya
McMaster University
1200 Main Street West
Hamilton
Ontario L8N 3Z5
Canada

L. Devoto
Institute of Maternal & Child Research
Department of Obstetrics & Gynecology
School of Medicine
University of Chile
PO Box 226–3
Santiago
Chile

D. de Ziegler
Columbia Laboratories
19 rue du Général Foy
75008 Paris
France

A. Faúndes
Centro de Pesquisas das Doencas
Materno-Infantis de Campinas (CEMICAMP)
Caixa Postal 6181
13081-970 Campinas
São Paulo
Brazil

J. Frick
Department of Urology
Landeskrankenanstalten Salzburg
Urologische Abteilung
Anton-Rauchstrasse 8d
6020 Innsbruck
Austria

A. R. Genazzani
Department of Reproductive Medicine and
    Child Development
University of Pisa
Via Roma 57
56100 Pisa
Italy

J. Guillebaud
Margaret Pyke Family Planning Centre
73 Charlotte Street
London W1P 1LB
UK

E. D. B. Johansson
The Population Council
Center for Biomedical Research
1230 York Avenue
New York
New York 10021
USA

F. Labrie
Department of Medicine & Laboratory of
    Molecular Endocrinology
CHUL Research Center
2705 Laurier Boulevard
Québec G1V 4G2
Canada

O. A. Ladipo
Department of Obstetrics & Gynaecology
The Royal Gwent Hospital
Newport
Gwent NP9 2UB
UK

B. Lunenfeld
7, Harav Ashi Street
Tel Aviv 69395
Israel

H. Maia
Endoscopy Unit
CEPARH
Rua Caetano Moura, 35
Salvador
40055-150 Bahia
Brazil

T. Maruo
Department of Obstetrics and Gynecology
Kobe University School of Medicine
7-5-1 Kusunoki-cho, Chuo-ku
Kobe 650-0017
Japan

L. Mettler
Department of Obstetrics & Gynecology
University of Kiel
Michaelisstr. 16
24105 Kiel
Germany

F. Petraglia
Department of Surgical Sciences
University of Udine
Piazz. le S Maria della Misericordia
33100 Udine
Italy

C. A. Petta
Caixa Postal 6181
13083-970, Campinas
São Paulo
Brazil

L. F. Pianowski
Hebron S/A
Rod. BR 232
Distrito Industrial
Caruaru
PE 55000-000
Brazil

M. M. Reidenberg
Weill Medical College of Cornell University
1300 York Avenue, Box 70
New York
New York 10021
USA

J. A. Rock
Department of Gynecology and Obstetrics
1639 Pierce Drive
Atlanta
Georgia 30322
USA

O. Rodriguez-Armas
Centro Medico de Caracas
Ed. Anexo, Cons. 8-A
San Bernardino
Caracas 14196
Venezuela

S. J. Segal
The Population Council
One Dag Hammarskyold Plaza
New York
New York 10017
USA

K. Semm
5160 East Oakmont Drive
Tucson
Arizona 85718
USA

M. Seppälä
Department of Obstetrics and Gynecology
Helsinki University Central Hospital
Haartmaninkatu 2
00290 Helsinki
Finland

R. Sitruk-Ware
Department of Medicine, Research &
    Development
Exelgyn Laboratories
6, Rue Christophe Colomb
75008 Paris
France

S. D. Spandorfer
The Center for Reproductive Medicine &
    Fertility
505 E. 70th Street, HMT-369
The New York Hospital – Cornell Medical
    Center
New York
New York 10021
USA

L. Speroff
Department of Obstetrics & Gynecology
Reproductive Endocrinology
School of Medicine
Oregon Health Sciences University
3181 SW, Sam Jackson Park Road, UHN 70
Portland
Oregon 97201-3098
USA

P. Spinola
Maternidade Climério de Oliveira
Federal University of Bahia
Rua do Limoeoiro No 1
Salvador
40055-150 Bahia
Brazil

J. F. Strauss, III
University of Pennsylvania Medical Center
Hospital of the University of Pennsylvania
778 Clinical Research Building
415 Curie Boulevard
Philadelphia
Pennsylvania 19104-6142
USA

G. P. Talwar
International Center for Genetic Engineering
    and Biotechnology
Aruna Asaf Ali Marg
New Delhi 110067
India

A. Watrelot
Centre de Recherche et d'Etude de la Sterilité
Clinique Sainte Anne Lumiere
85 cours Albert Thomas
69003 Lyon
France

Foreword

It is with great joy and personal satisfaction that I present this collection of selected papers to be delivered at the 10th World Congress on Human Reproduction, which is being held in Salvador, Bahia, Brazil, May 4–8, 1999. This congress closes a cycle of World Congresses on Human Reproduction, which started 25 years ago in Rio de Janeiro, and will be the last of the 20th century. The participants of the 10th World Congress will be taking stock of what has been accomplished so far in this area of medicine and will discuss their present work and their plans for the future. I am sure that this exercise will be enriching for everyone.

The second half of the 20th century has witnessed an extraordinary series of developments in reproductive medicine, which has created the impression that, in this area, anything is within the reach of scientists. The creation of life, considered by God-fearing mortals to be an exclusive privilege of the Almighty, seems to be just around the corner. The control of fertility by a pill almost free of side-effects is a triumph of reproductive medicine that is already 40 years old. Long-acting, injectable contraceptives, which have passed the test of time, are available everywhere in the world. The speed at which new discoveries in this area are made has fasci-

nated everyone but is a cause for concern for many of us. It is a fact that some of the new technologies to be presented during the 10th World Congress are so accessible that even unskilled and inexperienced students may soon be able to use them. Although this danger should be recognized, most of the contributors to this book agree that it should not be used as an excuse for obstructive legislation, which would inevitably be more harmful than beneficial.

The present volume includes reviews of work carried out in the past, as well as the presentation of work in progress in the fields of assisted reproductive technology, contraception, endocrinology of reproduction, endoscopy, menopause and sexuality. The excellent work by Parthenon Publishing is responsible for the availability of this book at the time of the congress. The authors are also to be praised for their collaboration and their speedy handling of the proofs. A special acknowledgement for her dedicated work in coordinating authors, editors, printers and publisher is due to Lesley Hanson de Moura.

Salvador
Bahia, Brazil
May, 1999

Elsimar M. Coutinho

Section I
Assisted reproductive technology

Reproductive medicine: past, present and future

Jean Cohen

Introduction

The occurrence of the first human birth by *in vitro* fertilization (IVF) 20 years ago was the outcome of a long process of development from times when a child was the product of chance to the situation today when birth is nearly under total control. Today, techniques of reproductive medicine allow the treatment of nearly all forms of infertility in a couple. Several hundreds of thousands of children have been born as a result of these techniques. Although worries still persist about the possible dangers, it is obvious that we will not stop progress and advancement in this field.

Reproductive medicine in the past

Study of the history of reproductive medicine is important because it can yield many lessons for the future[1]. Though medical knowledge on human reproduction is usually attributed to Hippocrates, we know that in the 5th Century B.C. people thought that males and females produced two seminal liquors, one stronger than the other: blending with the former would produce a male offspring, and blending with the latter a female one. In the following century Aristotle believed that the first stage of a human being was an egg found in females. The sperm had the power of giving it its shape. The male would bring the immaterial strength and the female the material substance.

For centuries people lived with this concept of pre-formation, even after De Graaf described the follicle in 1672 and Leuwenhoek the spermatozoa at the same time. Only in 1875 would Hertwig demonstrate in the urchin that one spermatozoa penetrates the egg. In 1833 Van Beneden, the cytologist, demonstrated that

gametes had only two chromosomes in the ascaria. The two chromosomes of the male nucleus would join the two of the female to form the nucleus of a new zygote. In 1903 a Danish pharmacist Johannsen coined the expression 'gene', from which Batesum in 1906 derived 'genetics', the new science. It was in 1953 that Watson, Crick and Wilkins discovered the helical structure of DNA and in 1956 that Tijo and Levan determined there to be 46 chromosomes in man.

Gynecologists made tremendous progress. While observing the effects of ovariectomy, they developed an understanding of the role of the ovary; menstrual cycles were understood and by injection of tissue extracts the first treatments were developed. In 1904 the notion of a hormone, as suggested by Baylin, was developed. The perfection of the different hormone treatments took many decades, and cannot be detailed here, but has resulted today in recombinant gonadotropins and antagonists of gonadotropin-releasing hormone (GnRH).

Studies on animal and then human fertilization took place in the second half of the 20th Century. The studies of Thibaut (1947), Chang (1957) and Edwards (1966) led to the birth of the first child conceived *in vitro* in 1978.

Reproductive medicine today

Twenty years after Louise Brown was born, the techniques of reproductive medicine have spread all over the world; several hundred thousand children have been born to infertile couples thanks to IVF, and many thousands thanks to intracytoplasmic sperm injection (ICSI). Rates of clinical pregnancies stand at 30% per

"

cycle with fresh embryos and at 50% if we also include frozen embryos. The rates of birth do not exceed 25% in the best cases.

ICSI applied to epididymal or testicular sperm in cases of azoospermia permits infertile men to become fathers. Concerns have been expressed about the potential and long-term hazards faced by IVF and ICSI children. These hazards include genetic damage, cytoplasmic changes, contamination of sperm, and other damage caused by the technique itself. So far, most reports on the incidence of malformations have been reassuring[2]. Similarly, fears about hazardous experiments in reproductive medicine have not been realized.

Techniques of reproductive medicine have become the most efficient treatment for infertile couples. Moreover, they allow the diagnosis as well as the prevention of certain hereditary transmitted diseases. However, we have to acknowledge that these techniques stress the distinction between sexuality and reproduction. They promote the development of pregnancies obtained by donor gametes. We shall examine later why these developments are so important for the future.

Even if the results of reproductive medicine have improved in terms of numbers of pregnancies in the last 20 years, it is still striking that it is necessary to use stimulation which sometimes leads to hyperstimulation and multiple pregnancies, that embryo development *in vitro* is still limited, and that implantation only occurs for less than 25% of embryos. The pregnancy rates currently obtained with IVF are at the most similar to those occurring *in vivo*. We still need to improve techniques to gain IVF pregnancy rates approaching 50% per embryo.

The immediate future

Less aggressive and much simpler ovarian stimulation

Since the birth of the first test-tube baby in 1978, assisted reproduction has developed a great deal (Steptoe and Edwards, 1978). While at that time only the natural cycle was considered able to allow fertilization of the oocyte, controlled ovarian hyperstimulation (COH) using urinary human menopausal gonadotropin (HMG) was a major step forward (Edwards, 1981; Trounson and co-workers 1981; Trounson, 1983). More oocytes to be rescued meant more oocytes to be fertilized *in vitro* and more embryos to be transferred during each attempt at treatment. This greatly raised the success rate in terms of pregnancies achieved.

However, the incidence of ovarian hyperstimulation syndrome (OHSS), the frequency of multiple pregnancies, and the concerns about ovarian cancer bring a demand for milder forms of ovarian stimulation. Different isoforms of recombinant follicle-stimulating hormone (FSH) seemingly stimulating follicles in different stages of growth may contribute to the solution of this problem. Recombinant luteinizing hormone (LH) will permit safer stimulation, because the half-life of LH is shorter than that of hMG.

The most promising aspect of introducing GnRH antagonists into COH may be the possibility of making this treatment less aggressive and much gentler than an agonistic long protocol, using old-fashioned schemes of stimulation such as clomiphene citrate (CC) in combination with hMG. It has been proved that ovarian stimulation with only CC for the purpose of ICSI is perfectly feasible, applying the simplest, least aggressive and least expensive form of stimulation (Ludwig and colleagues, 1997; Diedrich and associates, 1998)[3]. However, these results have been ignored. This could change very rapidly, if it could be shown that CC/hMG under the coverage of midcycle GnRH antagonist treatment (soft protocol) will allow the rescue of three to five mature metaphase II oocytes to be treated by ICSI. This would reduce the risk of OHSS to almost zero. The first feasibility studies using cetrorelix for this purpose are in progress at the moment.

The development of these new protocols for ovarian stimulation will permit less expensive, less aggressive treatments with a decrease of OHSS and multiple pregnancies.

In vitro maturation of gametes

Oocytes

Immature human oocytes in non-atretic pre-ovulatory follicles, like those in other mammals, can achieve maturation *in vitro* from germinal vesicle breakdown to the metaphase II arrest. *In vitro* maturation of mammalian oocytes was first reported in rabbits by Pincus and Enzmann (1935). *In vitro* maturation (IVM) and *in vitro* fertilization (IVF) of immature oocytes recovered from non-stimulated ovaries have been successfully performed in farm animals, resulting in pregnancy and birth (Goto *et al.*, 1988; Fukuda *et al.*, 1990). In humans, *in vitro* maturation studies were first performed by Pincus and Saunders (1939). During the 1960s, Edwards further demonstrated that *in vitro* matured human oocytes could be fertilized *in vitro* (Edwards *et al.*, 1969). Recently, the use of immature human eggs for the initiation of pregnancy has been achieved, (Cha *et al.*, 1991; Trounson *et al.*, 1994; Porcu *et al.*, 1998)[4–6] although the developmental competence of embryos resulting from *in vitro* matured and fertilized (IVM/IVF) human oocytes has rarely been reported. These techniques will suit women with polycystic ovaries where large numbers of oocytes can be recovered from follicles of 5–15 mm in diameter without any need for FSH treatment to stimulate follicle growth. Trounson and colleagues[6] observed that IVM/IVF embryos from polycystic ovary syndrome (PCOS) patients can be cultured for up to 68 h after insemination. In a case report, one early blastocyst was produced 110 h after intracytoplasmic sperm injection from IVM oocytes of a PCOS patient. The embryo was transferred to the patient's uterus and resulted in the birth of a baby.

Spermatocytes and spermatids

Spermatogenesis is a complex procedure of multiplication and in particular cellular diversification, the regulation of which is still imperfectly understood. Co-cultures of somatic and germinal cells, allowing more or less thorough spermatogenesis *in vitro*, have been tried with rats and mice.

Blastocyst culture

The goal of IVF and embryo culture is to provide high-quality embryos capable of continued development and implantation, and resulting in viable birth. Embryos are routinely transferred to the patient on day 2 or 3 of development, in order to avoid extended culture *in vitro*. Since the initial embryo culture studies, considerable progress has been made in culturing pre-implantation embryos.

New physiologically-based serum-free culture media have permitted the achievement of high rates of human blastocyst development. With the background information on embryo metabolic requirements and the need to avoid inhibiting conditions, a culture system involving biphasic media and the growth of embryos to blastocysts has been designed by Jones and associates[7]. More than 50% of zygotes develop to nascent blastocysts with a clearly defined trophoblast and inner cell mass in these culture conditions. Implantation rates of individual embryos are between 23 and 28% so that the transfer of two blastocysts will result in birth rates in excess of 40%. The pregnancy rate is significantly influenced by the number of embryos transferred, the morphology of the leading embryo transferred, and the mean morphology score of the transferred embryos. Maternal age, etiology of infertility and number of previous IVF cycles do not significantly influence the pregnancy rate.

Transfer of blastocysts leads to higher implantation and pregnancy rates and will therefore reduce the number of embryos required for transfer in order to achieve a pregnancy. Furthermore, the extended culture of human embryos will facilitate the identification of the most viable embryos by both natural selection during culture and by the application of new non-invasive tests of blastocyst viability.

However, we must take into consideration the very important results obtained by Scott and Smith[8]. They performed transfers 24–26 h post-insemination using two to six embryos (pronuclear stage) with the highest score. The score was based on alignment of pronuclei and nucleoli and the appearance of the cytoplasm. The best embryo score resulted in a 28%

implantation and 65% delivery rate. These data show that pronuclear embryos with good morphology can produce a very good pregnancy rate. The authors attempted to alter stimulation protocols of patients who routinely produced embryos with poor pronuclear morphology in an attempt to increase their chance of conception.

We must remember that embryo quality depends on the genetics of each individual embryo and its local environment.

Improvement of implantation rates

It is a disappointment when 85% of transferred human embryos resulting from IVF fail to implant in the uterus. Low implantation rates have been the largest obstacle to the success of IVF and its derivatives. The situation stands in stark contrast to the high implantation rates found after the transfer of embryos in domestic and laboratory animal species. New insights into the factors regulating implantation rates have now arisen.

Although the exact time of implantation remains unknown, in humans the process starts from day 7 after the LH peak. At the beginning of implantation the blastocyst has 100–120 cells. Of course, the blastocyst needs to have a normal development in order to permit its implantation. Three chronological stages precede implantation. First, opposition of the blastocyst resulting from myometrial activity (pinopodes); then adhesion of the blastocyst. A close functional relationship is formed between the outer membrane of the trophoblast cells and the luminal (surface) epithelium. Lastly, invasion of the trophoblast occurs. The second of these stages is the major event. We know now that molecular mechanisms permit apposition. These mechanisms include adhesion molecules or cell surface adhesion receptors: integrins, cadherins, selective and immunoglobulin superfamily. Cytokines exert their action locally by autocrine, paracrine and juxtacrine mechanisms (interleukin-1, LIF, CSF-1). Details of the cytokine cascade must be clarified as the first stage of implantation blends into successive stages of trophoblast penetration and implantation. The paracrine dialog between uterine epithelium and blastocyst is essential for implantation.

The suboptimal expression of some factors such as integrins in certain groups of women suffering from reproduction failure, either unexplained infertility, endometriosis or luteal phase defect, indicates that defective uterine receptivity and implantation failure may be the explanation for the infertility in these groups of women.

When these questions are answered we shall be able to apply the molecular aspects of implantation to clinical practice and improve the implantation rates of assisted reproductive techniques.

Further progress concerning the human embryo

Pre-implantation diagnosis

Pre-implantation genetic diagnosis (PGD) offers an alternative to prenatal diagnosis for couples at risk of transmitting a genetic defect and avoids the difficult decision of whether or not to terminate a pregnancy Liebaers, 1992; Handyside, 1997. PGD involving IVF allows the transfer of unaffected embryos to the uterus. During this procedure one or two blastomeres are biopsied and analyzed either by the polymerase chain reaction (PCR), allowing sexing of the embryos or the detection of a specific mutation, or by fluorescent *in situ* hybridization (FISH), allowing sexing of the embryos or the detection of some aneuploidies.

The identification of chromosome aneuploidies in some IVF patients by FISH for chromosomes X, Y, 13, 16, 18 and 21 show that 55–57% of all embryos at day 3 are abnormal[9]. Their identification and removal from the cohort of embryos growing to blastocysts will further increase the successful implantation and development to term of cleavage-stage embryos and blastocysts chosen for transfer.

Trophoblast biopsy of blastocysts enables the sampling of a relatively large number of cells[10]. These blastocysts can be DNA fingerprinted to identify individual embryos and screened for one or several mutations by fluorescent PCR techniques[11]. Genetic diagnosis at the blastocyst stage would involve screening less embryos. It is likely that preimplantation diagnosis will eventually become the first choice for couples who are at risk of transmitting serious genetic disease.

Actually 30 centers in the world offer this diagnostic procedure. The list of conditions for which PGD is performed is rapidly being extended and currently concerns genetic diseases but also age-related aneuploides. In the future PGD may also be of particular significance for assisted reproduction practices to improve the efficiency of IVF in couples of advanced maternal age.

Genetic therapy

Two levels can be considered. Incorporation of a foreign gene into the genoma by injection into one of the pronuclei after fertilization allows one to obtain transgenic animals. For the time being results are very disappointing in animals and will not adapt to humans. Transformed cells carrying the missing gene can be integrated into a deficient embryo: the individual which will result will be cured of the deficiency. For the time being successful experiments have only been carried out in mice, but it is not too early to foresee the application of this technique in humans. This new therapeutic approach constitutes a unique challenge for the third millenium. First of all, patients suffering from a fatal illness will find reason to hope. Also, scientists will be able to see new options for their research, with the prospect of creating new therapies, for example in the fields of cancer or vaccination.

Research on zygotes (pre-embryos)

Zygote research has already facilitated many advances in infertility treatments and diagnosis of inherited disorders. In the future, an area of research will be a better understanding of mechanisms of reproduction and early development.

One of the most promising areas of research concerns the fact that oocytes and fertilized eggs have a distinct polarity and their expression of RNA and proteins is highly polarized. Identification of numerous biochemical coumpounds and factors may provide a clue to understanding unexplained infertility. Understanding the mechanisms by which cells divide and differentiate in early development will be of great interest to our comprehension of cell growth and differentiation, and even cancer and more generally embryonic development.

Another promising area of research concerns embryonic stem cells. Human embryos can be grown in culture to the blastocyst stage and they will attach to the surface of plastic tissue culture dishes to form differentiated outgrowths. When grown under conditions that include fetal fibroblast feeder cells (STO cells), the inner cell mass cells will remain in a primary undifferentiated state and can be cultured to retain this apparent multipotential state for many months[12].

Genuine embryonic stem cells in mice will contribute to all the tissue types of the body, including undifferentiated germ cells and hence gametes. The multipotency of human and monkey embryonic stem cell lines have yet to be fully characterized. Actually the efficacy is very poor[13]. Given the multifactorial influences on lineage formation, it might be considered difficult to control embryonic stem cell differentiation into stable somatic cell types that could be multiplied for use in drug evaluation, transplantation and genetic manipulation. However, closely related human embryonal carcinoma cells have been stably differentiated into neuronal cells that are functional when transplanted. Cloned transgenic bovine embryos have been used to derive dopamine cells that are able to reverse abnormal motor performance in immunosuppressed parkinsonian rats. As a result, there is considerable interest in the derivation of multipotential human embryonic stem cells from human embryos for controlled differentiation and potential transplantation, gene therapy and drug evaluation purposes.

Nuclear transfer could be used to correct mitochondrial genetic disease. The nucleus of cells of the early developing embryo could be isolated from cytoplasmic mitochondrial elements and introduced into the enucleated cytoplasm of a donor oocyte known to have functionally normal mitochondria. The use of nuclear transfer for this purpose would be arguably ethical and experimental studies are likely to confirm the potential to eradicate the inheritance of mitochondrial defects for women.

Nuclear transfer can also be used to multiply ruminant embryos and these techniques can be used to produce offspring for nonhuman primates. This involves the disaggregation of cleaving embryos and fusion with mature enucleated oocytes. A source of donor oocytes is needed to act as surrogate cytoplasts for the embryonic nuclei. While this is feasible and the production of a restricted number of embryos could be considered to help patients who produce few of their own, ethical concerns are likely to be raised about this approach because of the close association with somatic cell cloning.

Human cloning

There are two kinds of cloning:

(1) Reproductive cloning is rejected by most people and is very difficult to imagine. Cloning a human being by somatic cell nuclear transfer, for example, would require a consenting person as a source of DNA, eggs to be enucleated and then fused with the DNA, a woman who would carry and deliver the child, and a person to raise the child. It should be clear that a cloned human may have the same appearance as his predecessor but not necessarily his nature, his mental ability, character or capacity for achievement.

(2) Cellular cloning is much more interesting. It could allow:

   (a) Understanding of the mechanisms of genetic diseases;

   (b) Better production of transgenic animals; and

   (c) By cloning up to the embryo stage, a possible source of stem cells or tissue for therapeutic means.

Conclusion

The future of assisted reproductive technology will progress in two fields; human reproduction will improve qualitatively, and social aspects such as parenthood and the status of the woman and the child will also improve.

We have already examined the increase of efficacy of assisted reproductive techniques and how to avoid the transmission of many hereditary illnesses. Though these techniques only apply to a minority (3% of births in France), we can foresee that the desire to control births will lead to a greater diffusion of these techniques.

We must keep in mind that humans are unique mammals. Evolution has been such that they do not resemble the other mammals and at each step we must wonder:

(1) Why do human oocytes and spermatozoans have such a high proportion of malformations?

(2) Why is the implantation rate so low and the abortion rate so high?

(3) Why does a woman hide her ovulation?

(4) Why does a human mother not recognize her own child?

(5) Why is the probability of birth only 25% per cycle?

Progress made in IVF may not allow us to answer these questions but at least we can attempt to overcome difficulties in order to reach the reproductive rates of other animal species.

Questioning the quality of the results of assisted reproductive techniques will lead to more interest in the child. Will the conditions of the birth give the child a new status and image? It seems that we can already answer that the child's behavior will be determined more by the attention, protection and affection of his parents. This emerges from the first studies on children resulting from IVF.

Society will have to examine the problems of the beginning of life. We are already informed of all the ethical, moral and religious problems concerning the beginning of human life and we know that the answers brought to these questions are not satisfactory. With time, and because we will have experimented on embryos, treated embryos, and replaced embryos or their genes, we will have to find an expression that is compatible with physiology rather than based on myths.

The future status of women seems strongly linked to the science of reproduction which allows them to master their femininity. The woman of tomorrow will rule with a growing influence the future of man, and a new relationship will develop between men and women, as well as with the family and jobs. The balance of masculine and feminine functions in society will change. We have not yet fully appreciated the consequences deriving from this liberation for all the different trends of social life.

References

1. Cohen J. Petite histoire des découvertes sur la fertilité humaine. *Contracept Fertil Sex* 1995;5: 315–9
2. Simpson JL. Are anomalies increased after ART and ICSI? In Kempers RD, Cohen J, Haney AF, Younger JB, eds. *Fertility and Reproductive Medicine*, Excerpta Medica Congress Series 1998; 1183:199–209
3. Felberbaum R, Diedrich K. Ovarian stimulation in ART: use of GnRH antagonist. In Kempers RD, Cohen J, Haney AF, Younger JB, eds. *Fertility and Reproductive Medicine*, Excerpta Medica Congress Series 1998;1183:113–25
4. Porcu E, Fabbri R, Savelti L, *et al.* Cryopreservation of human oocytes: state of the art. In Kempers RD, Cohen J, Haney AF, Younger JB, eds. *Fertility and Reproductive Medicine*, Excerpta Medica Congress Series 1998;1183:599–613
5. Cha KY, Koo JJ, Ko JJ, *et al.* Pregnancy after IVF of human follicular oocytes collected from non stimulated cycles. *Fertil Steril* 1991;55:109–13
6. Trounson A, Ward C, Kausche A. *In vitro* maturation and developmental competence of oocytes recovered from untreated PCO patients. *Fertil Steril* 1994;62:352–62
7. Jones GM, Trounson AO, Gardner DK, *et al.* Evolution of a culture protocol for successful blastocyst development and pregnancy. *Hum Reprod* 1998;13:169–77
8. Scott L, Smith S. The successful use of pronuclear embryo transfers the day following oocyte retrieval. *Hum Reprod* 1998;13:1003–13
9. Gianaroli L, Magli MC, Ferraretti AP, *et al.* PID increases the implantation rate in human IVF. *Fertil Steril* 1997;68:1128–31
10. Tarin J, Trounson AO. Embryo biopsy for PID. In Trouson AO, Gardner DK, eds. *Handbook of IVF*. CRC Press, 1993:115–29
11. Findlay I, Ray P, Quirke P, *et al.* Allelic drop-out and preferential amplification in single cells and human blastomeres: implications for preimplantation diagnosis of sex and cystic fibrosis. *Hum Reprod* 1995;10:1609–18
12. Trounson A. New developments in human embryology offer a new dimension to clinical reproductive medicine. In Kempers RD, Cohen J, Haney AF, Younger JB, eds. *Fertility and Reproductive Medicine*, Excerpta Medica Congress Series, 1998;1183:39–49
13. Thomson JA, Itskovitz-Eldor J, Shapiro SS, *et al.* Embryonic stem cell lines derived from human blastocysts. *Science* 1998;282:1145–7

Ovarian hyperstimulation in poor responders to artificial reproductive technologies

2

Z. Ben-Rafael, R. Orvieto and D. Feldberg

Introduction

Controlled ovarian hyperstimulation (COH) seems to be one of the key factors for the success of artificial reproductive technology (ART). The purpose of COH for *in vitro* fertilization–embryo transfer (IVF–ET) is the recruitment of multiple, fertilizable oocytes of optimal quality, since transfer of multiple embryos results in a better success rate. However, the extreme variability between women in the ovarian response to COH may result in the recruitment of only a small number of follicles, if any at all, in some patients. Therefore, the detection and treatment of these poor responder patients by IVF–ET is often unsuccessful and disappointing.

Ovarian steroidogenesis and folliculogenesis are now recognized to be modulated by autocrine, paracrine and endocrine factors[1]. Proliferation and differentiation of granulosa cells are greatly dependent on the hormonal environment, mainly follicle stimulating hormone (FSH) and estradiol.

FSH is the major physiological regulator of estradiol biosynthesis, acting through its stimulation of the aromatase cytochrome P-450[2]. Resistance or non-responsiveness to gonadotropin might be due to a circulatory antagonist[3], abnormalities in a signal transduction pathway (anywhere along the transmembrane pathway from a mutant gonadotropin receptor or a defective G protein to abnormalities in adenylate cyclase or cyclic AMP-dependent protein kinase A) or abnormal intraovarian modulatory mechanisms, of which the roles of several growth factors have been the subject of intense investigation.

Definition of a poor-responder cohort

Women treated in IVF–ET programs represent a heterogeneous group with a wide divergence in their responses to exogenous gonadotropin stimulation. Differences in peak estradiol levels and the number of follicles that develop may be used to categorize patients as low, normal or high responders. Each group responds differently to various protocols of gonadotropin stimulation and has distinct pregnancy rates. However, determining an individual patient's response can be carried out retrospectively, preventing optimal stimulation during the initial attempt.

The definition of poor-responder patients in an IVF program is controversial; nevertheless, during recent years, an effort has been made to define this specific cohort of patients. This was done due to the tremendous impact of elderly women seeking IVF therapy, who have a poor ovarian response to induction of ovulation, and also because of a fraction of younger patients with borderline ovarian reserve. Serafini and Kerin defined poor responders as a group of patients that presented less than three mature follicles on an increasing dose of human menopausal gonadotropin (hMG) and a poor estradiol profile[4]. Muasher and colleagues defined poor responders as patients who failed to recruit more than two follicles on an increasing dose of hMG stimulation[5]. The definition of poor responders given by Fenichel and colleagues combined this phenomenon with levels of estradiol lower than 300 pg/ml during aggressive induction by menotropins[6]. Hershlag and associates combined both factors into a definition scheme of poor-responder groups and found that a low response occurred in 9% of all IVF patients in all age groups[7].

Ben Rafael and colleagues[8] summarized the criteria of poor-responder groups into three main variables responsible for scant ovarian output on an increasing dose of hMG:

(1) Failure to develop more than 1–2 pre-ovulatory follicles;

(2) Estradiol levels not higher than 300 pg/ml;

(3) Triggering of a premature luteinizing hormone (LH) surge.

Predictive endocrine parameters

The outcome of IVF–ET and ovulation induction is strongly dependent on ovarian responsiveness to exogenous stimulation with menotropins and on the patient's age. It is common knowledge that the human menstrual cycle and ovarian activity are unstable during the last few years of reproductive life. Furthermore, a striking decrease in female fecundity in women over the age of 30 years has been reported[9]. This decline has also been observed during ovulation induction and IVF–ET[10].

However, chronological age has only a limited value in assessing female fecundity, since some women conceive with minimal effort even in their 40s, whilst follicle stimulation in women in their 30s is often hampered by a consistent lack of response. This observation implies an intrinsic change in the ovarian reserve capacity of humans – the well-recognized 'biological age'. Increasing age, however, is just one of many important processes that reduces the number of follicles[11]. It is possible that, like the menopause, the age-related reduction in fecundity may occur at different rates in different women. An index of such a reduction would be useful for the prognosis of ART therapy. One such indicator may be basal FSH level, which is established during infertility evaluation. It has been shown that the serum FSH level increases as ovarian function declines[12].

Muasher and colleagues have reported that elevated FSH levels on cycle day 3 are associated with a poor response to ovulation induction in ART[5]. Scott and associates have found that basal levels of FSH on day 3 can effectively predict the outcome of IVF–ET[13]. Licciardi and co-workers published data indicating that the day 3 estradiol levels were a prognostic factor of ovarian stimulation response and pregnancy outcome and found these levels to be, together with day 3 FSH levels, predictive parameters of ART results and success[14]. Looking for even more sensitive parameters, Mukherjee and Grunfeld discovered that an elevated day 3 FSH/LH ratio in the presence of a normal day 3 FSH level predicted a poor response to COH prior to ART[15]. Tambo and associates have performed a clomiphene citrate challenge test[16] based on the criteria of Navot and colleagues[17]. The test was performed by measuring serum concentrations of estradiol, FSH and LH on cycle days 2–3 and then on cycle days 9–11 after treatment of the women with 100 mg/day of clomiphene citrate for 5 days, starting on day 5 of the cycle. An excessive FSH response to clomiphene citrate predicted a poor response outcome to subsequent COH for ART, with 85% accuracy. Fenichel and co-workers have found an association between low responders and increased age, and high basal and clomiphene citrate-stimulated FSH levels[6]. Padilla and colleagues presented an additional test for the prediction of ovarian response, which used the estradiol response to leuprolide acetate as a prognostic assessment of the response to COH and IVF–ET treatment outcome[18]. Recently, Seifer and co-workers have published their data on day 3 serum inhibin-B levels and have found them to be sensitive and predictive for the outcome of ART and pregnancies resulting from those technologies[19]. All these associations may suggest a premenopausal state with reduced follicular and ovarian reserves.

Induction of ovulation protocols for poor responders

Clomiphene citrate plus hMG

Clomiphene citrate and hMG were originally combined for the induction of ovulation in IVF–ET by Edwards and associates[20] who added clomiphene citrate to hMG to amplify the response that occurred by hMG alone. Seppala developed this protocol extensively for ART cycles, with excellent results for the majority of his patients[21].

Trounson and Leeton stressed the benefit of this protocol in a poor-responder group who failed on the hMG-only strategy[22]. Pantos and colleagues[23], in an attempt to assess the traditional approach to a poor response to the first treatment cycle by increasing the dose of hMG after clomiphene citrate in the second treatment cycle, have found that increasing the hMG dosage above 150 IU does not increase the number of the follicles and oocytes retrieved. They suggested that this may be due to inherent differences in follicular development that cannot be overcome by increasing hMG dosage.

Ferrier and Berkely[24] compared the clomiphene citrate and hMG protocol with the hMG and gonadotropin releasing hormone (GnRH) analog protocol for IVF–ET and gamete intra-Fallopian transfer procedures. Among their patients were a selected group of poor responders that had better ongoing pregnancy rates with clomiphene citrate and hMG compared to the analog pretreatment strategy. Prak and Tiemessen found that, in 319 cycles induced by clomiphene citrate and hMG, the poor-responder group showed a better response on this protocol compared to the one utilizing GnRH agonist pretreatment[25]. Furthermore, our unpublished data from a group of poor responders cancelled on different protocols indicate that, in older poor-responder patients, treatment with clomiphene citrate and hMG is cost-effective and should be the first-line attempt.

It can be concluded that the clomiphene citrate and hMG protocol is effective and less expensive than protocols including analogs for GnRH. Although data are still scant and inconclusive, clinically it is logical to employ this protocol before reverting to more expensive ones.

High-dose hMG

The greatest experience in using hMG for ART cycles comes from the Norfolk program that used high and low doses of hMG for induction of ovulation in various cohorts of women[26]. Laufer and co-workers advocated the use of the high-dose hMG protocol, starting with three ampules of hMG for all IVF–ET patients[27]. Ben-Rafael and colleagues[28] found a direct correlation between the dose of hMG and FSH levels reached in the blood; they also found that FSH levels started to rise from day 1 of hMG administration, reaching a plateau after several days in normal responders, but continuing to rise in the high-responder group. Because the FSH in the blood of hMG-treated patients was derived from an exogenous source, it was suggested that differences in the metabolism of injected hMG predicted the various gonadal reactions. Based on these findings, it seems logical to increase the dosage of hMG in poor responders to try to overcome the metabolic 'lag' of blood FSH levels. This assumes that the extent of FSH accumulation in the circulation is a principal factor in determining an individual response to hMG therapy.

Van-Hooff and Leerentveld[29] have evaluated the effect of doubling the hMG dose in the same treatment cycle in which the ovarian response after 5 days of ovarian stimulation with three ampules of hMG was low. Doubling the hMG dose to six ampules was found to have no effect on the length of ovarian stimulation, peak estradiol levels, number of follicles, cancelled cycles and number of oocytes retrieved. This group concluded that doubling the hMG dose in the course of IVF–ET treatment cycle is ineffective in enhancing ovarian response in low responders. This is in accordance with current knowledge on follicular recruitment, which occurs only in the late luteal and early follicular phases of the menstrual cycle.

Nevertheless, in poor responders, the situation is different from that in a cohort of normal responders. It is conceivable that, in poor responders, a very high dose of hMG (more than five ampules/day) might result in the recruitment of a satisfactory number of follicles. In fact, Jones and associates[26] found that, in a group of very-low-responder patients with elevated basal FSH levels in whom exogenous FSH was increased up to a dose of six ampules per day, they were able to 'recruit an extra oocyte or two, and thereby improve the pregnancy rate, which is quite unsatisfactory with ordinary amounts of hMG'. Hofmann and colleagues[30] have investigated the use of high-dose FSH for ovarian hyperstimulation in ART in women with a previous poor response to stimulation with four ampules per day. They found that raising and maintaining FSH levels during stimulation by high-dose FSH in low responders reduces treatment cancellations and may improve the outcome of ART. Our impression is that the low-responder patients are a heterogeneous group that should be subdivided into several categories according to various basal and dynamic endocrine markers. The very-high-dose hMG protocol should be tailored according to these criteria.

GnRH agonists in protocols for poor responders

GnRH agonists can be used in a long-suppression protocol or a short flare-up protocol, which takes advantage of the initial agonistic stimulatory effect of GnRH agonists on endogenous FSH and LH secretion.

Feldberg and co-workers showed that the long protocol of Decapeptyl® administration in the mid-luteal phase is superior to other GnRH-agonist protocols and control group results[31]. Meldrum and Huynn[32] suggested that GnRH agonists should be used in the majority of patients enrolled on ART programs in order to avoid high cancellation rates in non-agonist cycles and to improve follicular recruitment in poor-responder groups. Since then, the issue of poor-responder patients and the use of various protocols which combine hMG with GnRH agonists has been discussed by several investigators, who focused their interest on this most problematic cohort of IVF patients.

Ben Rafael and associates found that the ovarian hyporesponsiveness associated with the use of a GnRH analog is due to the lack of endogenous FSH secretion[28]. Low circulating FSH levels were the cause of this lack of response. However, increasing the dose of hMG could overcome this problem. In another study, it was found that true low responders did not

benefit from the use of regular protocols employing GnRH analogs[29].

Serafini and Kerin[4] treated 27 patients who were categorized as poor responders and whose treatment on the standard hMG protocol of induction for IVF–ET was cancelled. In the subsequent treatment cycle, the GnRH analog was administered in the early follicular phase using the short flare-up protocol. A pregnancy rate per cycle of 33.3% was established in this poor-responder group after they were pretreated with the analog.

Droesh and Muasher[33] reported their experience with cohort of poor responders whose treatment on a regular hMG induction protocol was cancelled. They achieved a 37.5% clinical pregnancy rate per cycle in this unique, complicated population using the leuprolide acetate short-protocol strategy.

Other groups have reported less enthusiastic results concerning poor responders treated with a short protocol of leuprolide acetate. Muasher and colleagues were unable to demonstrate any beneficial effects from the use of GnRH-agonist suppression in low-responder patients[5]. In these patients, he found that the use of a flare-up GnRH-agonist protocol significantly improved stimulation characteristics and pregnancy rates.

In conclusion, it is obvious that application of GnRH agonists is the treatment of choice in a selected population of poor-responder patients, but, according to existing data, this group is heterogeneous with different prognoses for the various subgroups. It seems that the short GnRH agonist protocols with mild desensitization are superior to the longer ones with their profound downregulation of pituitary gonadotropin secretion. The leuprolide acetate screening test[18] is suggested as a possible tool for assessing and predicting the response in low-responder ART patients.

Co-treatment with human growth hormone and hMG for induction of ovulation

Adashi and Van Wyk[34] recognized the role of the insulin-like growth factor 1 (IGF-1) in follicular development. It has been shown that

IGF-1 has an important role to play in the development of ovarian follicles, and its synergistic effect with FSH on the differentiation of the granulosa has been demonstrated through stimulation of aromatase activity, induction of the LH receptor, synthesis of progestins and proteoglycans, and the evaluation of cyclic adenosine monophosphate accumulation.

Several studies suggest that pituitary growth hormone reserves, as judged by the growth hormone response to oral clonidine, may be impaired in patients displaying requirements for a high dose of hMG[35]. Based on these results, Homburg and Jacobs introduced the rationale for the use of growth hormone *in vivo* to facilitate ovulation induction by hMG[36]. In a subsequent study, this group also found that women treated with growth hormone and hMG, as compared to hMG alone, had a significant reduction in the required dose of hMG, duration of treatment and the daily effective dose of gonadotropins. Furthermore, serum IGF-1 rose during treatment with growth hormone, but not with placebo. Coukos and Volpe found an improved response in young poor-responder patients co-treated with growth hormone and hMG[37]. They demonstrated that intrafollicular levels of growth homone, estradiol and progesterone were significantly higher in these poor-responder patients than in normal responders stimulated with gonadotropins only. Volpe and co-workers[38] examined the efficacy of combined growth hormone and hMG therapy applied to normally cycling women, who were judged to be resistant to hMG therapy in an IVF–ET program. It appeared that concurrent administration of growth hormone and gonadotropin promoted superovulation and may therefore improve ovarian responsiveness in young gondotropin- resistant women.

Owen and Jacobs investigated 20 poor-responder patients treated for ART by clomiphene citrate and hMG, with the addition of a placebo or single injections of growth hormone (24 IU)[39]. Overall, there was no improvement in ovarian response to stimulation by the growth hormone-augmented regimens, although there was a tendency for the development of more follicles. Only a subgroup of poor-responder patients who presented with a polycystic ovary pattern of ovarian structure on ultrasonography benefited from the growth hormone therapy in terms of more follicles recruited and higher estradiol levels on the day of hCG administration.

In conclusion, these controlled studies have shown that co-treatment with growth hormone sensitizes the human ovary to stimulation by gonadotropins. Further studies to select the most appropriate groups of patients to be treated, explore the mechanism of action of growth hormone, define the role of IGF-1 in human follicular development and determine the minimum dose of growth hormone required to sensitize the human ovary are, however, still required.

Minidose GnRH agonist protocol for poor responders with elevated basal FSH levels

The combined GnRH agonist–menotropin stimulation protocol has now become a most efficient tool in IVF–ET and has been discussed here at length. However, we recently proposed that the hyposensitivity associated with GnRH analog use in poor responders can be alleviated by decreasing the dose of GnRH analog administered. Decreased GnRH analog dose can still prevent a premature LH surge, but does not inhibit endogenous FSH levels to the same extent as a full dose. This is consistent with our suggestion that hyposensitivity might be due to low peripheral FSH levels[30]. In our study, we investigated a group of 106 poor responders whose treatment on a standard regimen of menotropins in two consecutive cycles was cancelled and who were exposed to changing pretreatment dosages of GnRH agonists, which comprised:

(1) A single dose 3.75-mg microcapsule of Decapeptyl in the mid-luteal phase;

(2) Daily subcutaneous injections of 0.5 mg Decapeptyl in the mid-luteal phase, followed by 0.1 mg Decapeptyl from day 2 of the menstrual cycle until hCG administration;

Table 1 Pertinent laboratory data of all study groups

Parameter	Group I (n = 29)	Group II (n = 41)	Group III (n = 36)
Cancellation rate*	13/29 (44.8)	9/41 (21.9)	4/36 (11.1)[†]
Estradiol on hCG days[††] (ng/ml)	413 ± 67	676 ± 104	841 ± 233[‡]
Progesterone on hCG days[††] (ng/ml)	1.21 ± 0.34	0.89 ± 0.29	0.67 ± 0.31[†]
No. of oocytes[††] per retrieval	1.4 ± 0.6	3.6 ± 1.1	4.1 ± 1.3[‡]
Fertilization rate (%)	43.9	59.7	66.8[§]
No. of embryos per transfer[††]	1.2 ± 0.6	2.2 ± 0.3	3.1 ± 0.4[‡]
No. of hMG ampules[††]	46.1 ± 8.4	42.3 ± 8.6	36.9 ± 6.1[§]
No. days with stimulation periods[††]	14.8 ± 1.5	12.7 ± 0.8	11.7 ± 1.1[‡]

* values in parentheses are percentages; hCG, human chorionic gonadotropin; [†] $p < 0.05$ for group I versus groups II and III; [††] values are given as mean ± SD; [‡]$p < 0.05$ for group III versus groups I and II; [§]$p < 0.05$ for group I versus group III

Table 2 Clinical pregnancy and miscarriage rates in the study and control groups

Group	Pregnancy rate per transfer	Pregnancy rate per embryo (implantation)	Miscarriage rate
Group I (n = 29)	1/16 (6.3%)	1/20 (5%)	1/1 (100%)
Group II (n = 41)	5/32 (15.6%)	5/106 (4.7%)	2/5 (40%)
Group III (n = 36)	9/32 (28.1%)	12/132 (9.1%)	2/9 (22.2%)

There were no significant differences between groups I, II and III

(3) Daily subcutaneous injections of 0.1 mg Decapeptyl from day 21 of the mid-luteal phase, followed by 0.05 mg Decapeptyl daily from day 2 of the menstrual cycle until hCG administration.

All patients were stimulated using Metrodin® from day 3 of the cycle for 5 days, followed by an individually adjusted dose of hMG.

The group of patients treated by minidose Decapeptyl had a lower cancellation rate and an obvious superiority compared to the other groups in terms of peak estradiol levels, number of oocytes and embryos transferred, and pregnancy rates.

In summary, it is well established that in poor responders the ovary with reduced ovarian out- put has rising FSH levels on cycle day 3. It is well documented that such a perimenopausal profile can result in profound ovarian suppression by administration of a regular dose of Decapeptyl with continuous release[28].

In this study, we suggest that a minidose of GnRH agonist started in the mid-luteal phase offers the optimal treatment for low responders and, furthermore, it can prevent an untimely LH surge while avoiding excess inhibition. The improved implantation rate per embryo suggests that, in low responders, a minidose of GnRH agonist provides a superior stimulation protocol over the regular dose strategy. The results might be due to better embryo quality, endometrial receptivity, or both.

References

1. Ben Rafael Z, Orvieto R. Cytokines – involvement in reproduction. *Fertil Steril* 1992;58:1093–6

2. Erickson GF, Quigley ME, Yen SSC. Functional studies of aromatase activity in human granulosa cells from normal and polycystic ovaries. *J Clin Endocrinol Metab* 1979;49:514–21

3. Meyer WR, De Cherney AH. Evidence of gonadal and gonadotropin antibodies in women with a suboptimal ovarian response to exogenous gonadotropin. *Obstet Gynecol* 1990;75:795–9

4. Serafini P, Kerin J. An alternate approach to COH in 'poor responders': pretreatment with a GnRH analog. *Fertil Steril* 1988;49:90–6

5. Muasher SJ, Oehninger S, Jones GS, *et al.* The value of basal and or stimulated serum gonadotropin levels in prediction of stimulation response and IVF outcome. *Fertil Steril* 1988;50:298–302

6. Fenichel P, Gimaldi M, Olivero JF. Predictive value of hormonal profiles before stimulation for IVF. *Fertil Steril* 1989;51:845–9

7. Hershlag A, Assis MC, De Cherney A. The predictive value and the management of cycles with low initial estradiol levels. *Fertil Steril* 1990;53:1064–9

8. Ben Rafael Z, Bider D, Mashiach S. Ovarian hyporesponsiveness in combined GnRH agonist and menotropin therapy is associated with low serum FSH levels. *Fertil Steril* 1991;55:272–7

9. Federation CEOS, Shwatz D, Mayaux MJ. Female fecundity as a function of age: results of artificial insemination in 2193 multiparous women with azoospermic husbands. *N Engl J Med* 1982;306:404–6

10. Stoval D, Toma SK, Hammoud MG, *et al.* The effect of age on female fecundity. *Obstet Gynecol* 1991;77:36–8

11. Lenton EA, Sexton LL, Cooke ID. Progressive changes in LH and FSH and LH : FSH ratio in women through reproductive life. *Maturitas* 1988;10:35–8

12. Cameron IT, Healy DL. Occult ovarian failure: a syndrome of infertility, regular menses and elevated FSH concentrations. *J Clin Endocrinol Metab* 1988;67:1190–4

13. Scott TR, Robinson S, Rosenwaks Z. FSH levels on cycle day 3 are predictive of IVF outcome. *Fertil Steril* 1989;51:651–5

14. Lucciardi F, Liu HCH, Rosenwaks Z. Day 3 estradiol serum concentrations as prognosticators of ovarian stimulation response and pregnancy outcome in patients undergoing IVF. *Fertil Steril* 1995;64:991–9

15. Mukherjee T, Grunfeld L. An elevated day three FSH : LH ratio in the presence of normal day 3 FSH predicts a poor response to COH. *Fertil Steril* 1996;65:588–91

16. Tambo T, Dale PO, Abyholm J. Prediction of response to COH: a comparison of basal and CC stimulated FSH levels. *Fertil Steril* 1992;57:819–23

17. Navot D, Rosenwaks Z, Margalioth EJ. Prognostic assessment of female fecundity. *Lancet* 1987:645–9

18. Padilla SL, Bayat J, Garsia J. Prognostic value of the early serum estradiol response to leuprolide acetate in IVF. *Fertil Steril* 1990;53:288–91

19. Seifer DB, Blazar AS, Berk CH. Day 3 serum inhibin-B is predictive in assisted reproductive technologies outcome. *Fertil Steril* 1997;67:110–13

20. Edwards RG, Steptoe PC, Purdy JM. Establishing full term human pregnancies using cleaving embryos grown *in vitro*. *Br J Obstet Gynaecol* 1980;87:757–9

21. Seppala M. The World Collaborative Report on IVF and ET. Current state-of-the-art. *Ann NY Acad Sci* 1985;442:558–62

22. Trounson AO, Leeton JF. The endocrinology of clomiphene stimulation. In Edwards RC, Purdy JM, eds. *Human Conception In Vitro*. New York: Academic Press, 1982

23. Pantos C, Spiers A, Johnston J. Increasing the human menopausal gonadotropin dose – does the response really improve? *Fertil Steril* 1990;53:436–40

24. Ferrier A, Berkely AS. Evaluation of leuprolide acetate and gonadotropins versus CC and gonadotropins for IVF or GIFT. *Fertil Steril* 1990;54:90–6

25. Prak FM, Tiemessen CH. Clomiphene citrate and hMG in routine IVF: still a cost-effective treatment in 1992. Presented at the *8th Meeting of ESHRE*, The Hague, The Netherlands, July 1992

26. Jones HW, Rosenwaks Z, Veek LL. Three years of IVF at Norfolk. *Fertil Steril* 1984;42:826–30

27. Laufer N, De Cherney AH, Naftolin F. The association between pre-ovulatory serum 17 beta-estradiol pattern and conception in hMG–hCG stimulation. *Fertil Steril* 1986;46:73–7

28. Ben-Rafael Z, Mastroianni L, Flickinger GL. Differences in ovarian stimulation in human menopausal gonadotropin treated women may be related to FSH accumulation. *Fertil Steril* 1986;46:582–6

29. Van-Hooff MH, Leerentveld RA. Doubling the human menopausal gonadotropin dose in the course of an IVF treatment cycle in low responders: a randomized study. *Hum Reprod* 1993;8:369

30. Feldberg D, Dicker D, Goldman J. The value of Gn-RH agonists in the treatment of failed cycles

in the IVF-E program: a comparative study. *Eur J Obstet Gynecol* 1990;103:34–7

31. Meldrum DR, Huynn D. Routine pituitary suppression with leuprolide acetate before ovarian stimulation for oocyte retrieval. *Fertil Steril* 1989;51:455

32. Droesh K, Muasher ST. Value of suppression with a Gn-RH agonist prior to gonadotropin stimulation for IVF. *Fertil Steril* 1989;51:292

33. Adashi EY, Van Wyk JJ. Insulin-like growth factors as intra-ovarian regulators of granulosa cell growth and function. *Endocrin Rev* 1985;6:400

34. Menashe Y, Lunenfeld B, Mashiach S. Can GH increase after clonidine administration predict the dose of human menopausal hormone needed for induction of ovulation? *Fertil Steril* 1990;53:765–8

35. Homburg R, Jacobs HS. Growth hormone facilitates ovulation induction by gonadotropins. *Clin Endocrinol* 1988;29:113–16

36. Coukos G, Volpe A, Genazzani AR. Improvement of ovarian response to induction of superovulation with combined growth hormone-gonadotropin treatment. In Mashiach S, Ben-Rafael Z, Laufer N, *et al.*, eds. *Advances in Assisted Reproductive Technologies.* London: Plenum Press, 1990:389–95

37. Volpe A, Giozdana G, Genazzani AR. Ovarian response to combined GH–gonadotropin treatment in patients resistant to induction of superovulation. *Gynecol Endocrinol* 1989;3:125–8

38. Owen EJ, Jacobs HS. Co-treatment with growth hormone in sub-optimal responders in IVF–ET. *Hum Reprod* 1991;6:52–6

39. De-Fazio J, Meldrum DR, Chang RJ. Acute ovarian response to a long acting agonist of GnRH in ovulatory women and women with polycystic ovarian disease. *Fertil Steril* 1985;44:453–5

Intracytoplasmic sperm injection: challenges and prospects

3

R. Abdelmassih

Introduction

During the past 15 years, *in vitro* fertilization (IVF) has been successful in the treatment of long-term infertility caused by tubal disease, and idiopathic and male-factor infertility. It is a well-documented fact that the results of IVF in male infertility are not as good as those for patients with normal semen parameters. In a 3-year survey comparing IVF in male and tubal infertilities, we observed that, with andrological infertility, only 20–30% of the inseminated cumulus–oocyte complexes are normally fertilized; this is much lower than the 60–70% fertilization rate in patients with tubal infertility[1]. An absence of fertilization may occur in about one-third of cycles in couples with infertility using standards for IVF. It has been the experience of all centers for reproductive medicine, including our own, that a certain number of patients with andrological infertility cannot be helped by standard IVF treatment. Furthermore, a sizeable proportion of couples cannot be accepted for IVF if the number of progressively motile spermatozoa with normal morphology available for insemination is below a certain threshold (i.e. 500 000).

Over the past 6 years, assisted fertilization procedures have been developed to circumvent the barriers that prevent sperm access to the ooplasm, namely the zona pellucida and the ooplasmic membrane. Successful fertilization, embryo development, pregnancies and births have been reported after partial zona dissection and subzonal insemination (SUZI)[2–4].

In 1992, the first pregnancies and births obtained by a novel procedure of assisted fertilization, intracytoplasmic sperm injection (ICSI), were reported by a Brussels group[5]. In rabbits and cattle, embryos obtained by ICSI have been transferred to recipient mothers, and live offspring have resulted[6]. Recently, ICSI was also successful in the mouse, when a piezo-driven micropipette was used instead of a mechanically driven conventional pipette[7]. The results of the first 600 cycles of assisted fertilization by SUZI and ICSI at the Brussels Free University center, as well as a controlled comparison of 144 oocytes in 11 cycles, indicated that the mean fertilization rate after ICSI was substantially higher than after SUZI, while further *in vitro* development to transferable or freezable embryos was similar for the two procedures. The higher fertilization rate and similar cleavage rate resulted in more embryos for replacement after ICSI, and high implantation rates have been obtained[8–11]. These results were also confirmed in the review of 1275 consecutive ICSI treatment cycles carried out between October 1991 and December 1993[12].

Progress of ICSI

Since publication of the first papers on the use of ICSI for oligozoospermia in 1992 and 1993, an intense flurry of scientific effort has been dedicated to extending its application to virtually every type of male infertility (Table 1)[5,11,13]. The first extension came when Nagy and colleagues[14] confirmed that the most severe cases of oligoasthenoteratozoospermia produced the same pregnancy rates as mild cases of male-factor infertility, which were no different from those of men with normal spermatozoa undergoing conventional IVF.

Liu and co-workers[15] then demonstrated that the way in which the spermatozoa are pretreated, prior to ICSI, is immaterial, and that

Table 1 Current indications for intracytoplasmic sperm injection (ICSI)

Ejaculated spermatozoa
Oligozoospermia
Teratozoospermia (< 4% normal morphology
  using strict criteria – caveat for
  globozoospermia)
Asthenozoospermia (caveat for 100% immotile
  spermatozoa)
High titers of antisperm antibodies
Repeated fertilization failure after conventional
  in vitro fertilization
Auto-conserved frozen sperm from cancer patients
  in remission
Ejaculatory disorders (e.g. electroejaculation,
  retrograde ejaculation)

Epididymal spermatozoa
Congenital bilateral absence of vas deferens
Young syndrome
Failed vaso-epididymostomy
Failed vasovasostomy
Azoospermia after bilateral herniorrhaphy
Obstruction of both ejaculatory ducts

Testicular spermatozoa
All indications for epididymal spermatozoa
Extensive scar tissue preventing aspiration of
  spermatozoa from the epididymis
Azoospermia caused by testicular failure
Necrozoospermia

---

any method for aspirating the spermatozoa into an injection pipette and transferring them into the oocytes is adequate.

Liu and co-workers[15] also demonstrated that fertilization failure was always related to poor egg quality or to sperm non-viability. It appeared that the most severe morphological defect, the most severe motility defect or the tiniest number of spermatozoa in the ejaculate had no negative effect on the pregnancy rate with ICSI. Only absolute immotility of ejaculated or epididymal spermatozoa lowered the fertilization rate, and this was found to be not a result of the immotility *per se* but rather the non-viability of the sperm[14].

ICSI then took another leap forward with the development of sperm aspiration and extraction techniques, allowing couples who were absolutely azoospermic to have pregnancy rates no different from those in whom the male had a normal sperm count[13,14].

The first successful attempts at sperm aspiration combined with ICSI were reported by Silber and colleagues[16] and Tournaye and associates[17] in 1994: the procedure was carried out using microsurgical epididymal sperm aspiration (MESA). To facilitate the MESA procedure, it was discovered that percutaneous epididymal sperm aspiration (PESA) was possible.

Conventional IVF with aspirated epididymal spermatozoa yielded a pregnancy rate of only 9% and a delivery rate of 4.5%, whereas ICSI with aspirated epididymal spermatozoa in men with congenital absence of the vas deferens yielded a pregnancy rate of 47% and a delivery rate of 33%.

After the MESA–ICSI procedure was developed in 1994, it was discovered that testicular sperm could fertilize as efficiently as ejaculated spermatozoa, and also result in normal pregnancies[13,18,19]. This procedure was named testicular epididymal sperm extraction (TESE). TESE revolutionized the treatment of infertile couples with azoospermia, and created the possibility for parents with zero motility of epididymal or ejaculated spermatozoa, or even for men with no epididymis, to have their own genetic child, as long as there was normal spermatogenesis.

In the majority of cases of patients with testicular failure due to maturation arrest, Sertoli cell-only syndrome, cryptorchid testicular atrophy, post-chemotherapy azoospermia or even Klinefelter's syndrome, or only a very tiny number of spermatozoa or spermatids, some sperm can usually be extracted from extensive biopsies of the testicle and utilized for ICSI.

The following describes some points relating to the ICSI procedure and prospects for the future.

Are ICSI babies normal?

Genetics

If the most important refinement of ICSI in 1994 and 1995 was the development of TESE–ICSI for cases of non-obstructive azoospermia, the major development in 1996 was the detailed follow-up study of ICSI babies and the information it provided about the genetics of infertility. Liebaers and Bonduelle[20,21] have described the extensive follow-up studies of ICSI babies who underwent chromosomal evaluation at amniocentesis or chorionic villus sampling (CVS), as well as a detailed 2-year pediatric follow-up. In the first 877 consecutive ICSI babies born in the Brussels Dutch-speaking Free University program, to date there has been no greater incidence of major or minor congenital abnormalities than is seen in routine screenings of normal large populations. The chromsomal studies of ICSI pregnancies are similarly reassuring. First, of the 877 ICSI babies who underwent detailed pediatric follow-up, 448 were male and 429 were female, indicating no significant difference in sex ratio[20,21]. The overall incidence of major congenital malformations in these 877 children was 2.6%, which is no different from the incidence of similar major malformations in many studies involving very large samples of normal populations (from 2.1 to 3.6%). In 1995, the ICSI task force reported 18 major malformations in 763 children, which corresponds to the figure reported by Liebaers and Bonduelle of 2.6%[22-25].

The incidence of autosomal chromosomal abnormalities inherited from parents was 1.0%[20,21]. All were paternally transmitted chromosomal aberrations seen in the father prior to ICSI during initial counselling. The transmission of these abnormalities from the father to the child was not of serious concern to most of the parents. These inherited structural chromosomal anomalies included three inversions and two balanced translocations. Thus, the results of detailed follow-up of ICSI pregnancies and delivered babies are very reassuring, but suggest that there may be a very slightly higher risk (1%) than normal of sex chromosomal abnormalities in these children. Furthermore, attention must be given to the possibility of the occasional balanced translocation in the father giving rise to a rare unbalanced translocation in the fetus.

Cystic fibrosis

The genetics of cystic fibrosis and congenital male obstructive infertility have been studied in great detail as a result of the introduction of ICSI[26-29]. Previously, there was no evidence to suggest that congenital absence of the vas might be a genetic condition transmitted via the cystic fibrosis gene. The only clue was the clinical observation that all men with cystic fibrosis also have congenital absence of the vas deferens. However, the majority of men visiting fertility clinics because of azoospermia caused by congenital absence of the vas deferens had normal sweat chloride test results and no clinical signs of cystic fibrosis. Yet, genetic studies showed that 70% of these men had common cystic fibrosis mutations on one allele, and 10% had common cystic fibrosis mutations on both alleles. In those cases where both alleles were affected, one of the mutations was always extremely mild. Today, men with frank cystic fibrosis, with both alleles having strong mutations, are also presenting at fertility clinics to attempt to achieve pregnancy with MESA–ICSI.

The big mystery has been why 30% of cases show no cystic fibrosis mutations, while 60% have only one affected allele. Studies performed by the Cystic Fibrosis Consortium in Europe[30,31], in which the entire coding region of the cystic fibrosis genes was scanned, revealed absolutely no mutations in these men, meaning that the problem was not one of a hidden, undiscovered mutation in any of the exons or coding regions. However, a splicing error in intron 8, called the T_5 allele, was found to be on the opposite allele of a patient who was heterozygous for cystic fibrosis, but in both alleles of those who showed no mutations. This resulted in a defective production of cystic fibrosis (CFTR) protein that was adequate to prevent cystic fibrosis but inadequate to prevent congenital absence of the vas deferens.

Thus, use of ICSI for treatment of the most severe cases of male-factor infertility is leading to major molecular genetic discoveries that would never have been anticipated in the era of classical andrology.

Y chromosome and male infertility

Two characteristics distinguish the Y chromosome from all other chromosomes in the nuclei of human cells: it is specific to males, and the bulk of the chromosome does not undergo recombination. It is also among the smallest of human chromosomes, with its euchromatic or functional portion spanning roughly 30 million base pairs of DNA, or about 1% of the human genome. In 1992, comprehensive physical maps of the human Y chromosome were reported[32,33]. These maps incorporated hundreds of polymerase chain reaction (PCR)-detectable Y-DNA landmarks, sometimes referred to as sequence-tagged sites (STSs). These maps continue to be refined, and it is anticipated that they will provide a framework for determining the DNA sequence of the chromosome.

Investigators in many countries have used the maps, and the STSs on which they are based, to explore the hypothesis that some cases of spermatogenic failure are caused by Y chromosome defects. These studies have demonstrated that deletion of a particular segment of the Y chromosome, a segment often referred to as the AZFc region, is the most common molecularly defined cause of spermatogenic failure. It was found that the AZFc region of the Y chromosome is deleted *de novo* in 13% of men with non-obstructive azoospermia, and in a smaller percentage of men with severe oligozoospermia. These deletions define a region in which one or more genes required for spermatogenesis should be found, hence the term azoospermia factor, or AZF. Although infertile, AZFc-deleted men are otherwise healthy, suggesting that AZFc is a 'pure sterile' locus required only for germ cell development. In the absence of AZFc, spermatogenic output is greatly diminished, and in some cases the testes contain no germ cells. It was speculated that AZFc facilitates differentiation of primordial germ cells into spermatogonial stem cells or influences the destiny of these stem cells which, in normal males, confront three alternative fates: proliferation, degeneration or differentiation. AZFc deletions encompass a cluster of virtually identical *DAZ* (deleted in azoospermia) genes, which are expressed specifically in spermatogonia (and their immediate descendants, primary spermatocytes) and encode a putative RNA-binding protein. The absence of

DAZ may cause the severe spermatogenic defects observed in men in whom the gene cluster is deleted. In fruit flies and in mice, a gene homologous to *DAZ* is required for male germ cell development. It can be supposed that *DAZ* is AZFc.

Although less frequent than deletions of the AZFc region, *de novo* deletions of other portions of the Y chromosome are also observed in some men with severe spermatogenic defects, and in these Y regions investigators around the world are searching for genes that play critical roles in male germ cell development. Indeed, the whole of the Y chromosome has been systematically searched for transcription units, and it has been discovered that the majority of genes are members of Y-amplified families expressed specifically in testes. (Most other human Y genes are shared with the X chromosome and are ubiquitously expressed.) The association of Y deletions with male infertility, and the abundance of testis-specific gene families, suggest that, over evolutionary time, the Y chromosome may have acquired a specialized role in male germ cell development.

Cloning 'Dolly': implications for human medicine

The technique of nuclear transfer was originally proposed by Spemann[34] as a method of studying cellular differentiation. By transferring nuclei from increasingly advanced developmental stages to an egg from which the genetic material had been removed, any restrictions on development owing to loss or irreversible inactivation of the genome would be elucidated. These experiments were carried out by Briggs and King[35], who obtained development using embryonic blastomeres as nuclear donors, and then by Gurdon[36,37], who produced adult frogs after transferring nuclei from tadpole intestinal epithelial cells; however, no adults were produced where somatic nuclei from adult animals were used as nuclear donors. In mammals, the techniques for embryo reconstruction were not developed until the early 1980s when McGrath and Solter[38] demonstrated pronuclear exchange in mouse zygotes. Subsequently,

Willadsen[39] produced live lambs after transferring nuclei from 8–16-cell sheep embryos to enucleated MII oocytes.

Methodology of nuclear transfer

In mammalian species, enucleated MII oocytes have now become the recipient cell of choice, owing to the lack of development obtained when using enucleated zygotes (in cattle and pigs). This restriction may be a result of the removal of zygotic factors, essential for early development, which may be associated with the pronuclei. MII oocytes to be used as nuclear donors may be obtained from a variety of sources dependent upon species. In ruminants, particularly cattle, oocytes may be aspirated from ovarian follicles following slaughter, and matured *in vitro*. Additionally, matured oocytes may be flushed from the oviducts of donor animals following superovulation regimens, and immature oocytes may be aspirated from follicles *in vitro* or following ovariectomy. Having obtained a suitable donor oocyte, the genetic material located on the meiotic spindle is removed by microsurgery. Briefly, a small amount of cytoplasm is aspirated from directly beneath the first polar body using a fine glass pipette. Fluidity of the cell membranes allows both the oocyte and the aspirated karyoplast to reseal following manipulation. The enucleation procedure can be monitored by staining the aspirated karyoplast with a DNA-specific fluorochrome, for example Hoechst 3332. Following enucleation, the genetic material from the donor cell is introduced by fusion of the donor cell (karyoplast) to the enucleated oocyte (cytoplast). In farm animal species, electrofusion has become the method of choice although viral and chemical methods have been used, which have proved less reproducible and, in the case of chemical fusion, may be toxic. At this point, the reconstructed embryo is able to begin development; however, many factors are involved in the successful development of such reconstructed embryos. These include other techniques associated with the methods of activation (induction of fertilization responses), culture and, in addition, biological factors relating to both the cytoplast and the karyoplast. Of great importance for successful development is co-ordination of the nuclear and cytoplasmic cell cycle phases of both donor and recipient cells.

Uses of genetic modification in human medicine

The ability to carry out precise genetic modification of cells in culture not only provides a method for the improvement of present transgenic technology but also facilitates previously improbable genetic modifications.

Transgenic animals can play a role in a range of human therapies and these are discussed below in relation to present and future therapies.

Biopharmaceuticals

Human proteins may be produced in a range of tissues and body fluids including blood, urine and milk. Although each of these may play a particular ole, the value of biopharmaceutical production in transgenic animals lies in the high volume that can potentially be produced at relatively low cost. To this end, the production of proteins in the milk of sheep, goats and cattle provides a useful route, although for products required in small amounts, transgenic rabbits may also be used. A range of therapeutic proteins are being produced in the milk of transgenic animals including α-1-antitrypsin (for treatment of cystic fibrosis) and factor IX (for treatment of hemophilia B). Nuclear transfer will facilitate the removal of endogenous genes to aid purification, for example the replacement of bovine serum albumin with human serum albumin (HSA), to produce large amounts of HSA for the treatment of burns.

Nutraceuticals

Animal milk may be modified to enhance the nutritional value, or for the removal of allergens (for example β-lactoglobulin in cattle).

Xenotransplantation

Animal organs and other tissues can potentially be used in the future for human transplantation. Physiologically, pig organs are similar to those of humans and are considered suitable for transplantation. However, there is a major problem with organ rejection. Although all the mechanisms involved in this rejection are not completely understood, it is known that a major antigen involved is α-1,3-galactose. This is present in pig cells but is not found in humans, who therefore mount an immune response. Nuclear transfer from cultured cells will facilitate knock-out of the pig gene coding for α-1,3-galactosyl transferase. Potential organs and tissues for transplantation include the heart, lungs, kidneys, liver and islets (treatment of diabetes).

Disease models

At present, many of the animal models used for the study of human genetic disorders are only available in mice. This species may not manifest the same clinical symptoms as do humans. Nuclear transfer technology will allow the production of disease models in species physiologically more similar to the human, to enable the monitoring of disease progression or to assess the benefits of any potential new therapies (including gene therapy). An example of this is cystic fibrosis; in mice, this disease manifests in the gut and not the chest.

Examples with indirect effects on human health

Genetic modification of farm animals may be used to improve various production or nutritional traits. In addition, improvement of animal health by the introduction of genes for disease resistance or removal of genes for disease susceptibility (for example the *PrP* gene involved in scrapie and bovine spongiform encephalopathy, BSE) may have long-term implications for human health.

Other uses of nuclear transfer technology

The production of 'Dolly' by nuclear transfer from an adult somatic cell demonstrates that the differentiated state of the genetic material may be reversed. In humans, there are many diseases or traumas which result in the loss of specific cell types or tissues. Nuclear transfer offers a route whereby the phenotype of a single differentiated cell may be removed and undifferentiated cells produced. With a greater understanding of cellular differentiation, it may be possible to remove cells from a patient, produce undifferentiated cells by nuclear transfer and then differentiate these cells in culture to specific phenotypes. Such cells may then be returned to the patient, avoiding the problems of rejection owing to mismatching of tissue types. Such cells may be used to replace lost populations such as in nerve damage or Parkinson's disease, possibly as a treatment for immune disorders, leukemias and other blood diseases or as a vector for gene therapy.

ICSI with immature sperm

In patients with non-obstructive azoospermia due to germ-cell failure or maturation arrest, recovery of mature testicular spermatozoa or late elongated spermatids with regard to ICSI is only possible in about 50% of patients, even when multiple testicular biopsies are taken. None of the clinical parameters, such as testicular volume, semen analysis, serum follicle stimulating hormone (FSH) level or testicular histology can reliably predict whether testicular spermatozoa will be found. Recently, there have been a few reports in the literature describing ICSI with immature sperm cells such as round spermatids[40]. The fertilization and pregnancy rates, however, generally remain far below those obtained with mature spermatozoa and elongated spermatids. The use of round spermatids in ICSI raises several concerns such as DNA immaturity, genomic imprinting normality of the centrosome and presence of sperm-derived oocyte-activating factor. Furthermore, the correct identification of the round spermatids within a heterogeneous population of testicular cells has not received enough attention. Identification of round spermatids is problematic when conventional Hoffman modulation contrast systems are used on the inverted microscope. If appropriate phase-contrast optics are used on an inverted microscope, reliable recognition of the round spermatids in a cell suspension smeared at the bottom of a glass dish is possible. However, exploration of several biopsies from patients with non-obstructive azoospermia showing no spermatozoa after extensive search have never, in our experience, revealed round spermatids. This observation first questions whether enough effort is spent, in general, searching for mature spermatozoa or later spermatids. Furthermore, it casts some doubt on the existence of a real target for round spermatid injection. In any case, experimental investigations should precede the introduction of round spermatid injection into the clinical practice of any assisted reproductive technology (ART) center.

Preimplantation genetic diagnosis

Preimplantation genetic diagnosis (PGD) is a recent development which became possible as a result of ART and progress in molecular genetics. PGD can be offered to couples at risk of having a child with a genetic disease. Indications for PGD are similar to those for prenatal diagnosis by CVS or amniocentesis. PGD is usually carried out by molecular genetic procedures (fluorescent *in situ* hybridization, FISH or PCR) on one or preferentially two blastomeres from a day-3 cleaving embryo (with usually about eight blastomeres). PGD involves genetic counselling and preparation of the couple, an ART procedure (conventional IVF or ICSI), biopsy of one or two blastomeres by micromanipulation on a day-3 embryo, the diagnostic procedure on the biopsied blastomere(s) and replacement of non-affected embryos (maximum two or three). In PCR, contamination by extraneous DNA may be a problem and could arise during the embryo biopsy procedure if sperm DNA is adhering to the zona pellucida. This contamination can be prevented by using ICSI as the ART procedure in PGD cycles. This

policy is followed world-wide by all centers that practice PGD. The clinical experimental nature of this early form of prenatal diagnosis, and the resulting pregnancies and the health of children born after PGD are carefully monitored.

Cytoplasmic transfer

Cytoplasmic transfer, also known as cytoplasmic donation or transplantation, is an assisted reproduction procedure that involves the injection of a small amount of cytoplasm – the portion of the egg surrounding the nucleus – from a donor egg directly into the patient's egg. The injected cytoplasm replaces missing or abnormally functioning components of the recipient egg, while the genetic blueprints of the parents are retained.

The goal of cytoplasmic transfer is to overcome any problems that may exist in the cytoplasm of the egg. Every cell in the body consists of two components: a nucleus, which provides the genetic material; and cytoplasm, which is best described as the fuel that enables development. By transferring cytoplasm from a healthy donor egg, some of the problems that exist in the patient's cytoplasm may be alleviated, while allowing the mother's own genetic material to remain intact.

Until now, women with recurrent poor embryo development and failed implantation had no options for having their own genetic children. This process enables embryologists and physicians selectively to correct problems in the eggs, which then allows for the conception of children with the genes of both parents. Approximately 70% of eggs are anatomically impaired. Other eggs do not produce sufficient energy or lack crucial proteins. For some women, cytoplasmic transfer may correct or repair some of these abnormalities. If done early enough, before egg maturation, some genetic abnormalities may also be corrected.

The egg is a very large cell, larger than any other cell. Most of the cytoplasm is not needed and sometimes the egg or its daughter cells split into two or three, as is the case with identical twins or triplets. Although it is not known precisely how much donor cytoplasm should be added, or indeed whether all the cytoplasm should be removed first and replaced with that from a donor, the amount of cytoplasm injected in these patients is considerably more than the volume of regular body cells.

Culture of viable human blastocysts

In human IVF, embryos are routinely transferred to the uterus on either day 2 or day 3 of development, resulting in a 10–15% implantation rate. However, in other mammalian species, the transfer of cleavage-stage embryos, which normally reside in the oviduct, to the uterus results in a significantly lower implantation rate, compared to that achieved with blastocysts. It is therefore proposed that, to increase implantation rates in human IVF, the move is made to extended culture and transfer at the blastocyst stage. The transfer of blastocysts will not only help synchronize the embryo with the female tract, but will also facilitate the identification of those embryos with little or no development potential. To culture viable blastocysts, it is important to use more than one culture medium to cater for the changing requirements of the preimplantation embryo as it develops and differentiates. If sequential culture media are not used, one can obtain blastocysts but their resultant viability is low. The use of sequential serum-free media in human IVF has resulted in more than 50% of embryos becoming blastocysts with an implantation rate of approximately 50%. Further advances in human embryo culture should come from the replacement of protein with the glycosaminoglycan hyaluronate, which is more suitable than albumin for supporting implantation in the mouse, and which will eliminate biological variation and possible contamination from blood products. With the routine culture of human blastocysts will come the introduction of non-invasive tests of embryo viability, capable of identifying those blastocysts most likely to develop from a given cohort. As the implantation rate of the blastocyst is higher than that of the cleavage-stage embryo, fewer embryos will be required for transfer to establish a successful pregnancy, thereby reducing the number of multiple gestations and increasing the overall efficiency of human IVF.

References

1. Tournaye H, Devroey P, Camus M, *et al.* Comparison of *in vitro* fertilization in male and tubal infertility: a 3 year survey. *Hum. Reprod* 1992;7:218–22
2. Ng SC, Bongso A, Ratnam SS. Microinjection of human oocytes: a technique for severe oligoasthenoteratozoospermia. *Fertil Steril* 1991;56:1117–23
3. Cohen J. Zona pellucida micromanipulation and consequences for embryonic development and implantation. In Cohen J, Malter HF, Talansky BE, Grifa J, eds. *Micromanipulation of Human Gametes and Embryos.* New York: Raven Press, 1992:191–219
4. Fishel S, Timson J, Lisi F, Rinaldi L. Evaluation of 225 patients undergoing subzonal insemination for the procurement of fertilization *in vitro*. *Fertil Steril* 1992;57:840–9
5. Palermo G, Joris H, Devroey P, Van Steirteghem AC. Pregnancies after intracytoplasmic injection of single spermatozoon into an oocyte. *Lancet* 1992;342:17–18
6. Iritani A. Micromanipulation of gametes for *in vitro* assisted fertilization. *Mol Reprod Develop* 1991;28:199–207
7. Kimura Y, Yamagimachi R. Mouse oocytes injected with testicular spermatozoa and round spermatids can develop into normal offspring development. *Development* 1995;121:2397–405
8. Palermo G, Camus M, Joris H, *et al.* Sperm characteristics and outcome of human assisted fertilization by subzonal insemination and intracytoplasmic sperm injection. *Fertil Steril* 1993;59:826–35
9. Van Steirteghem AC, Liu J, Joris H *et al.* Higher success rate by intracytoplasmic sperm injection than by subzonal insemination. Report of a second series of 300 consecutive treatment cycles. *Hum Reprod* 1993;8:1055–60
10. Van Steirteghem AC, Liu J, Joris H, *et al.* Higher fertilization and implantation rates after intracytoplasmic sperm injection. *Hum Reprod* 1993;8:1061–6

11. Van Steirteghem AC, Nagy ZP, Liu J, *et al.* Intracytoplasmic sperm injection. *Assist Reprod Rev* 1993;3:160–3

12. Tournaye H, Silber S, Van Steirteghem A. Normal fertilization of human oocytes after testicular sperm extraction and intracytoplasmic sperm injection. *Fertil Steril* 1995;63:639–41

13. Silber SJ, Nagy ZP, Liu J, *et al.* The use of epididymal and testicular spermatozoa for intracytoplasmic sperm injection: the genetic implications for male infertility. *Hum Reprod* 1995;10:2031–43

14. Nagy ZP, *et al.* The result of intracytoplasmic sperm injection is not related to any of three basic sperm parameters. *Hum Reprod* 1995;May

15. Liu J, Lissens W, Silber SJ, *et al.* Birth after pre-implantation diagnosis of the cystic fibrosis ∆F508 mutation by the polymerase chain reaction in human embryos resulting from intracytoplasmic sperm injection with epididymal sperm. *J Am Med Assoc* 1994;272:1858–60

16. Silber SJ, Nagy ZP, Liu J, *et al.* Conventional *in-vitro* fertilization versus intracytoplasmic sperm injection for patients requiring microsurgical sperm aspiration. *Hum Reprod* 1994;9:1705–9

17. Tournaye H, Devroey P, Liu J, *et al.* Microsurgical epididymal sperm aspiration and intracytoplasmic sperm injection. A new effective approach to infertility as a result of congenital bilateral absence of the vas deferens. *Fertil Steril* 1994;61:1045–51

18. Schoysman R, *et al.* Pregnancy after fertilization with human testicular spermatozoa (letter, comment). *Lancet* 1993;Nov

19. Devroey P, Liu J, Nagy ZP, *et al.* Pregnancies after testicular sperm extraction and intracytoplasmic sperm injection in non-obstructive azoospermia. *Hum Reprod* 1995;10:1457–60

20. Bonduelle M, Legein J, Buysse A, *et al.* Prospective follow-up study of 423 children born after intracytoplasmic sperm injection. *Hum Reprod* 1996;11:1558–64

21. Bonduelle M, Wilikens A, Buysse A, *et al.* Prospective follow-up study of 877 children born after intracytoplasmic sperm injection (ICSI), with ejaculated, epididymal and testicular spermatozoa and after replacement of cryopreserved embryos obtained after ICSI. *Hum Reprod* 1996;11(Suppl 4)

22. Office of Population Censuses and Surveys. *Mortality Statistics: Perinatal and Infant* (Serial and Biological Factors). London: HMSO, 1987–88, OPC series DH3, nrs 18 and 20

23. Office of Population Censuses. *Congenital Malformation Statistics 1979 to 1985.* London: HMSO, 1982–88, OPC series MB3

24. National Perinatal Statistics Unit and the Fertility Society of Australia. *IVF and GIFT Pregnancies, Australia and New Zealand.* National Perinatal Statistics Unit (NPSU), 1990

25. New York State Department of Health. *Congenital Malformations Registry Annual Report. Statistical Summary of Children Born in 1986 and Diagnosed through 1988.* New York: New York State Department of Health, USA, 1990

26. Silber SS, Ord T, Balmaceda J, *et al.* Congenital absence of the vas deferens. The fertilizing capacity of human epididymal sperm. *N Engl J Med* 1990;323:1788–92

27. Aneviano A, Dates RD, Amos JA, *et al.* Congenital bilateral absence of the vas deferens. A primarily genital form of cystic fibrosis. *J Am Med Assoc* 1992;267:1794–7

28. Chillon M, Casals T, Mercier B, *et al.* Mutations in the cystic fibrosis gene in patients with congenital absence of the vas deferens. *N Engl J Med* 1995;332:1475–80

29. Chillon M, Dork T, Casals T, *et al.* A novel splice site in intron 11 of the CFTR gene, created by mutation 1811 1.6 kbA → G. Produces a new exon: high frequency in Spanish cystic fibrosis chromosomes and association with severe phenotype. *Am J Hum Genet* 1995;56:623–9

30. Cystic Fibrosis Genetic Analysis Consortium. Population variation of common cystic fibrosis mutations. *Hum Mutat* 1994;4:167–77

31. Cystic Fibrosis Genotype–Phenotype Consortium. Correlation between genotype and phenotype in patients with cystic fibrosis. *N Engl J Med* 1993;329:1308–13

32. Vollrath D, Foote S, Hilton A, *et al.* The human Y chromosome. A 43-interval map based on naturally occurring deletions. *Science* 1992;258:52–9

33. Foote S, Vollrath D, Hilton A, Page DC, *et al.* The human Y chromosome: overlapping DNA clones spanning the euchromatic region. *Science* 1992;258:60–6

34. Spemann H. *Embryonic Development and Induction.* New York: Hafner Publishing, 1938;210–11

35. Briggs R, King T. Changes in the nuclei of differentiating cells as revealed by nuclear transfer. *J Morph* 1957;10:269–312

36. Gurdon JB. The development capacity of nuclei taken from intestinal epithelium cells of feeding tadpoles. *J Embryol Exp Morphol* 1962;10:622–40

37. Gurdon JB. Adult frogs from the nuclei of single somatic cells. *Dev Biol* 1962;4:256–73

38. McGrath I, Solter D. Nuclear transplantation in the mouse embryo by microsurgery and cell fusion. *Science* 1983;220:1300–2

39. Willadsen SM. Nuclear transplantation in sheep embryos. *Nature (London)* 1986;320:63–5

40. Tesarik J, Mendoza C. Spermatid injection into human oocytes. I. Laboratory techniques and special features of zygote development. *Hum Reprod* 1996;11:772–9

Fertility drugs and ovarian cancer 4

S. Daya

Introduction

Ovarian cancer is a highly fatal form of cancer that has a 5-year survival rate of 37%[1]. The life-time risk of ovarian cancer among Canadian women is 1.2% (i.e. 1 in 83 women will develop this disease in their lifetime)[1]. Even though ovarian cancer is relatively less common than breast cancer, which has a life-time risk of approximately 12%[2], its late presentation and the lack of effective screening make it the leading cause of death from gynecologic malignancy[3].

Although the etiology of ovarian cancer remains poorly understood, pregnancy and oral contraceptive use have consistently been recognized as being protective against the development of the disease. In a small proportion of cases, a genetic link is clearly evident and transmitted as an autosomal dominant trait[4]. Familial ovarian cancer is characterized by onset at an early age and affects approximately 50% of first-degree relatives. It is also associated with malignancies at other sites such as breast and endometrium[2]. Increased rates of ovarian cancer have been observed following exposure to environmental factors such as asbestos and talcum powder[5,6].

In contrast to the protective effects of increased parity, infertility has been implicated in several studies as a risk factor for ovarian cancer[7–9]. Recently, case reports and two US studies have implicated fertility drugs in the development of ovarian cancer[10,11]. Although these studies are not conclusive, their findings are of concern because the case reports involve young women with a rapid onset of ovarian cancer after ovulation induction, and the epidemiologic studies report large relative risks associated with fertility drug use. Whittemore and colleagues[10] reported a risk estimate for all women using fertility drugs of 2.8 (95% confidence interval (CI), 1.3–6.1), and Rossing and colleagues[11] reported a risk estimate of 11.1 (95% CI, 1.5–82.3) for clomiphene citrate use for 12 or more cycles. These observations are of concern particularly in light of the increasing demand for infertility services. Approximately 7–8% of couples desiring a pregnancy have difficulty conceiving. Among those seeking medical evaluation and therapy, it is estimated that 50% or more eventually take ovulation-inducing drugs at some time in their treatment plan. Similarly, the number of cycles of *in vitro* fertilization (IVF), in which high doses of ovarian stimulating fertility drugs are used, has increased dramatically over the last two decades. Annually, more than 35 000 cycles of treatment are provided in the United States[12] and over 100 000 cycles world-wide[13]. For these women and their health providers, information regarding the true risk associated with fertility drugs is required so that informed choices can be made regarding these treatment options. A causal relationship between fertility drugs and ovarian cancer, if verified, would have significant implications for clinical practice and public health.

Proposed hypotheses for ovarian cancer pathogenesis

Incessant ovulation

The suggestion that ovarian cancer is related to 'incessant ovulation' was first made in 1971[14]. It was hypothesized that human ovulation is 'extravagant', mostly purposeless and contributes to ovarian epithelial surface neoplasia via the healing process in response to the minor trauma associated with each ovulation. The

"

tears in the ovarian surface resulting from follicle rupture are repaired by cell division, which ceases when repair is complete. During this repair process, inclusion cysts may form from inward folding of the epithelium that becomes entrapped in the stroma. Malignant transformation of the epithelium lining these cysts might occur as a consequence of gonadotropin or estrogen stimulation or by gonadotropin-induced steroidogenesis[15]. Thus, the risk of ovarian cancer is directly proportional to the number of ovulatory cycles experienced by the woman. This hypothesis would explain the protective effect of pregnancy or oral contraceptive use, because both situations result in cessation of ovulation, thereby interrupting the process of repeated trauma and repair.

Genetic transmission

The genetic hypothesis has gained credibility in recent years with the increased reporting of familial ovarian cancers. Epithelial cells with a lack of genetic material on chromosome 17, possibly lacking tumor suppressor genes, have been found in over 80% of malignant ovarian tumors[16]. During the repair process following ovulation, cells in which tumor suppressor genes are absent will undergo uncontrolled cell division and malignant transformation.

Environmental factors

An environmental hypothesis, relating primarily to asbestos and talc exposure, may also fit with the incessant ovulation theory in that repeated defects induced in the surface epithelium of the ovary by ovulation would allow easy entry of these carcinogenic factors[17]. The incidence of ovarian cancer is higher among asbestos workers. Also, the practice of regular application to the perineum of dusting talc, thought to be possibly contaminated by asbestos, has been associated with an increased risk of ovarian cancer. In addition, one study reported the finding of talc particles in 75% of ovarian tumors[18].

Dietary factors

Dietary risk factors such as high fat and caffeine intake are believed to play a causal role in ovarian cancer development. However, to date the published evidence suggests that these factors may produce a small increase in the probability of the disease, but the results from the various studies are inconsistent.

Infertility and ovarian cancer

Nulliparity and infertility have both been shown to increase the risk of ovarian cancer, but are difficult to separate from each other. Women who develop ovarian cancer are more frequently nulliparous, have a later age at first pregnancy and have smaller families[8,19]. The observations of a greater risk of ovarian cancer in never-married–never pregnant women compared to never-married women, or in women who had tried and failed to become pregnant, led to the suggestion that a gonadal status predisposed to both ovarian cancer and low fertility[8]. Although decreased parity predisposes to ovarian cancer, many studies suggest that there may be something more about infertility than decreased parity that accounts for the association with ovarian cancer. There are several possible suggestions including:

(1) An underlying hormonal or gonadal defect causing infertility also predisposes to ovarian cancer[8];

(2) An underlying cancer also predisposes to infertility[15]; and

(3) Fertility drugs either cause cancer[20] or stimulate pre-existing cancers[21].

Although there is presently no conclusive evidence to support the gonadal status theory, the reports of an increased prevalence of ovarian cancer in infertile women suggest that this possibility should be entertained. In one study, women who had not conceived after greater than 10 years of having unprotected intercourse were observed to have a 6.5-fold increase in the risk (95% CI, 2.1–20.4) of developing ovarian cancer, compared with nulliparous women with fewer than 3 months of unprotected intercourse[7].

The possibility that a pre-existing ovarian tumor may cause infertility was suggested by the finding of an increased prevalence of ovarian cancer in women undergoing microsurgery for infertility compared to women undergoing other abdominal surgery such as cholecystectomy and appendectomy[22].

The results from a cohort study of 10 358 women referred for IVF treatment in Victoria, Australia between 1978 and 1992 demonstrated that unexplained infertility was a significant risk factor for invasive ovarian cancer (relative risk, 19.9; 95% CI, 2.23–165)[23].

The safety of fertility drugs has been widely debated since the publication of the Whittemore overview[10]. In order to clarify the issue, the available evidence should be subjected to critical appraisal before a causal association between fertility drugs and ovarian cancer can be established.

Review of the evidence purporting a causal relationship between fertility drugs and ovarian cancer

Any allegation of a causal association between an exposure risk factor (such as fertility drug use) and an outcome (such as ovarian cancer) should stand up to certain diagnostic criteria before it can be accepted[24].

Is there evidence from true experiments in humans?

The strongest evidence for causation can be obtained from randomized controlled trials comparing fertility drugs with no treatment. Unfortunately, to date, there has been no study of this high quality published. Therefore, the answer to this question is 'no' because no randomized controlled trials have been conducted with long-term follow-up to evaluate the risk of ovarian cancer in women previously exposed to fertility drugs. The next level of evidence in descending order is provided by cohort studies (either prospective or retrospective). Using this study design, women who have been exposed to

fertility drugs are followed for a long period of time, as are those who have not been exposed to the drugs, to determine if there is a significant difference in the incidences of ovarian cancer in the two groups. Because the rate of ovarian cancer is very low, a large number of subjects is required for the study to demonstrate significant differences. Consequently, the time and expense involved are often prohibitive. Nevertheless, there have been two publications recently that have addressed this issue.

In a relatively short-term follow-up period of a cohort of women who had registered for IVF treatment in Australia, there were 5564 women who had undergone ovarian stimulation and 4794 who had been referred for IVF, but were untreated or had had 'natural cycle' treatment without ovarian stimulation[23]. The standardized incidence ratios (SIR) for ovarian cancer were 1.70 (95% CI, 0.55–5.27) and 1.62 (95% CI, 0.52–5.02) in the exposed and unexposed groups, respectively, indicating no increased risk of disease with the use of fertility drugs.

In another cohort study of infertile Israeli women treated between 1964 and 1974 with ovulation-inducing drugs, the SIR for ovarian cancer was 1.6 (95% CI, 0.8–2.9)[25].

Is the association strong?

The quality of evidence that is presently available is very poor and precludes one from answering that question in the affirmative. The odds ratios for invasive ovarian cancer associated with fertility drug use range from 0.8 (i.e. potential benefit) to 2.8 (i.e. potential harm). However, because of the small sample sizes in the studies, the precision of the estimate of the true risk is very poor. By undertaking subgroup analyses (e.g. restricting the analysis to infertile women who took the drug but remained infertile), the risk estimate increases at the expense of precision of this estimate, thereby reducing the confidence with which the findings can be interpreted. In the case–cohort study of 3837 women published by Rossing and colleagues[11], the elevated risk associated with exposure to 12 or more cycles of clomiphene citrate is not statistically significant (relative risk 6.7; 95% CI,

0.8–58.8) when one focuses only on epithelial ovarian tumors (i.e. after excluding the two cases of granulosa cell tumors)[26].

Is the association consistent from study to study?

The demonstration by different investigators in different populations of an association between fertility drug exposure and ovarian cancer would strengthen an inference of a causal association. The findings of an Italian case–control study in which the odds ratio of ovarian cancer with exposure to fertility drugs was 0.84 (95% CI, 0.2–3.7)[27] are diametrically opposite to the conclusion from other reported studies, thereby raising doubts about a causal association.

Is the temporal relationship correct?

A temporal sequence in which fertility drug exposure is followed by detection of ovarian malignancy is strong evidence of a causal effect. Because the data in the case–control studies are collected retrospectively, it is difficult to answer this question with certainty. However, in the Whittemore study[10], the fertility drugs included estrogens, diethylstilbestrol, progesterone, thyroid hormone, dextro-amphetamine and amobarbital[26]. Also, the great majority of women in this study were treated in the 1960s when ovulation-inducing drugs were either not readily available or had not been registered. In contrast, an Italian study[27], which was performed at a time when the drugs were readily available, demonstrated no risk of ovarian cancer. Similarly, no increase in risk was observed in the two cohort studies in which the subjects were likely to have been disease-free prior to commencing treatment with fertility drugs[23,25]. Thus, with the more recent data which are more likely to have the appropriate temporal relationship between exposure and outcome, there does not appear to be much support for a causal association between fertility drugs and ovarian cancer.

Is there a dose–response gradient?

A dose–response gradient (i.e. a higher risk of disease with a higher level of exposure to the risk factor) is an important criterion for a causal association between exposure and outcome. Apart from the Rossing study[11], in which a dose–response gradient was observed when all types of ovarian tumor were considered, no information is provided on doses or duration of therapy in the other studies. Also, the drugs specified are varied and do not reflect the current approach to infertility treatment[28]. In the study by Rossing and colleagues[11], the higher risk of disease with 12 or more cycles of treatment with clomiphene is not statistically significant when the analysis is restricted only to epithelial ovarian tumors[26]. Thus, no dose–response gradient is evident in the currently available data.

Does the association make epidemiological sense?

Fertility drugs have been widely available for 20 years, during which time there has been no associated increase in the incidence of ovarian cancer. In fact, in Finland the incidence of ovarian granulosa cell tumors (which are believed to possibly be linked to fertility drug use[29]) has declined by nearly 40% during the same time period, when a dramatic increase in the use of clomiphene citrate (13-fold increase in use) and human menopausal gonadotropin (200-fold increase in use) had occurred[30]. Thus, the association between fertility drug use and ovarian cancer does not make epidemiological sense. However, ovarian cancer is a relatively rare malignancy and any appreciable change in its incidence may not be perceptible until very large numbers of women are followed over a long period of time.

Does the association make biological sense?

The incessant ovulation theory is supported by the observation of a protective effect of oral contraceptive use and pregnancy, because ovulation is halted in these situations. However, in a woman who has had one pregnancy and breast-fed, the resulting reduction in the number of ovulations occurring during her reproductive life span is only 3%, whereas a single pregnancy is associated with a 50% reduction in ovarian cancer incidence[31]. Thus, the incessant ovarian theory alone does not explain the mechanism of ovarian cancer. Consequently, the association between fertility drugs and ovarian cancer does not make biological sense.

Is the association specific?

A specific association between a single cause and effect has not been established. Studies suggest that environmental, endocrine and genetic factors also play an important role in the etiology of ovarian cancer.

Is the association analogous to a previously proven causal association?

Although reproductive tract cancers have occurred in response to hormonal exposure, the analogy is imperfect at best. To date, fertility drugs have not been shown to have a causal association with other cancers.

Conclusion

A causal association between fertility drug use and ovarian cancer has not been established. The published data demonstrate a relationship that is not consistent and that lacks a temporal dose–response gradient. The association does not make sense epidemiologically or biologically. The older studies included some drugs which are currently not used in infertility treatment. More recent cohort studies indicate that there may be no significant risk. The question of a possible causal association between fertility drugs and ovarian cancer can only be answered by large prospective studies with carefully selected controls and appropriate duration of follow-up. The multifactorial etiology, the unknown natural history of ovarian cancer and its low prevalence are major challenges to such an undertaking. The need for a national registry for post-market surveillance of fertility drugs to monitor and evaluate their long-term effect is clearly evident.

References

1. National Canadian Institute of Canada. *Canadian Cancer Statistics*, 1990. Toronto: Canadian Cancer Society, 1990
2. Miller BA, Gloecker Reis LA, Hankey BF. SEER cancer statistics review 1973–1990. Bethesda, MD: National Institutes of Health, 1993;93:2789
3. Heintz AP, Hacker NF, Lagasse LD. Epidemiology and etiology of ovarian cancer: a review. *Obstet Gynecol* 1985;66:127–35
4. Lynch HT, Schuelke GS, Wells IC, Cheng SC, Kimberling WJ, Biscone KA. Hereditary ovarian carcinoma: biomarker study. *Cancer* 1985;55: 410–15
5. Newhouse ML, Pearson RM, Fullerton JM, Boesen EA, Shannon HS. A case–control study of carcinoma of the ovary. *Br J Prev Soc Med* 1977; 31:148–53
6. Whittemore AS, Wu ML, Paffenbarger RS. Personal and environmental characteristics related to epithelial ovarian cancer. II. Exposures to talcum powder, tobacco, alcohol and coffee. *Am J Epidemiol* 1988;128:1228–40
7. Booth M, Beral V, Smith P. Risk factors for ovarian cancer: a case–control study. *Cancer* 1989;60: 592–8
8. Joly DJ, Lilienfeld AM, Diamond EL, Bross ID. An epidemiologic study of the relationship of reproductive experience to cancer of the ovary. *Am J Epidemiol* 1974;99:190–209
9. Risch H, Jain M, Marrett LD, Howe GR. Parity, contraception, infertility and the risk of epithelial ovarian cancer. *Am J Epidemiol* 1994;140: 585–97
10. Whittemore AS, Harris R, Itnyre J and the Collaborative Ovarian Cancer Group. Characteristics relating to ovarian cancer risk: collaborative analysis of 12 US case–control studies. II. Invasive epithelial ovarian cancers in women. *Am J Epidemiol* 1992;136:1184–203
11. Rossing MA, Daling JR, Weiss NS, Moore DE, Self SG. Ovarian tumors in a cohort of infertile women. *N Engl J Med* 1994;331:771–6
12. The American Fertility Society, Society for Assisted Reproductive Technology. Assisted

reproductive technology in the United States and Canada: 1992 results generated from the American Fertility Society/Society for Assisted Reproductive Technology Registry. *Fertil Steril* 1994;62:1121–8

13. Testart J, Plachot M, Mandelbaum J, Salat-Baroux J, Frydman R, Cohen J. World collaborative report on IVF–ET and GIFT: 1989 results. *Hum Reprod* 1992;7:362–9

14. Fathalla MF. Incessant ovulation – a factor in ovarian neoplasia? *Lancet* 1971;2:163

15. Balasch J, Barri PN. Follicular stimulation and ovarian cancer? *Hum Reprod* 1993;8:990–6

16. Russell SEH, Hickey GI, Lowry WS, White P, Atkinson RJ. Allele loss from chromosome 17 in ovarian cancer. *Oncogene* 1990;5:1581–3

17. Piver MS, Bake T, Piedmonte M, Sandecki A. Epidemiology and etiology of ovarian cancer. *Semin Oncol* 1991;18:177–85

18. Henderson W, Joslin C, Turnbull A, Griffiths K. Talc and carcinoma of the ovary and cervix. *Obstet Gynecol* 1971;78:266

19. DiSaia PJ. Ovarian disorders. In Scott JR, DiSaia RJ, Hammond CD, Spellacy WN, eds. *Danforth's Obstetrics and Gynecology*, 6th edn. Philadelphia: JB Lippincott Co: 1067–20

20. Whittemore AS. Fertility drugs and risk of ovarian cancer. *Hum Reprod* 1993;8:999–1000

21. Bessigher K, Eshkol A, Brinsden P, Edwards RG. Follicular stimulation: is it safe? *Br Med J* 1989;289:916

22. Lais CW, Williams TJ, Gaffey TA. Prevalence of ovarian cancer found at time of infertility microsurgery. *Fertil Steril* 1988;49:551–3

23. Venn A, Watson L, Lumley J, Giles G, King C, Healy D. Breast and ovarian cancer incidence after infertility and *in vitro* fertilisation. *Lancet* 1995;346:995–1000

24. Department of Clinical Epidemiology and Biostatistics, McMaster University Health Sciences Centre. How to read clinical journals. IV. To determine etiology or causation. *Can Med Assoc J* 1981;124:985–90

25. Modan B, Ron E, Lerner-Gera L, Blumstein T, Menczer J, Rabinovici J, Delsner G, Freedman L, Mashiach S, Lunenfeld B. Cancer incidence in a cohort of infertile women. *Am J Epidemiol* 1998;147:1038–42

26. Rossing MA, Daling JR, Weiss NS. Risk of ovarian cancer after treatment for infertility. *N Engl J Med* 1995;332:1302

27. Franceschi S. Fertility drugs and the risk of epithelial ovarian cancer in Italy. *Hum Reprod* 1994;9:1673–5

28. Shapiro S. Risk of ovarian cancer after treatment for infertility. *N Engl J Med* 1995;332:1301

29. Willemsen W, Kruitwagen R, Bastiaans B, *et al.* Ovarian stimulation and granulosa-cell tumour. *Lancet* 1993;341:986–8

30. Unkila-Kallio L, Leminen A, Tiitinen A, Ylikorkala O. Nationwide data on falling incidence of ovarian granulosa cell tumours concomitant with increasing use of ovulation inducers. *Hum Reprod* 1998;13:2828–30

31. Scott JS. How to induce ovarian cancer and how not to. *Br Med J* 1984;289:781–2

Section II
Contraception

New Stericlip and other prospective technologies for sterilization of women

5

J. Guillebaud

Introduction

World-wide, the most common surgical procedure today is minilaparotomy, in which the Fallopian tubes are approached from a small cut in the abdomen[1].

The advent of fiber-optic technology led to the introduction of the laparoscope in the 1960s, and this was soon followed by techniques of electrocoagulation and of applying clips and rings to the Fallopian tubes to block them. There have been improvements in the design of devices for blocking the tubes, but gains in safety and efficacy have been small. Efforts to reach the Fallopian tubes through the vagina rather than the abdomen increased in the 1970s, but there was a high rate of failure to complete the operation coupled with a significant number of complications. The possibility of reaching the tubes via the uterus (the transcervical approach) was first recognized in the 19th century, but efforts to perform female sterilization by this method have had mixed success. Nevertheless, the transcervical approach remains promising for development[1].

Abdominal route for tubal occlusion

The Fallopian tubes can be reached through laparotomy, minilaparotomy or laparoscopy. Minilaparotomy is considered ideal for sterilization performed within a few days of delivery. Laparoscopy is usually faster and gives endoscopic access to the tubes, and the woman normally recovers slightly more quickly than with laparotomy or minilaparotomy.

The first method of sterilization developed using the laparoscope was electrocoagulation in which a segment of the tube is blocked by burning it electrically. One method of electrocoagulation, unipolar diathermy, was found to cause significant morbidity, and even mortality, as a result of burns. So bipolar diathermy is recommended as a safer alternative (although now less favored owing to a high failure rate and a particularly high ectopic pregnancy rate in the Collaborative Review of Sterilization (CREST) study[2].

A variety of clips and rings can be applied to the tube via all three abdominal approaches. The Falope ring is a silicone rubber band that is fitted around a loop of the tube. The ring destroys about 3 cm of tube, so reversal is likely to be difficult. Also, there are reports of more postoperative pain with this method than with clips, which is in all cases best abolished by use of local anesthetic applied directly to the site of application, advantageous postoperatively even if general anesthesia is primarily used.

Clips have the advantage of causing the least damage to the tube (about 1 cm destroyed), thus offering the greatest potential for reversal. The original spring-loaded clip performed poorly in CREST[2]. The Filshie clip, which has a silicone rubber lining, was designed to overcome this problem.

One disadvantage with all mechanical devices for occluding the tube is that there is scope for operator error. Where the person applying the device is inexperienced, there is the risk that it may be applied incompletely across the tube or even to the wrong structure such as a ligament. If not applied with care, clips may close prematurely or fall off the applicator

transcervical methods researched seemed to fall short of the safety and efficacy levels required.

Work on transcervical methods of female sterilization, however, has continued in various parts of the world, as more fully reported in the present volume. China has reported near-complete success and a low rate of complications from blind injection of *phenol–mucilage* into the tubes using a simple cannula and catheter. Although some positive results have been shown in research into this method in Hong Kong, there remain concerns about the approach. Toxicological testing of this method is still required. More promising is the STOP device, a solid intratubal plug of unique design (Conceptus Inc., USA), which is inserted hysteroscopically under local anesthesia and currently undergoing international trials.

The sclerosing property of the antimalaria drug *quinacrine* for sterilization has been widely exploited, usually by (repeatedly) placing pellets of the drug in the uterus by means of a special inserter. The WHO Program's Toxicology Panel and the Scientific and Ethical Review Group recommended in 1995 that further clinical studies with quinacrine should not be undertaken until proper toxicological testing had been done, but interesting research into the method continues, as the concept is so attractive. However, efficacy issues (including efficacy against ectopic pregnancies) also need resolving, given the accumulating data on the amazing efficacy and longevity of banded copper intrauterine devices (IUDs) such as the TCu 380 and GyneFIX[7,8].

Recommendations for research into female sterilization methods

Participants in the WHO 1994 consultation on the development of new technologies for female sterilization agreed on a number of recommendations for future research into new methods of female sterilization. They concluded that the ideal methods would be safe, simple and effective one-time procedures for occlusion of the Fallopian tubes that cost little, involve only local anesthesia, cause minimum damage and are both individually and culturally acceptable, whether used postpartum, postabortion or as interval procedures. There should also be more operational research to increase acceptability of local anesthesia, to develop indicators to measure quality of services and to test approaches to training[1]. These remain significant, highly relevant objectives.

None of the current procedures meets all the criteria.

References

1. Anon. Advances in female sterilization research. *Progress* in human reproduction research (WHO) 1995;36:1–8
2. Peterson HB, Zhisen X, Hughes JM, *et al.* The risk of pregnancy after tubal sterilization: findings from the US Collaborative Review of Sterilization. *Am J Obstet Gynecol* 1996;174:1161–70
3. Royal College of Obstetricians and Gynaecologists. *Male and Female Sterilization: Evidence-Based Guidelines no 5*. London: RCOG, 1999;in press
4. Philp T, Guillebaud J, Budd D. Late failure of vasectomy after two documented analyses showing azoospermic semen. *Br Med J* 1994;289:77–9
5. Guillebaud J, Johnson J, Mansour D, Bounds W, Casey D. Laparoscopic sterilisation with a new polycarbonate/silicone rubber clip. *Br J Fam Plann* 1997;23:3–4
6. Mackenzie IZ, Turner E, O'Sullivan GM, Guillebaud J. Two hundred out-patient laparoscopic sterilisations using local anaesthesia. *Br J Obstet Gynaecol* 1987;94:449–53
7. Guillebaud J. Contraception. In McPherson A, Waller D, eds. *Women's Health in General Practice*. Oxford: Oxford University Press, 1997:128–216
8. Guillebaud J. Modern intrauterine contraception: closer than ever to reversible sterilization without an abdominal scar? *Middle East Fertil Soc J* 1999;4:1–5

The risk of cardiovascular disease in women aged over 35 years and using oral contraception

P. G. Crosignani

Introduction

The use of oral contraception has been associated in the past with an increased risk of myocardial infarction, while more recently the combination of estrogens and progestogens has been associated with an increased risk of venous thromboembolism. Since the incidence of cardiovascular disease tends to increase with age, it is of particular interest to look in some detail at the vascular events occurring during oral contraception use in women aged over 40 years.

Venous thromboembolism

Venous thromboemboli are rare among apparently normal non-pregnant women (Table 1), while their incidence increases during pregnancy, being approximately 6 : 10 000 pregnancies[1,2]. Approximately 10% of cases of venous thrombosis progress to pulmonary embolism. The case–mortality rate of venous thrombosis and/or pulmonary embolism is approximately 1%[3].

A literature search located 14 epidemiological studies which properly assessed the risk of venous thromboembolism in oral contraceptive users compared with non-users. Five cohort and nine case–control studies involving 1429 venous cases in oral contraceptive users were examined[4] to estimate the rise of venous thromboembolism in relation to oral contraceptive use[5–18]. Venous thromboembolism rates are 3.89 times higher (95% confidence interval 3.22–4.70) for women using oral contraceptives than for non-users. Age-specific relative risks were reported in four studies[6,9,14,18] and the oral contraceptive-associated risk for venous thromboembolism appears to be constant throughout the reproductive years. Three studies reported risks according to estrogen dose, $< 50\,\mu g$ versus $\geq 50\,\mu g$. The first estimate involved 10 exposed cases and the venous thromboembolism risk was 20 times higher in women using pills containing more than $50\,\mu g$ estrogen[1]. The second estimate involved 32 exposed cases, where the venous thromboembolism risk was double for doses $\geq 50\,\mu g$[16]. The third study involved 435 exposed cases and found no effect of the estrogen dose[18].

Third-generation progestins

The risk of venous thromboembolism was 5.97 (3.72–9.60) for users of oral contraceptives containing third-generation progestins[5,7,10,19], compared with 3.58 (2.91–4.41) for users of oral contraceptives containing other progestins. The average risk for third-generation progestin users was 1.80 times greater than the risk with oral contraceptives containing other progestins

Table 1 Incidence of venous thromboembolism among non-pregnant women not using oral contraceptives[1,2]

Age (years)	Cases (per 100 000 women per year)
20	2
25	3
30	4
40	8

$(1.02–3.16)$[10]. There is still disagreement about this increase[20].

Conclusions

The risk for venous thromboembolism associated with oral contraceptives is very low[21]. Women with histories of venous thromboembolism should not use oral contraceptives[22]. For women not at increased risk, the likelihood of venous thromboembolism should not be a deterrent to the use of oral contraceptives, nor a reason to change from an otherwise satisfactory product. The mechanism whereby the third-generation progestins are associated with an increased risk for venous thromboembolism is unknown.

Myocardial infarction

When oral contraceptive formulations with more than 35 μg ethinyl estradiol were given to women who smoked, their risk of myocardial infarction was markedly greater than that of women smokers who did not take oral contraceptives[23]. Myocardial infarction in oral contraceptive users was due mainly to coronary artery thrombosis. The angiographic studies by Engel and colleagues of 173 women under the age of 50 years who had had a myocardial infarction indicated that 60% of the oral contraceptive users of this series did not have the typical features of coronary atherosclerosis[24]. In contrast, 75% of young women not taking oral contraceptives who had had a myocardial infarction had evidence of coronary atherosclerosis[24].

Other indirect evidence that the major cause of myocardial infarction in oral contraceptive users is thrombosis and not atherosclerosis is the fact that former oral contraceptive users have no greater risk of myocardial infarction than never users[25].

Epidemiological studies have shown that the observed-to-expected ratio for myocardial infarction is higher in women taking oral contraceptives with 50 μg ethinyl estradiol than in those taking 30 μg ethinyl estradiol[26]. Analysis of women developing myocardial infarction during the first 20 years of the Royal College of General Practitioners' cohort study of oral contraceptive use found there was no change in risk with oral contraceptive use for non-smokers but nearly a 30-times higher risk in oral contraceptives users who were heavy cigarette smokers[27]. Their level of risk was much greater than that of smokers not using oral contraceptives. An American case–control study reported similar findings[28]. The increase in risk of myocardial infarction in oral contraceptive users is therefore limited to women who smoke cigarettes, especially if they are over 35 years old. One mechanism by which oral contraceptives may act synergistically with cigarette smoking is that the inhaled nicotine reduces the excretion of prostacyclin metabolites in women using oral contraceptives, while this does not happen in smokers not taking oral contraceptives[29].

In recent years and in current practice most smokers over the age of 35 years do not take oral contraceptives and epidemiological studies in this decade have found no significant increase in the risk of myocardial infarction among women using oral contraceptives[30]. One such study suggests that women taking formulations with less than 50 μg ethinyl estradiol and either gestodene or desogestrel had one-third the risk of myocardial infarction compared with women taking formulations with a similar amount of estrogen and levonorgestrel, and that the adverse effects of oral contraceptives in smokers may be less in those taking the newer pills[31]. Because this was an observational study, the findings may be the result of prescribing bias and may not reflect a true causal relationship between the formulations and the risk of myocardial infarction[4].

Cerebrovascular disease

After the first case reports of a possible link between oral contraceptives and stroke in the early 1960s, several case–control and cohort investigations were conducted during the 1960s and 1970s[32]. The first case–control studies were essentially related to high-dose estrogen and progestogen pills, and showed relative risk ratios of the order of 5–15 for ischemic stroke and around 1.5–2 for hemorrhagic stroke[32]. It was also clear that there was an important interaction between oral contraceptives and smoking, the relative risk being grossly elevated in women exposed to both risk factors. Cohort studies included about 60 cases of stroke, and gave an excess absolute risk of between 3 and 7 per 100 000 women[32]. Most episodes occurred in women aged over 35 years. These observations thus made it possible to avoid the excess risk of cerebrovascular diseases by restricting the use of oral contraceptives in women over the age of 35 years who also smoked or had hypertension[32]. At least four studies provided information on newer patterns of use with lower-dose oral contraceptives. In a Danish study of 320 cases with various cerebrovascular events and 1297 controls without predisposing factors[33], the multivariate relative risk ratio was 2.9 (95% confidence interval 1.6–5.4) for users of pills containing 50 µg estrogen, 1.8 (1.1–2.9) for users of pills containing 30–40 µg ethinyl estradiol, and 0.3 for users of progestogen-only oral contraceptives. The fraction of all cerebrovascular events attributable to oral contraceptive use was estimated at 15%.

The World Health Organization Collaborative Study of Cardiovascular Disease and Steroid Hormone Contraceptives was conducted between 1989 and 1993 in 21 centers from 17 developed and developing countries. The risk ratios for ischemic stroke and oral contraceptive use[34], based on 697 cases and 1962 controls, were 3.0 (1.7–5.6) in Europe and 2.9 (3.2–4.0) in developing countries, compared to no oral contraceptive use, and reached 7.2 and 4.8, respectively, for smokers and 10.7 and 14.5 for hypertensive women. The risk ratio for users of lower-dose pills (< 50 µg estrogen) was 1.5 (0.7–3.3) in Europe compared to 5.3 for users of higher-dose oral contraceptives.

A total of 1068 cases and 2910 controls were considered in the same study with reference to hemorrhagic stroke[35]. The risk ratio for oral contraceptive use was 1.8 (1.3–2.3) in developing countries, and 1.4 (0.8–2.3) in Europe. Furthermore, use of oral contraceptives before the age of 35 years was not related to hemorrhagic stroke risk in either group of countries, and use of low-dose preparations was not significantly associated with hemorrhagic stroke in Europe.

Likewise, in a study of 144 cases of ischemic stroke, 151 cases of hemorrhagic stroke and 744 controls conducted at the California Kaiser Permanente Medical Care Program[36], the risk ratio for current oral contraceptive users was 1.2 (0.5–2.6) for ischemic and 1.1 (0.6–2.2) for hemorrhagic stroke. Current oral contraceptive users and smokers had a risk ratio of 3.6 (1.0–13.9).

Hemostasis

Many studies show the activation of coagulation and fibrinolysis during the use of estrogen and progestogen. The coagulation system relies on factor Xa formed through both the intrinsic and extrinsic pathways for thrombin formation. Thrombin, in turn, regulates the conversion of fibrinogen to form the fibrin clot. The coagulatory system maintains a feedback system with factors having anticoagulatory potential. These include protein C, protein S and antithrombin III. In opposition to the coagulatory system is the fibrinolytic system, which is similarly regulated by factors with stimulatory and inhibitory potential.

Oral contraceptives appear to influence both the coagulatory and the fibrinolytic systems. The studies, however, lend themselves to some criticism because the cases were few, apparently healthy and in a static hemostatic situation when blood samples were taken.

Recently a new proposition has been put forward to explain the hypercoagulability observed in a subpopulation of oral contraceptive users based upon a cross-sectional population study. The study showed an interaction between oral contraceptive use and a mutation in a gene regulating the action of factor V (factor V Leiden mutation)[37]. This causes hypercoagulability by inducing resistance to the anticoagulant action of activated protein C. The factor V Leiden mutation increases the baseline risk of venous thromboembolism by eight times, for oral contraceptive users and non-users[38]. Since the factor V mutation is found frequently in Caucasian populations (2–5%)[37], the question arises whether women should be screened before they take oral contraceptives. Such a policy, however, might deny effective contraception to 2–5% of women, while preventing only a small number of venous thromboembolism episodes[39]. Hence, the presence of a genetic defect such as the factor V mutation is not an absolute contraindication to use of oral contraceptives, but should always be considered in the assessment of individual risk.

The thrombophilic effects of low-dose oral contraceptives still increase the risk of venous thromboembolism about three-fold, about half the thrombophilic risk induced by pregnancy.

References

1. Farmer RDT, Preston TD. The risk of venous thromboembolism associated with low-oestrogen oral contraceptives. *J Obstet Gynaecol* 1995;15:195–200
2. Lis Y, Spitzer WO, Mann RD, *et al.* A concurrent cohort study of oral contraceptive users from the VAMP research bank. *Pharmacoepidemiol Drug Safety* 1993;2:51–63
3. Stadel BV. Oral contraceptives and cardiovascular disease (Part I). *N Engl J Med* 1981;305:612–18
4. The ESHRE Capri Workshop Group. Hormones and cardiovascular diseases: oral contraceptives and hormonal replacement therapy: differential effects on coronary heart disease, deep venous thrombosis and stroke. *Hum Reprod* 1998;13:2325–33
5. Bloemenkamp KWM, Rosendaal FR, Helmerhorst FM, *et al.* Enhancement by factor V Leiden mutation of risk of deep vein thrombosis associated with oral contraceptives containing a third-generation progestagen. *Lancet* 1995;346:1593–6
6. Boston Collaborative Drug Surveillance Program. Oral contraceptives and venous thromboembolic disease, surgically confirmed gallbladder disease, and breast tumours. *Lancet* 1973;1:1399–404
7. Farmer RDT. Oral contraceptives and thromboembolism. *Lancet* 1996;347:259
8. Fuertes-de la Haba A, Curet JO, Pelegrina I, *et al.* Thrombophlebitis among oral and normal contraceptive users. *Obstet Gynecol* 1971;38:259–63
9. Helmrich SP, Rosenberg L, Kaufman DW, *et al.* Venous thromboembolism in relation to oral contraceptive use. *Obstet Gynecol* 1987;69:91–5
10. Lewis MA, Heinemann LAJ, MacRae KD, *et al.* The increased risk of venous thromboembolism and the use of third-generation progestagens: role of bias in observational research. *Contraception* 1996;54:5–13
11. Ludwing H. Anovulatory agents and venous disease. *Ergebnisse der Angologie und Phlebologie* 1970;4:81–102
12. Maguire MG, Tonascia J, Sartwell PE, *et al.* Increased risk of thrombosis due to oral contraceptives: A further report. *Am J Epidemiol* 1979;110:188–95
13. Petitti DB, Wingerd J, Pellegrin F, *et al.* Risk of vascular disease in women. Smoking, oral contraceptives, noncontraceptive estrogens, and other factors. *J Am Med Assoc* 1979;242:1150–4
14. Porter J, Hunter J, Jick H, *et al.* Oral contraceptives and nonfatal vascular disease. *Obstet Gynecol* 1985;66:1–4
15. Royal College of General Practitioners' Oral Contraception Study. Oral contraceptives, venous thrombosis, and varicose veins. *J R Coll Pract* 1978;28:392–9
16. Vessey MP. Epidemiologic studies of oral contraception. *Int J Fertil* 1989;34:64–70
17. Vessey MP, Doll R. Investigation of relation between use of oral contraceptives and thromboembolic disease. A further report. *Br Med J* 1969;2:651–7
18. World Health Organization Collaborative Study of Cardiovascular Disease and Steroid Hormone Contraception. Venous thromboembolic disease and combined oral contraceptives: results of international multicentre case– control study. *Lancet* 1995;346:1575–82
19. World Health Organization Collaborative Study of Cardiovascular Disease and Steroid Hormone Contraception. Effect of different progestogens in low-oestrogen oral contraceptives on venous thromboembolic disease. *Lancet* 1995;346:1586–8
20. Farmer RDT, Lawrenson RA, Thompson CR, *et al.* Population-based study of risk of venous thromboembolism associated with various oral contraceptives. *Lancet* 1997;349:83–8

21. World Health Organization. *World Health Statistics Annual 1995*. Geneva: World Health Organization, 1996:B-625

22. Lee DH, Henderson PA, Blajchman MA. Prevalence of factor V Leiden in a Canadian blood donor population. *Can Med Assoc J* 1996;155:285–9

23. World Health Organization Collaborative Study of Cardiovascular Disease and Steroid Hormone Contraception. Acute myocardial infarction and combined oral contraceptives: results of an international multicentre case–control study. *Lancet* 1997;349:1202–9

24. Engel HJ, Engel E, Lichtlen PR. Coronary atherosclerosis and myocardial infarction in young women – role of oral contraceptives. *Eur Heart J* 1983;4:1

25. Stampfer MJ, Willett WC, Colditz GA, *et al.* A prospective study of past use of oral contraceptive agents and risk of cardiovascular diseases. *N Engl J Med* 1988;319:1313

26. Meade TW, Greenberg G, Thompson SG. Progestogens and cardiovascular reactions associated with oral contraceptives and a comparison of the safety of 50- and 30-µg oestrogen preparations. *Br Med J* 1980;280:1157–61

27. Croft P, Hannaford PC. Risk factors for acute myocardial infarction in women: evidence from the Royal College of General Practitioners' Oral Contraception Study. *Br Med J* 1989;298:165–8

28. Rosenberg L, Palmer JR, Lesko SM, *et al.* Oral contraceptive use and the risk of myocardial infarction. *Am J Epidemiol* 1990;131:1009–16

29. Mileikowski GN, Nadler JL, Huey F, *et al.* Evidence that smoking alters prostacyclin formation and platelet aggregation in women who use oral contraceptives. *Am J Obstet Gynecol* 1988;159:1547–52

30. Sidney S, Petitti DB, Quesenberry Jr CP, *et al.* Myocardial infarction in users of low-dose oral contraceptives. *Obstet Gynecol* 1996;88:939–44

31. Lewis MA, Spitzer WO, Heineman LAJ, *et al.* Third-generation oral contraceptives and risk of myocardial infarction: an international case–control study. *Br Med J* 1996;312:88–90

32. Longstreth Jr WT, Swanson PD. Oral contraceptives and stroke. *Stroke* 1984;15:747–50

33. Lidegaard O. Oral contraception and risk of a cerebral thromboembolic attack: results of a case–control study. *Br Med J* 1993;306:956–63

34. World Health Organization Collaborative Study of Cardiovascular Disease and Steroid Hormone Contraception. Ischaemic stroke and combined oral contraceptives: results of an international multicentre case–control study. *Lancet* 1996;348:498–505

35. World Health Organization Collaborative Study of Cardiovascular Disease and Steroid Hormone Contraception. Ischaemic stroke and combined oral contraceptives: results of an international multicentre case–control study. *Lancet* 1996;348:505–10

36. Petitti DB, Sidney S, Bernstein A, *et al.* Stroke in users of low-dose oral contraceptives. *N Engl J Med* 1996;335:8–15

37. Helmerhorst FM, Bloemenkamp KWM, Rosendaal FR, *et al.* Oral contraceptives and thrombotic risk: risk of venous thromboembolism. *Thromb Haemostat* 1997;77:327–33

38. Vandenbroucke JP, Koster T, Briët E, *et al.* Increased risk of venous thrombosis in oral contraceptive users who are carriers of factor V Leiden mutation. *Lancet* 1994;344:1453–7

39. Chae CU, Ridker PM, Manson JE. Postmenopausal hormone replacement therapy and cardiovascular disease. *Thromb Haemostat* 1997;77:770–80

Oral contraceptives and thrombosis 7

L. Speroff

Introduction

In October, 1995, the United Kingdom Committee on Safety of Medicines sent a letter to all UK physicians and pharmacists stating that women taking oral contraceptives containing desogestrel or gestodene should be urged to complete their current cycle and to continue with a formulation with these progestins only if prepared to accept an increased risk of venous thromboembolism. The Committee on Safety of Medicines took this action because of observational studies that indicated a 2-fold increase in the risk of venous thromboembolism when desogestrel- and gestodene-containing contraceptives were compared to products with other progestins (mostly levonorgestrel). This action and the studies upon which it was based immediately became controversial. The controversy went beyond the validity of the epidemiologic data. The publicity surrounding these events reverberated throughout Europe, leading to an immediate overall decrease in oral contraceptive use, an increase in unwanted pregnancies, and an increase in induced abortions[1,2].

The controversy involving new progestin oral contraceptives that began in late 1995 continued through 1996, and began to reach resolution in 1997. The fundamental question is whether oral contraceptives containing desogestrel and gestodene have a different risk of thrombosis when compared with oral contraceptives containing older progestins.

Thrombosis can be divided into two major categories, venous thromboembolism and arterial thrombosis. Venous thromboembolism includes both deep vein thrombosis and pulmonary embolism. Arterial thrombosis includes acute myocardial infarction and stroke.

Venous thromboembolism

Conventional wisdom

Is there still a risk of venous thromboembolism with the current low-dose formulations of oral contraceptives? In the first years of oral contraception, the available products, containing 80 and 100 µg ethinyl estradiol (a very high dose), were associated with a 6-fold increased risk of venous thrombosis[3]. Because of the increased risks for venous thrombosis, myocardial infarction and stroke, lower dose formulations (less than 50 µg estrogen) came to dominate the market, and clinicians became more careful in their screening of patients and prescribing of oral contraception. Two forces, therefore, were at work simultaneously to bring greater safety to women utilizing oral contraception: the use of lower dose formulations, and the avoidance of oral contraception by high-risk patients. Because of these two forces, the Puget Sound study in the USA documented a reduction in venous thrombosis risk to 2-fold, although this is still an increased risk[4]. The new studies to be reviewed also reflect the importance of these two forces, and also still indicate an increased risk.

Controversial studies

The World Health Organization Collaborative Study of Cardiovascular Disease and Steroid Hormone Contraception[5] was a hospital-based, case–control study with subjects collected from 21 centers in 17 countries in Africa, Asia, Europe and Latin America[5]. As part of this study, the risk of idiopathic venous thromboembolism associated with a formulation containing 30 µg ethinyl estradiol and levonorgestrel (doses ranging from 125 µg to 250 µg) was compared to the risk with preparations containing 20 or 30 µg ethinyl estradiol and either desogestrel or gestodene (data from 10 centers in nine countries)[6]. The increased risk for desogestrel and gestodene was 2.6 times that of levonorgestrel, when adjusted for body weight and height.

The second case–control study (from an international team of epidemiologists), the Transnational Study on Oral Contraceptives and the Health of Young Women, analyzed 471 cases of deep vein thrombosis and/or venous thromboembolism from the UK and Germany[7]. Comparing users of second-generation products to non-users, the odds ratio was 3.2 (confidence interval 2.3–4.3). Comparing users of desogestrel and gestodene products to users of second-generation oral contraceptives, the risk of venous thromboembolism was 1.5-fold greater. The third study was from Boston University, but the data were derived from the General Practice Research Database, a computerized system involving the general practitioners in the UK[8]. Using this cohort, the authors calculated the death rate from pulmonary embolism, stroke and acute myocardial infarction in the users of levonorgestrel, desogestrel and gestodene low-dose oral contraceptives. Over a 3-year period, they collected a total of 15 unexpected idiopathic cardiovascular deaths in users of these products, a non-significant change, and no difference in the risk comparing desogestrel and gestodene to levonorgestrel. The risk estimates (adjusted for smoking and body size) were 2.2 for desogestrel (30 cases; confidence interval 1.1–4.4) and 2.1 for gestodene (22 cases; 1.0–4.4), compared to levonorgestrel users. Similar results were reported when women with deep vein thrombosis in the Leiden Thrombophilia Study in the Netherlands were reanalyzed for their use of oral contraceptives[9]. As expected, the risk of deep vein thrombosis was markedly higher in women who were carriers of the factor V Leiden mutation and in women with a family history of thrombosis.

Smoking, well recognized as a risk factor for arterial thrombosis, does not affect the risk estimates in these studies. This is not a new observation; older studies of venous thromboembolism also failed to identify smoking as a risk factor[10,11].

Subsequent studies

In Denmark, Lidegaard and colleagues performed a hospital-based, case–control study of 492 women with confirmed diagnoses of venous thromboembolism in 1994 and 1995 (in Denmark, all women with this diagnosis are hospitalized, and therefore very few, if any, cases were missed)[12]. A 2- to 3-fold increased risk of venous thromboembolism was found in current users of oral contraceptives, regardless of estrogen doses ranging from 20 to 50 µg. The increased risk was concentrated in the first year of use. Because there were more short-term users of the new progestins and more long-term users of the older progestins, adjustment for duration of use resulted in no significant differences between the different types of progestins.

A case–control study using 83 cases of venous thromboembolism derived from the computer records of general practices in the UK concluded that the increased risk associated with oral contraceptives was the same for all types, and that the pattern of risk with specific oral contraceptives suggested confounding because of 'preferential prescribing' (defined later)[13]. In this study, matching cases and controls by exact year of birth eliminated differences between different types of oral contraceptives. A similar analysis based upon 42 cases from a German database again found no difference between new progestin and older progestin oral contraceptives[14]. Thus, in these two studies, more precise adjustments for age eliminated a confounding bias. A reanalysis of the Transnational Case–Control Study considered the duration and patterns of oral contraceptive use[15]. This reanalysis focused on first-time users of second- and third-generation oral contraceptives. Sophisticated statistical analysis with adjustment for duration of use in 105 cases who were first-time users could find no differences between second- and third-generation products.

Former users discontinue oral contraceptives for a variety of reasons, and often are switched to what clinicians perceive to be 'safer' products ('preferential prescribing')[16,17]. Individuals who do well with a product tend to remain with that product. Thus at any one point in time, individuals on an older product will be relatively healthy and free of side-effects ('healthy user effect'). This is also called 'attrition of susceptibles' because higher-risk individuals with problems are gradually eliminated from the group[18]. Comparing users of older and newer products, therefore, can involve disparate cohorts of individuals.

Because desogestrel- and gestodene-containing products were marketed as less androgenic and therefore 'better' (a marketing claim not substantiated by epidemiologic studies), clinicians chose to provide these products to higher-risk patients and older women[16,17]. In addition, clinicians switched patients perceived to be at greater risk for thrombosis from older oral contraceptives to the newer formulations with desogestrel and gestodene. Furthermore, these products were prescribed more often to young women who were starting oral contraception for the first time (these young women will not have experienced the test of pregnancy or previous oral contraceptive use to help identify those who have a congenital predisposition to venous thrombosis). These changing practice patterns exert different effects over the lifetime of a product, and analytical adjustments are extremely difficult. The Transnational Group believes it accomplished an appropriate adjustment by focusing on first-time users and duration of use[15]. It is also unlikely that the 'healthy user effect' will be dominant in first-time users. Of course, this analysis found no differences between second- and third-generation oral contraceptives.

The challenge for a clinician is to make a decision: is an observational study with statistically significant results clinically (biologically) real? This controversy illustrates how difficult this can be. When faced with results from observational studies, clinicians want to see uniformity, consistency and agreement – all arguing in favor of a real clinical effect. Examples are the protective effect of oral contraceptives on the risk of ovarian cancer, and the benefits of postmenopausal estrogen therapy on cardiovascular disease. The initial studies were impressive in their agreement. All indicated increased relative risks associated with desogestrel and gestodene compared to levonorgestrel. Nevertheless, all of the early studies, somewhat similar in design, were influenced by the same unrecognized biases. Persistent errors will produce consistent conclusions.

The apparent differences associated with the new progestins, it is now clear, were due to two major factors: the marketing and prescribing of new products, and the characteristics of the patients for whom the new products were prescribed. Most impressive and important is the fact that there is no evidence of an increase in mortality due to venous thromboembolism since the introduction of new progestin oral contraceptives[8,19].

Venous thromboembolism and the factor V Leiden mutation

The new studies indicate that a risk of idiopathic venous thrombosis persists with low-dose oral contraceptives, at a level of approximately 3–4-fold greater than the normal, general incidence[6–9,20]. However, an inherited resistance to activated protein C, the factor V Leiden mutation, may account for a significant portion of the patients who experience venous thrombosis while taking oral contraceptives.

Several European centers have argued that screening for the factor V Leiden mutation should be routine prior to prescribing contraceptives. The carrier frequencies of the Leiden mutation in the American population (the percentages are similar in men and women) are given in Table 1[21]. These estimates are consistent with the European assessments, indicating that this is a trait carried in people of European origin. In the USA, of the 10 million women currently using oral contraceptives, about 423 000 are likely to carry the factor V mutation. However, because the incidence rate of venous thromboembolism is so low (4–5 per 10 000 young women per year)[21,22], the number of women required to be screened to prevent one death is tremendously large (Table 2). Furthermore, because only a small number of women even with the Leiden mutation have a clinical event, the finding of a positive screening test would be a barrier to the use of oral contraceptives, and a subsequent increase in unwanted pregnancies would likely follow. Most experts believe that screening for the Leiden mutation should only be pursued in women with a previous episode of venous thromboembolism or a positive family history for venous thrombosis.

Arterial thrombosis

Myocardial infarction

A population-based, case–control study analyzed 187 cases of myocardial infarction in users of low-dose oral contraceptives in the Kaiser Permanente Medical Care Program[23]. There was no statistically significant increase in the odds ratio for myocardial infarction in current oral contraceptive users compared with past or never users. A transnational case–control study of 182 cases of myocardial infarction collected from 16 centers in Austria, France, Germany, Switzerland and the UK obtained the results shown in Table 3[24]. These data were interpreted as indicating no increased risk of myocardial infarction associated with oral contraceptives containing desogestrel or gestodene. However, the reduced risk with the new progestin oral contraceptives was also emphasized (the comparison of third-generation products to second-generation products yielded a reduced risk that was statistically significant), suggesting a possible saving of deaths from myocardial infarction with desogestrel and gestodene. The problem is that the small actual incidence makes it difficult to acquire sufficient numbers. The conclusion was based on only seven cases and 49 controls using third-generation oral contraceptives and 28 cases and 71 controls using second-generation products, and, in the view of this author, the power is too limited to make any conclusion regarding the new progestin oral contraceptives. This is a good example of a conclusion that may be mathematically significant, but clinically not real.

The same study found that cigarette smoking carried a higher risk for myocardial infarction

Table 1 Carrier frequencies of the Leiden mutation in the American population[21]

Caucasian	5.27%
Hispanic	2.21%
Native American	1.25%
African	1.23%
Asian	0.45%

Table 2 Relative risk and actual incidence of venous thromboembolism[21,22]

Population	Relative risk	Incidence (per 10 000 per year)
General population of young women	1	4–5
Pregnant women	12	60
High-dose oral contraceptive users	6–10	24–50
Low-dose oral contraceptive users	3–4	12–20
Leiden mutation carriers	6–8	24–40
Leiden carriers and oral contraceptive users	30	120–150
Leiden mutation homozygous carriers	80	320–400

Table 3 Results of a transnational case–control study of myocardial infarction and oral contraceptive use[24]

Type of oral contraceptive	Number of cases	Number of controls	Odds ratio	Confidence interval
All oral contraceptives	57	156	2.35	1.42–3.89
50 µg estrogen	14	22	4.32	1.59–11.74
Old progestins	28	71	2.96	1.54–5.66
New progestins	7	49	0.82	0.29–2.31

than oral contraceptives, and that non-smoking users of oral contraceptives had no evidence of an increased risk[24]. In addition, there was an indication that patient screening is important in minimizing the impact of hypertension on the risk of myocardial infarction.

In the World Health Organization multicenter study, there were 368 cases of acute myocardial infarction[25]. Although there was about a 5-fold overall increased odds ratio of myocardial infarction in current users of oral contraceptives, essentially all cases occurred in women with cardiovascular risk factors. There was no apparent effect of increasing age on risk; however, there were only 12 cases among oral contraceptive users less than 35 years old. There was no apparent relationship with estrogen dose, and there was no apparent influence of type or dose of progestin. In the view of this author, the rare occurrence of this condition produced such small numbers that there was insufficient statistical power to accurately assess the effects of progestin type, and estrogen and progestin doses. The conclusion of this study was that the risk of myocardial infarction in women who use oral contraceptives is increased only in smokers (Table 4). In a Danish case–control study of 102 cases of acute myocardial infarction in young women, a statistically significant increase in risk was noted only in current users of 50 µg ethinyl estradiol[12].

Stroke

Older case–control and cohort studies indicated an increased risk of cerebral thrombosis among current users of high-dose oral contraceptives[27–29]. However, thrombotic stroke did not appear to be increased in healthy, non-smoking women with the use of oral contraceptives containing less than 50 µg ethinyl estradiol[28,29]. A case–control study of all 794 women in Denmark who suffered a cerebral thromboembolic attack during 1985–1989 concluded that there was an almost 2-fold increased relative risk associated with oral contraceptives containing 30–40 µg estrogen, and the risk was significantly influenced by both smoking and the dose of estrogen in additive (non-

Table 4 Incidence of myocardial infarction in reproductive-age women[25]

Population	Incidence (per 100 000 per year)
Overall incidence[26]	5
Women < 35 years old	
non-smokers	4
non-smokers and OC users	4
smokers	8
smokers and OC users	43
Women ≥ 35 years old	
non-smokers	10
non-smokers and OC users	40
smokers	88
smokers and OC users	485

Incidences are estimates based upon oral contraceptive use paired with cardiovascular risk factors prevalent in the general population. Effective screening would produce smaller numbers

synergistic) fashion[30]. A case–control analysis of data collected by the Royal College of General Practitioners' Oral Contraception Study concluded that current users were at increased risk of stroke (with a persisting effect in former users); however, this outcome was limited mainly to smokers and to formulations with 50 µg or more of estrogen[29].

A population-based, case–control study of 408 stroke patients from the California Kaiser Permanente Medical Care Program found no increase in risk for either ischemic stroke or hemorrhagic stroke[31]. Current users of low-dose oral contraceptives did not have an increased risk of ischemic or hemorrhagic stroke compared with former users and with never users. There was no evidence for an adverse effect of increasing age or smoking (for hemorrhagic stroke, there was a suggestion of a positive interaction between current oral contraceptive use and smoking, but the numbers were small, and the result was not statistically significant).

In a case–control study of 220 ischemic strokes in the UK, Germany, France, Switzerland and Austria[32], there was an overall 3-fold increase in the risk of ischemic stroke associated with the use of oral contraceptives, with higher risks observed in smokers (more than 10 cigarettes per day), in women with hypertension, and in users of higher-dose estrogen products. No differences were observed comparing second- and third-generation progestins.

The World Health Organization data on stroke come from the same collaborative study that yielded the publications on venous thromboembolism. The results with stroke were published as two separate reports, one on ischemic stroke and the other on hemorrhagic stroke[33,34]. The overall odds ratio for ischemic stroke indicated about a 3-fold increased risk. In Europe, however, the risk was statistically significant only for higher-dose products, and not for products with less than 50 µg ethinyl estradiol. In developing countries, there was no difference in risk with low- and higher-dose oral contraceptives. This is believed to be due to the strong influence of hypertension. In Europe, it was uncommon for women with a history of hypertension to be using oral contraceptives; however, this was not the case in developing countries. Duration of use and type of progestin had no impact, and past users did not have an increased risk, but smoking 10 or more cigarettes daily exerted a synergistic effect with oral contraceptives, increasing the risk of ischemic stroke, approximating the effect of hypertension and oral contraceptives. The risk was greater in women ≥ 35 years old; however, this too was believed to be due to an effect of hypertension. The conclusion of this study was therefore that the risk of ischemic stroke is extremely low, concentrated in those who use higher-dose products, smoke, and have hypertension.

Current use of oral contraceptives was associated with a slightly increased risk of hemorrhagic stroke only in developing countries, and not in Europe. This again probably reflects the presence of hypertension, because the greatest increased risk (about 10- to 15-fold) was identified in current users of oral contraceptives who had a history of hypertension. Current cigarette smoking also increased the risk in oral contraceptive users, but not as dramatically as hypertension. For hemorrhagic stroke, the dose of estrogen had no effect on risk, and neither did duration of use or type of progestin. This study concluded that the risk of hemorrhagic

stroke due to oral contraceptives is increased only slightly in older women, probably occurring only in women with risk factors such as hypertension.

The latest Danish case–control study included thrombotic strokes and transitory cerebral ischemic attacks analyzed together as cerebral thromboembolic attacks. Only users of second-generation oral contraceptives (levonorgestrel, norgestrel and norgestimate) had a statistically significant increased risk (about 2-fold). There was a dose–response relationship with estrogen in the dose range 20–50 µg ethinyl estradiol, although the number of 20-µg users (five cases, 22 controls) was not sufficient to establish a lower risk at this lower dose. This analysis claimed a reduced risk associated with desogestrel and gestodene; however, the odds ratio did not achieve statistical significance. Risk was increased with smoking, treated hypertension, diabetes, heart disease, frequent migraine, and a family history of myocardial infarction, but not with duration of use, or family history of venous thromboembolism.

The incidences of stroke in women of reproductive age, according to age and oral contraceptive use, are given in Table 5[26,31,33,34].

Conclusions

The large number of epidemiologic data in the last few years allows the construction of a clinical

Table 5 Incidence of stroke in reproductive-age women[26,31,33,34]

Population	Incidence (per 100 000 per year)
Ischemic stroke	
All women	5
women < 35 years old	1–3
women $\geq$ 35 years old	10
Hemorrhagic stroke	
All women	6
Excess cases due to oral contraceptives, including smokers and hypertensive patients	
low-dose oral contraceptives	2
low-dose oral contraceptives, age < 35 years	1
high-dose oral contraceptives	8

formulation that is evidence-based. The following conclusions are consistent with the recent reports.

(1) Pharmacologic estrogen increases the production of clotting factors.

(2) Progestins have no significant impact on clotting factors.

(3) Past users of oral contraceptives do not have an increased incidence of cardio-vascular disease.

(4) All low-dose oral contraceptives, regardless of progestin type, have an increased risk of venous thromboembolism. The actual risk of venous thrombosis with low-dose oral contraceptives is lower in the new studies compared to previous reports. Some have argued that this is due to preferential prescribing and the healthy user effect. However, it is also logical that the lower risk reflects better screening of patients and lower estrogen doses.

(5) Smoking has no effect on the risk of venous thrombosis.

(6) Smoking and estrogen have an additive effect on the risk of arterial thrombosis. Why is there a difference between venous and arterial clotting? The venous system has low flow with a state of high fibrinogen and low platelets, in contrast to the high flow state of the arterial system with low fibrinogen and high platelets. It is therefore understandable that these two different systems respond in different ways.

(7) Hypertension is a very important additive risk factor for stroke in oral contraceptive users.

(8) Low-dose oral contraceptives (less than 50 μg ethinyl estradiol) do not increase the risk of myocardial infarction or stroke in healthy, non-smoking women, regardless of age.

(9) Almost all myocardial infarctions and strokes in oral contraceptive users occur in users of high-dose products, or users with cardiovascular risk factors over the age of 35 years.

(10) Arterial thrombosis (myocardial infarction and stroke) has a dose–response relationship with the dose of estrogen, but there are insufficient data to determine whether there is a difference in risk with products that contain 20, 30 or 35 μg ethinyl estradiol.

The recent studies reinforce the belief that the risks of arterial and venous thrombosis are a consequence of the estrogen component of combination oral contraceptives. Current evidence does not support an advantage or disadvantage for any particular formulation, except for the greater safety associated with any product containing less than 50 μg ethinyl estradiol. Although it is logical to expect the greatest safety with the lowest dose of estrogen, the rare occurrence of arterial and venous thrombosis in healthy women makes it unlikely that there will be any measurable differences in the attributable incidence of clinical events with all low-dose products.

The new studies emphasize the importance of good patient screening. The occurrence of arterial thrombosis is essentially limited to older women who smoke or have cardiovascular risk factors, especially hypertension. The impact of good screening is evident in the repeated failure to detect an increase in mortality due to myocardial infarction or stroke in several studies[8,26]. Although the risk of venous thromboembolism is slightly increased, the actual incidence is still relatively low, and the mortality rate is about 1% (probably less with oral contraceptives, because most deaths from thromboembolism are associated with trauma, surgery, or a major illness). The minimal risk of venous thrombosis associated with oral contraceptive use does not justify the cost of routine screening for coagulation deficiencies.

If a patient has a family history or a previous episode of idiopathic thromboembolism, an evaluation to search for an underlying abnormality in the coagulation system is warranted[35]. A DNA-based test can be used to verify the presence of the factor V Leiden mutation. Other risk factors for thromboembolism that should be considered by clinicians include an acquired predisposition such as the presence of lupus anticoagulant or malignancy, and immobility or trauma. Varicose veins are not a risk factor unless they are very extensive[3].

Combination oral contraception is contra-indicated in women who have a history of idiopathic venous thromboembolism, and also in women who have a family history of idiopathic venous thromboembolism. These women will have a higher incidence of congenital deficiencies in important clotting measurements, especially antithrombin III, protein C and protein S, and resistance to activated protein C[36].

The conclusion once again is that low-dose oral contraceptives are very safe for healthy, young women. By effectively screening for the presence in older women of smoking and cardiovascular risk factors, especially hypertension, we can limit, if not eliminate, any increased risk for arterial disease associated with low-dose oral contraceptives. It is very important to emphasize that there is no increased risk of cardiovascular events associated with long-term use.

In the 1970s, as epidemiologic data first became available, we emphasized in our teaching and communication with patients the risks and dangers associated with oral contraceptives. In the 1990s, with better patient screening and epidemiologic data documenting the effects of low-dose products, we have appropriately emphasized the safety and benefits associated with modern oral contraceptives. The new studies summarized in this review should reinforce this message. The proper use of low-dose oral contraceptives is exceptionally safe, and oral contraceptives are associated with a collection of effects which yield an overall improvement in individual health. From a public health point of view, the combined impact leads to a decrease in the cost of healthcare. For both individual and public health, these impacts are especially significant in older women. These considerations allow the clinician to present oral contraception with a very positive attitude, an approach which makes an important contribution to a patient's ability to make appropriate health choices.

References

1. Child TJ, Rees M, MacKenzie IZ. Pregnancy terminations after oral contraception scare. *Lancet* 1996;347:1260–1

2. Skjeldestad FE. Increased number of induced abortions in Norway after media coverage of adverse vascular events from the use of third-generation oral contraceptives. *Contraception* 1997;55:11–14

3. Royal College of General Practitioners. Oral contraceptive study: oral contraceptives, venous thrombosis, and varicose veins. *J R Coll Gen Prac* 1978;28:393–9

4. Porter JB, Hershel J, Walker AM. Mortality among oral contraceptive users. *Obstet Gynecol* 1987;70:29–32

5. WHO Collaborative Study of Cardiovascular Disease and Steroid Hormone Contraception. Venous thromboembolic disease and combined oral contraceptives: results of international multicentre case–control study. *Lancet* 1995;348:1575–82

6. WHO Collaborative Study of Cardiovascular Disease and Steroid Hormone Contraception. Effect of different progestagens in low-oestrogen oral contraceptives on venous thromboembolic disease. *Lancet* 1995;348:1582–8

7. Spitzer WO, Lewis MA, Heinemann LAJ, *et al.* on behalf of the Transnational Research Group on Oral Contraceptives and the Health of Young Women. Third-generation oral contraceptives and risk of venous thromboembolic disorders: an international case–control study. *Br Med J* 1996;312:83–8

8. Jick H, Jick SS, Gurewich V, *et al.* Risk of idiopathic cardiovascular death and non-fatal venous thromboembolism in women using oral contraceptives with differing progestagen components. *Lancet* 1995;348:1589–93

9. Bloemenkammp KWM, Rosendaal FR, Helmerhorst FM, *et al.* Enhancement by factor V Leiden mutation of risk of deep vein thrombosis associated with oral contraceptives containing a

third-generation progestagen. *Lancet* 1995;348: 1593–6

10. Lawson DH, Davidson JF, Jick H. Oral contraceptive use and venous thromboembolism: absence of an effect of smoking. *Br Med J* 1977;2:729–30

11. Petitti DB, Wingerd J, Pellegrin F, *et al.* Oral contraceptives, smoking, and other factors in relation to risk of venous thromboembolic disease. *Am J Epidemiol* 1978;108:480–5

12. Lidegaard Ø, Edström B, Kreiner S. Oral contraceptives and venous thromboembolism. A case–control study. *Contraception* 1998;5:291–301

13. Farmer RDT, Lawrenson RA, Thompson CR, *et al.* Population-based study of risk of venous thromboembolism associated with various oral contraceptives. *Lancet* 1997;349:83–8

14. Farmer RDT, Todd J-C, Lewis MA, *et al.* The risks of venous thromboembolic disease among German women using oral contraceptives: a database study. *Contraception* 1998;57:67–70

15. Suissa S, Blais L, Spitzer WO, *et al.* First-time use of newer oral contraceptives and the risk of venous thromboembolism. *Contraception* 1997; 56:141–6

16. Heinemann LAJ, Lewis MA, Assman A, *et al.* Could preferential prescribing and referral behaviour of physicians explain the elevated thrombosis risk found to be associated with third-generation oral contraceptives? *Pharmacoepidemiol Drug Saf* 1996;5:285–94

17. Jamin C, de Mouzon J. Selective prescribing of third-generation oral contraceptives. *Contraception* 1996;54:55–6

18. Lewis MA, Heinemann LAJ, MacRae KD, *et al.* The increased risk of venous thromboembolism and the use of third-generation progestagens: role of bias in observational research. *Contraception* 1996;54:5–13

19. Farmer R, Lewis M. Oral contraceptives and mortality from venous thromboembolism. *Lancet* 1996;348:1095

20. Farmer RDT, Preston TD. The risk of venous thromboembolism associated with low-estrogen oral contraceptives. *J Obstet Gynaecol* 1995;15: 195–200

21. Ridker PM, Miletich JP, Hennekens CH, *et al.* Ethnic distribution of factor V Leiden in 4047 men and women: implications for venous thromboembolism screening. *J Am Med Assoc* 1997;277:1305–7

22. Vandenbroucke JP, van der Meer FJM, Helmerhorst FM, *et al.* Factor V Leiden. *Br Med J* 1996;313:1127–30

23. Sidney S, Petitti DB, Quesenberry CP, *et al.* Myocardial infarction in users of low-dose oral contraceptives. *Obstet Gynecol* 1996;88:939–44

24. Lewis MA, Heinemann LAJ, Spitzer WO, *et al.* for the Transnational Research Group on Oral Contraceptives and the Health of Young Women. The use of oral contraceptives and the occurrence of acute myocardial infarction in young women. Results from the Transnational Study on Oral Contraceptives and the Health of Young Women. *Contraception* 1997;56:129–40

25. WHO Collaborative Study of Cardiovascular Disease and Steroid Hormone Contraception. Acute myocardial infarction and combined oral contraceptives: results of an international multi-centre case–control study. *Lancet* 1997;349: 1202–9

26. Petitti DB, Sidney S, Quesenberry Jr CP, *et al.* Incidence of stroke and myocardial infarction in women of reproductive age. *Stroke* 1997;28:280–3

27. Jick H, Porter J, Rothman KJ. Oral contraceptives and non-fatal stroke in healthy young women. *Ann Int Med* 1978;89:58–60

28. Vessey MP, Lawless M, Yeates D. Oral contraceptives and stroke: findings in a large prospective study. *Br Med J* 1984;289:530

29. Hannaford PC, Croft PR, Kay CR. Oral contraception and stroke: evidence from the Royal College of General Practitioners' Oral Contraception Study. *Stroke* 1994;25:935–42

30. Lidegaard Ø. Oral contraception and risk of a cerebral thromboembolic attack: results of a case–control study. *Br Med J* 1993; 306:956–63

31. Petitti DB, Sidney S, Bernstein A, *et al.* Stroke in users of low-dose oral contraceptives. *N Engl J Med* 1996;335:8–15

32. Heinemann LAJ, Lewis MA, Spitzer WO, *et al.* Thromboembolic stroke in young women. A European case–control study on oral contraceptives. *Contraception* 1998;57:29–37

33. WHO Collaborative Study of Cardiovascular Disease and Steroid Hormone Contraception. Ischaemic stroke and combined oral contraceptives: results of an international, multicentre case–control study. *Lancet* 1996;348:498–505

34. WHO Collaborative Study of Cardiovascular Disease and Steroid Hormone Contraception. Haemorrhagic stroke, overall stroke risk, and combined oral contraceptives: results of an international, multicentre, case–control study. *Lancet* 1996;348:505–610

35. Vandenbroucke JP, Koster T, Briët E, *et al.* Increased risk of venous thrombosis in oral contraceptive users who are carriers of factor V Leiden mutation. *Lancet* 1994;344:1453–7

36. Pabinger I, Schneider B and the GTH Study Group. Thrombotic risk of women with hereditary antithrombin III, protein C, and protein S deficiency taking oral contraceptive medication. *Thromb Haemost* 1994;5:548–52

Abortion in adolescence 8

G. Benagiano, P. Franceschinis and A. Pera

Introduction

Induced abortion, or the voluntary termination of an already established pregnancy, is – for most women – a traumatic event. It may have psychological consequences, especially in those cultures where suppression of human life – after gestation has been proven – is considered ethically unacceptable, and it can have consequences for health and future fertility if it is performed under unsafe conditions.

There is wide international consensus that induced abortion should never be considered as a method of family planning. The Report of the 1994 Cairo Conference on Population and Development states clearly that 'In no case should abortion be promoted as a method of family planning'[1]. In spite of this official position of the United Nations, unavailability or the high cost of modern contraceptives has forced women, especially in the countries of the former socialist block, to rely upon easily accessible and free abortion facilities to meet their family planning needs[2].

These two considerations are particularly important when dealing with induced abortion in adolescence. In this eventuality, psychological consequences are often more serious, because the young woman will normally want to have children, and physical damage is more serious, especially if the intervention leads to pelvic infection and infertility.

It is therefore of paramount importance to educate girls regarding the consequences of abortions (especially in those countries where the interruption of a gestation is illegal and therefore the likelihood that a clandestine abortion be performed under unsafe conditions is greater), and regarding the contraceptive methods that are available in that particular setting.

Starting from updated statistics, this chapter briefly discusses the most common consequences of an induced abortion for adolescent girls and the work that needs to be carried out to educate and empower girls so that they can move from abortion to contraception.

The World Health Organization (WHO) defines an adolescent as a person between 10 and 19 years of age, and many studies throughout the world have adopted this age range as the standard. Defining adolescence by a particular age range may defy standardization, as various terms and age ranges are commonly encountered in the literature: 15–24 (youth) and 10–24 (young people)[3].

Size of the problem

Current estimates have identified 16 June 1999 as the 'official day' when the world population will reach the six billion mark[4]. The United Nations has estimated that more than half the world's population is under 25 and, by the year 2020, their total number will increase by more than 20%[5].

When, in less than a year from now, humanity will celebrate the beginning of the third millennium, another 90 million people will be added to the six billion figure, and about 17.5% (or more than one billion) will be aged 15–24[5].

Even utilizing WHO's definition, there are today more than one billion young men and women between the ages of 10 and 19 around the world, the largest generation of youth in history. A significant number of these adolescents are sexually active at early ages, and an increasing proportion of this sexual activity occurs outside marriage. A large number of sexually active adolescents, even those who are already married, do not utilize any method of protection against unwanted pregnancy, nor do they protect themselves against the risk of sexually transmitted diseases (STDs). As a consequence, each year, one in every 20 teenagers contracts a sexually transmitted infection, and about one-half of all the human immunodeficiency virus (HIV) infections have occurred in persons below age 25, their total number probably exceeding six million[6].

Because, globally, the number of adolescents is growing and the world-wide decrease in birth rates affects them less than it does other age groups (teenage pregnancies account for some 10% of the total), the absolute number of adolescent pregnancies is increasing[7], and it is calculated that, today, 15 million teenage girls give birth every year[6]. Details of the global situation are given in Table 1.

Referring more specifically to the voluntary interruption of gestation or voluntary abortion in adolescent women, current estimates indicate that their number is globally around 4.4 million world-wide[5], with two million unsafe abortions per year being performed in developing countries[8].

It must be stressed that, for adolescent girls of developing countries, with limited access to primary and secondary obstetric care facilities, pregnancy – irrespective of its outcome – carries an increased risk. Even when pregnancies are planned, there can be risks for both the young mother and her child: maternal mortality is two to four times higher below age 20 and infant death some 30% higher[6]. The World Bank has calculated that, in the absence of obstetric care, giving birth before the age of 18 increases three-fold the likelihood of dying in childbirth[9] and, indeed, pregnancy represents a source of inequity between adolescents: in Western, industrialized countries, where appropriate care exists for teenage mothers, no excessive risk has been observed[10,11].

Young and unmarried women, because of the social stigma of pregnancy before marriage, usually seek abortion under unsafe, clandestine conditions, even where voluntary interruption of gestation is legal and available through the health system. This, in turn, causes a higher than average (for a given country) incidence of complications among teenage girls.

Consequences of abortion for adolescents

Unsafe abortion in adolescent girls of developing countries is burdened by severe sequelae and deaths. A number of medical complications may be associated with voluntary interruption of gestation performed on adolescent girls, especially when the procedure is performed outside of obstetric facilities. The immediate results can be hemorrhage, septicemia, cervical and vaginal lacerations and pelvic abscess and, in the long term, there may be risk of ectopic pregnancy, chronic pelvic infection and secondary infertility[12].

Table 1 Teenagers and motherhood by world region[6]

Region	Population 15–19 1994 (million)	Ever married, female (%)	Giving birth each year (%)	Contraceptive prevalence rate, married (%)
Sub-Saharan Africa	62	33	14	—
North Africa	16	13	5	13
West Asia	16	—	6	—
South Asia	129	44	10	17
Southeast Asia	49	16	5	25
East Asia	116	4	1	15
Oceania	2	7	3	—
Latin America	48	17	8	36
North America	19	5	6	46
Europe	36	5	2	—
Former USSR	22	—	5	—
World	513	21	6	19

Generally, health consequences of abortion are particularly serious for adolescents; even where abortion is legal and unrestricted, as is the case for India, a number of studies indicate that unmarried adolescents, because of lack of awareness, cost, ignorance of services and fear of the social stigma[13] are more likely to delay the time of the voluntary interruption of gestation and therefore end up with a second-trimester voluntary abortion, not only a more complex procedure, but also a more hazardous one[14–19]. Indeed, studies suggest that almost 25% of all Indian adolescents who sought second-trimester abortions suffered complications, compared to 11% for the first trimester[17].

A tragedy within the drama is that, in certain countries, a substantial number of abortions are requested because of a pregnancy that resulted from rape or forced sex[20]. In this eventuality, there can be major psychological consequences, although it is rare that an abortion would not carry some mental imbalance.

Besides immediate severe bleeding, the most serious sequela of an abortion is pelvic infection; the consequences of such an infection will be very different, depending on the country and setting in which the adolescent lives. A major WHO study of the causes of infertility[21] indicates that, overall, more than 85% of the couples studied in Africa had diagnoses which could be attributed to infection, something that clearly involves a sexually transmitted origin. The rate of tubal occlusion in these women was more than three times that of other geographical areas. It must be stressed that, in Africa,

tubal occlusion is a non-curable condition, as the probability for a woman there to resort to *in vitro* fertilization and embryo transfer is close to zero.

Prevention of upper genital tract infections then becomes essential as, clearly, both STDs and infectious complications of pregnancy or abortion affect the level of bilateral tubal occlusion in a population. As indicated in Table 2, in all regions evaluated in the WHO-sponsored study, women with a history of STDs or pregnancy complications had higher rates of infection-related diagnoses, but Africa had the greatest problems.

Finally, we must not forget that, all over the world, a childless couple suffers the psychological trauma of a truncated family. The social consequences of infertility are, however, very different in different settings. If a young woman is condemned to infertility following a pelvic infection acquired after a voluntary interruption of gestation, she may – in a number of developing countries – be rejected by society, abandoned by her husband and end up marginalized, to say the least.

Educating adolescent women

In developed and developing countries, adolescents initiate sexual activity at about the same age. However, pregnancy rates are 5–20 times higher in developing countries, because sexual and contraceptive education and services are usually absent[22].

Table 2 Women with infection-related diagnoses, by history of sexually transmitted disease: pregnancy complications by regional group

	% Infection-related diagnoses			
	Developed	*Africa*	*Asia*	*Latin America*
History of STD in the woman				
yes	52.1	88.5	56.3	75.0*
no	26.8	61.4	32.2	34.2
History of postpartum/abortion complications				
yes	56.3	76.2	65.2	57.7
no	26.9	62.2	31.9	34.1

*Less than ten observations per cell. Adapted from WHO: infections, pregnancies and infertility: perspectives on prevention. *Fertil Steril* 1987;47:964–8

Almost without exception, adolescents of both sexes are poorly informed about ways to protect themselves from sex in general and unwanted pregnancy in particular; therefore, sexually active adolescent girls are often more exposed to pregnancy than adult women. In addition, voluntary interruption of gestation places a particularly high burden on adolescent women because, in the majority of settings, it will affect her future behavior, health and opportunities in life.

Changes in the economy of countries and increased urbanization have made formal-sector employment increasingly more important, and education more critical in finding work and advancing careers[23].

Formal education not only gives adolescents the skills that enable them to compete in a changing labor market, but also provides practical knowledge that can be applied in all areas of their lives. In addition, an educated woman will usually acquire a higher status in the family and the community, and a greater say in decisions such as when and whom she will marry[24]. For adolescent girls, the benefits are especially important and lasting, because an educated woman has a better chance of receiving medical care, and of having the knowledge necessary to maintain her own and her family's health[23]. She is better equipped to avoid unwanted pregnancy and therefore voluntary abortion, because she is more likely to use contraception; in turn, she will have a better chance of delaying having children until after 20 years of age[25]. Although we know of no data on the specific issue of the relationship between education and the likelihood of needing an abortion during adolescence, it is a fact that the countries where widespread sexual education and information about contraception make adolescents aware of the risks of unprotected sexual activities are those with the lowest abortion rates[26].

From abortion to contraception

The voluntary interruption of gestation was treated as a crime in most European countries until the 1960s and 1970s. Unfortunately, more often than not, this policy was coupled with restrictions on the use of contraceptives. This created a situation where, on the one hand, women could not prevent unwanted pregnancies and, on the other, they had to resort to clandestine voluntary abortion. An interesting insight into this situation was provided in a conversation held some 4 years ago in London, with the then President of the International Planned Parenthood Federation's Central Council, François Ekam of Togo. He explained that his interest in family planning dated back to when he was a student at the Sorbonne in Paris more than 30 years previously. He was then a member of the board of the student health-insurance plan, and this insurance group was chronically in the red; being an economics student, he started investigating the reasons for the deficit, and found out that female students purchased large quantities of antibiotics. He then discovered that this was a consequence of the fairly large number of clandestine abortions among these students, which, of course, carried complications necessitating treatment[27].

Therefore, the criminalization of abortion and the lack of access to contraception simply made termination of pregnancy a health hazard, not a procedure that young French women would not utilize.

Considering the period in life when women resort to voluntary abortion, in the industrialized Western countries, abortion rates are highest at around 20 years of age. In England and Wales, women below 25 years of age account for 56% of all abortions; this percentage increases to 61% in the case of the USA. One explanation is that young unmarried women often find access to contraception restricted and, even when they utilize a contraceptive modality, they utilize it less effectively. In addition, raising a child poses greater challenges to them than to a married woman[26].

As already stated, education and awareness about sex and family planning play a crucial role in avoiding voluntary interruption of gestation. Although the rates of premarital sex are similar in North America and in Western Europe, in some European countries such as The Netherlands or Finland, where the knowledge about contraception is widespread and the

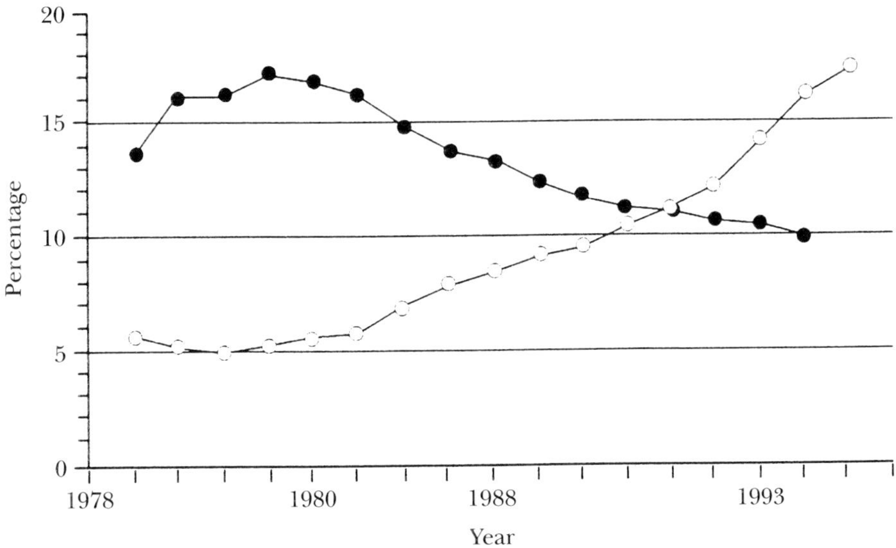

Figure 1 Relationship between voluntary pregnancy termination (black circles) and oral contraceptive use (white circles) in Italy

provision of family planning services for adolescents non-controversial, abortion rates are one-fifth those of the USA, where contraceptives are harder to obtain[26]. Abortion rates are also rising among adolescents in many urban areas of sub-Saharan Africa, where policies on contraception for single adolescent girls are ambiguous, to say the least[28].

The utilization of contraceptive methods by adolescents (irrespective of whether they are married or not) is increasing all over the world, although, in the majority of developing countries, it is still low. Surveys tell us that the majority of adolescent women have heard about contraceptives, but this does not translate into widespread use, because they often lack proper access to clinics and therefore do not know how to utilize them correctly, or fear their side-effects. Furthermore, often, family planning clinics do not offer the necessary confidentiality, and may expose them to the social stigma of being seen as practicing premarital sex. Finally, in the field of contraception, many young women have little negotiating power with their partners, and meager financial resources to secure the most effective methods.

For all these reasons, moving from abortion to contraception requires the positive intervention of governments. For example, in Estonia, where voluntary abortion is legal, the government has recently adopted a policy whereby women are charged for abortion services and this money is then used to subsidize contraceptives[27].

Another positive example is provided by Italy, where, following legalization, abortions decreased from about 235 000 in 1984 to some 150 000 in 1993. Also, the ratio of abortions/live births decreased from 38 to 27%. Finally, abortion rates among women of reproductive age decreased from 17 to a very low 10.5 per 1000[29]. The downward trend continues to this day, as a result of the active promotion of contraception (Figure 1).

A few years ago, the Ministry of Health of Italy launched a very good initiative called 'Women's Welfare'[30] (Figure 2). The text under the center diagram says: 'this young woman is happy not because she found the ideal shampoo against dandruff,...but because [right picture] she now knows that she will be able to avoid abortion with a contraceptive adapted to her needs'.

Thus, in Italy, it is family planning that has created the conditions for a major reduction in the need to resort to abortion, especially among adolescents, as shown in Figure 3[31].

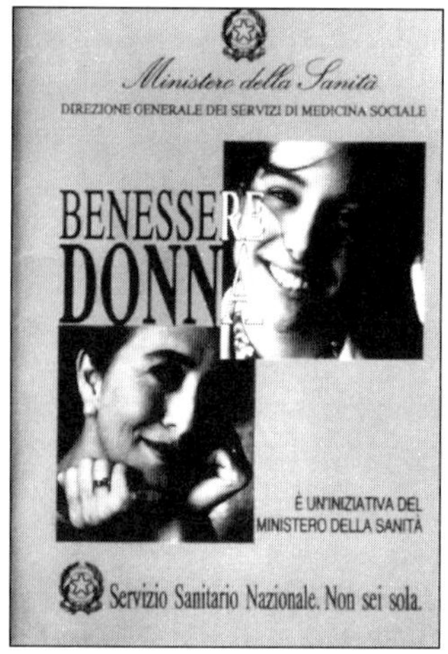
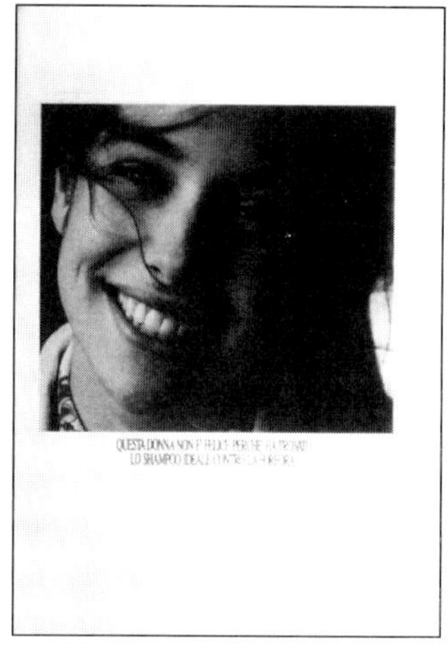
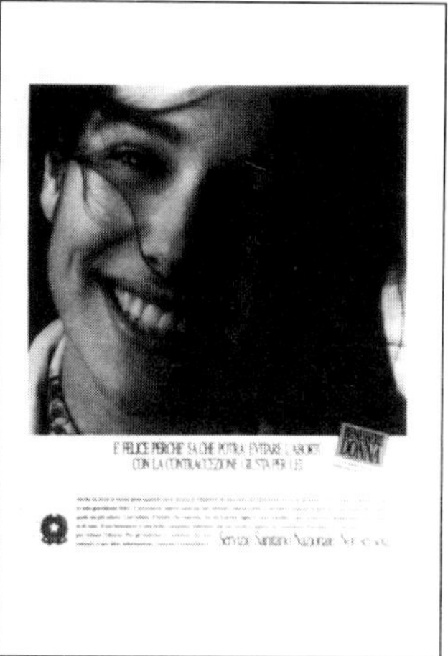

Figure 2   The 'Women Welfare' initiative of the Italian Ministry of Health

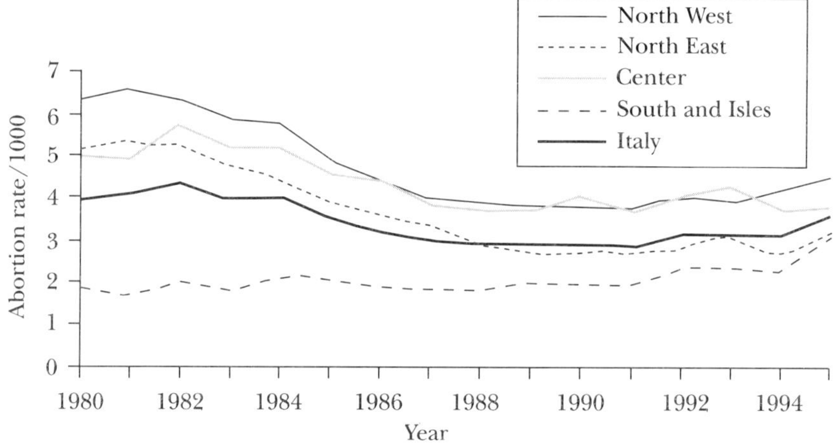

Figure 3   Voluntary pregnancy termination in Italy: abortion rates per 1000 adolescents in different areas

There is no question that contraception is the corner-stone of our fight to reduce abortion, although the relationship between contraception and abortion is fairly complex. As already stated, data from several industrialized countries tell us that, where contraception is well established and utilized by the vast majority of people and where it is associated with a proper sex education, the need to resort to an abortion has substantially decreased. France, Finland (and the other Scandinavian countries) and The Netherlands are the best examples of this[32].

Contraceptive prevalence is directly linked to method availability: the higher the number of methods available, the higher the contraceptive prevalence, as shown in Figure 4[24]. Indeed, the availability of a variety of methods encourages contraceptive continuation by allowing women and couples to switch to methods that better meet their changing needs.

Conclusion

The fight to reduce the need for an adolescent to resort to an abortion to eliminate an

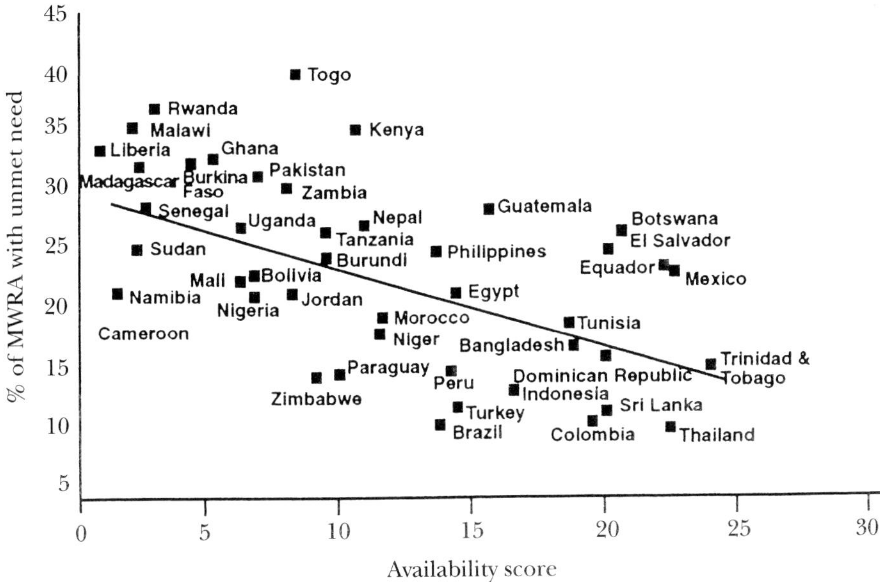

Figure 4 Relationship between number of methods available and unmet need for contraception: scores calculated on basis of judgements about availability of contraceptive methods by senior family personnel and observers in each country. MWRA, married women of reproductive age

unwanted pregnancy should be a unifying force in the world. Unfortuately, this is absolutely not the case, and the international community remains deeply divided on the subject.

One reason for this inability to unite in the fight against abortion is the rejection, or lukewarm support, that contraception receives among certain groups. Also, those opposed to premarital sex often prefer to stand firm on the rejection of contraception, and therefore refute the idea of sexual education programs that include knowledge of modern contraceptive modalities.

Under the circumstances, those committed to decreasing abortion among adolescent girls must continue their fight for appropriate education of adolescents, for easy availability of modern contraceptives and for prompt access to clinics, which not only provide updated information, but also guarantee the level of confidentiality that makes the adolescent comfortable.

References

1. United Nations. *Population and Development. Programme of Action Adopted at the International Conference on Population and Development.* New York: UN, 1995;1:30–1

2. Serbanescu F, Morris L, Stupp P, Stanescu A. The impact of recent policy changes on fertility, abortion and contraceptive use in Romania. *Stud Fam Plann* 1995;26:76–87

3. World Health Organization. *Young People's Health: a Challenge for Society.* Geneva: WHO, 1986

4. United Nations Population Fund. *UNFPA and Adolescents.* New York: UNFPA, 1998

5. United Nations. *The Sex and Age Distribution of the World Population.* New York: UN, 1994

6. Population Reference Bureau/Center for Population Options. *The World's Youth: a Special Focus on Reproductive Health.* New York: PRB, 1994

7. Family Health International. Adolescent reproductive health. *Network* 1997;17:9

8. Population Reference Bureau. *Chart of the World's Youth 1996*. Washington: PRB, 1996

9. The World Bank. *Investing in Health. World Development Report 1993*. New York: Oxford University Press, 1993

10. Morini A, Schwarzenberger L, Petronio E, *et al*. Il parto nelle adolescenti: casistiche del periodo 1976–1986 negli Istituti di Clinica Ostetrica e Ginecologica dell'Università 'La Sapienza' di Roma. In *Adolescenza: un Problema Sociale*. Rome: Pozzi, 1989:121–2

11. Alan Guttmacher Institute. *Risks and Realities of Early Childbearing Worldwide: Issues in Brief*. New York: Alan Guttmacher Institute, 1997

12. International Planned Parenthood Federation. *Understanding Adolescents*. London: IPPF, 1994

13. Jejeebhoy S. *Adolescent Sexual and Reproductive Behavior: a Review of the Evidence from India*. Washington: International Center for Research on Women, 1996

14. Chhabra S. A step towards helping mothers with unmarried pregnancies. *Indian J Maternal Child Health* 1992;3:41–2

15. Solapurkar ML, Sangam RN. Has the MTP act in India proved beneficial? *J Fam Welfare* 1985;31: 46–52

16. Diverkar SA, Natarajan G, Canguli AC, Purandare VN. Abortion in unmarried girls. *Health Pop Perspect Issues* 1979;2:308–21

17. Aras RY, Pai NP, Jain SG. Termination of pregnancy in adolescents. *J Postgrad Med* 1987;33: 120–4

18. Bhatt RV. An Indian study of the psychosocial behavior of pregnant teenage women. *J Reprod Med* 1978;21:275–8

19. Chhabra S, Gupte N, Mehta A, Shende A. Medical termination of pregnancy and concurrent contraceptive adoption in rural India. *Stud Fam Plann* 1988;19:244–7

20. De Silva WI. Socio-economic change and adolescent issues in the Asian and Pacific region. In *Report and Recommendations of the Expert Group Meeting on Adolescents: Implications of Population Trends, Environment, and Development*. New York: UN, 1998,46–70

21. Cates W, Farley TMM, Rowe PJ. Worldwide patterns of infertility: is Africa different? *Lancet* 1985;2:596–8

22. Ketting E. Meeting young people's sexual and reproductive health needs worldwide. *Planned Parenthood Challenges* 1995;1:28–31

23. United Nations Population Fund. *The State of World Population: the New Generation*. New York: UNFPA, 1998

24. Martin LG, Kinsella K. Research on the demography of aging in developing countries. In Martin LG, Preston SH, eds. *Demography of Aging*. Washington: National Academy Press, 1994

25. World Health Organization, Division of Family Health. *Health Benefits of Family Planning*. Geneva: WHO, 1995

26. Jones EF, Forrest JD, Henshaw SK, Silverman J, Torres A. *Pregnancy, Contraception and Family Planning Services in Industrialized Countries*. New Haven: Yale University Press, 1989

27. Benagiano G, Pera A. Decreasing abortion: the potential and the constraints. In Rabe T, Runnebaum B, eds. *Fertility Control Update and Trends*. Berlin, Heidelberg: Springer-Verlag, 1999

28. Coeytaux F. Induced abortion in sub-Saharan Africa: what we know and do not know. *Stud Fam Plann* 1988;19:186–90

29. Spinelli A. Italia. In Dalla Zuanna G, ed. *Contraccezione ed Aborto alle soglie del 2000*. Rome: Dipartimento di Scienze Demografiche, Università degli Studi di Roma 'la Sapienza', 1996:189–208

30. Ministero della Sanità, Servizio Sanitario Nazionale. *Benessere Donna*. Rome: Istituto Poligrafico dello Stato, 1994

31. Istituto Nazionale di Statistica. *L'interruzione volontaria di gravidanza in Italia*. Rome: ISTAT, 1997

32. Grunseit A, Kippax S. *Effects of sex education on young people's sexual behaviour*. Unpublished review commissioned by the Global Programme on AIDS. Geneva: WHO, 1993

Monthly injectable contraceptives: recent advances

9

P. Spinola

Introduction

Contraceptive steroid formulations are more easily delivered systemically than orally. The injectable approach fulfils many of the features of an ideal contraceptive as it is highly effective, long-acting, simple to use, non-invasive, unrelated to coitus, requires minimal motivation and is relatively inexpensive[1]. It is estimated that about 15 million women worldwide use injectable contraceptives to regulate their fertility. The most widely used injectable (by more than 12 million women) is depot-medroxyprogesterone acetate (DMPA)[2]. There is increasing interest in once-a-month injectables consisting of a combination of a long-acting progestin and estrogen, because they give rise to a monthly bleeding episode and to a lower frequency of bleeding irregularities than progestin-only injectables. The formulation most frequently tested during the period 1960–70 was a combination of 150 mg of dihydroxyprogesterone acetophenide (DHPA) with 10 mg estradiol enanthate. This combination proved later to give the most satisfactory cyclic bleeding, minimal side-effects and rapid return of ovulation after discontinuation. The combination of progestin and estrogen that became Cyclofem was originally developed in Brazil in 1968[3], and the combination that became Mesigyna was first tested in 1974[4]. Indeed, the first formulation tested as an injectable contraceptive was 17α-hydroxyprogesterone caproate 500 mg and estradiol valerate 10 mg in 1963[5]. The half-dose of this formulation has been extensively used in China as Chinese Injectable No. 1 or Gravibinon.

Monthly injectables currently available

There is an estimated total of at least three million women using the once-a-month injectables most widely used in Latin America and China (Table 1). When the clinical assessment of Cyclofem and Mesigyna was satisfactorily completed, the World Health Organization initiated a systematic program to introduce Cyclofem into the national family planning programs of several countries. The injection of all injectable contraceptives should be given intramuscularly because absorption may be too slow if the provider injects into fat. In contrast, massaging the injection site accelerates absorption and thus should also be avoided.

The advantages and disadvantages of once-a-month injectable contraceptives compared to progestin-only formulations are shown in Table 2. The main indication for the contraceptive use of monthly injectables includes women who do not tolerate or are unwilling or unable to use oral contraceptive pills, intrauterine devices or barrier methods. Also, those who prefer a long-acting method and accept some menstrual irregularities are possible candidates for the use of these injections. Contraindications are the same as those of combined oral contraceptives[1].

The combination of DHPA 150 mg with estradiol enanthate 10 mg is probably the most widely used injectable contraceptive in Latin

Table 1 Brand names, formulations and injection schedules of various injectable contraceptives commonly used in Latin America and China

Brand name	Formulation	Injection schedule
Perlutan, Unociclo, Ciclovular, Perlutal, Topasel, Agurin, Horpotral	DHPA 150 mg + EEN 10 mg	every month between the 7th and 10th days of each menstrual cycle
Anafertin, Yectames	DHPA 75 mg + EEN 5 mg	every month between the 7th and 10th days of each menstrual cycle
Cyclofem, Cyclofemina, Cycloprovera, Cyclogeston	DMPA 25 mg + ECYP 5 mg	every month; first injection 1st to 5th day of the menstrual cycle; subsequently every 30 ± 3 days
Mesigyna	NEE 50 mg + EVAL 5 mg	every month; first injection 1st to 5th day of the menstrual cycle; subsequently every 30 ± 3 days
Gravibinon, Chinese Injectable No. 1	17-OH-PC 250 mg + EVAL 5 mg	every month; two injections in the first month; subsequently at 28-day intervals

DHPA, dihydroxyprogesterone acetophenide; EEN, estradiol enanthate; DMPA, depot-medroxyprogesterone acetate; ECYP, estradiol cypionate; NEE, norethindrone enanthate; EVAL, estradiol valerate; 17-OH-PC, 17-hydroxyprogesterone caproate

Table 2 Relative advantages and disadvantages of once-a-month injectables compared to long-acting progestin-only formulations

Advantages	Disadvantages
Better cycle control	not suitable for lactating women
Less endometrial suppression	shorter-acting and more injections
More rapid return of fertility	not for women with contraindications to use of estrogens
More contact with health personnel	presence of estrogen side-effects
Shorter inconvenience if side-effects occur	
Half of the progestin dose	
Similar or higher contraceptive efficacy and acceptability	

America, being used by at least one million women[6]. Despite the good acceptability of the combination, some investigators believe that the doses of both components could be reduced without loss of efficacy[7]. Recently, a clinical trial was carried out in nine family planning centers in Brazil[8]. The study was a comparative, double-blind clinical trial in which a combination containing DHPA 90 mg with estradiol enanthate 6 mg was compared with the regular combination of DHPA 150 mg with estradiol enanthate 10 mg. The study showed that intramuscular injection of the low dose given at approximately 24-day intervals is as effective in preventing conception in women as the higher dose injection, and the study also showed that the total number of subjects who discontinued the use of either one of the two combinations was approximately the same. One of the important aspects of this trial is the fact that the women in the study had constant access to other methods of contraception. During their monthly visits to the family planning clinics, they met with women using other methods of contraception such as intrauterine devices and other long-acting methods such as subdermal implants or sterilization. As these methods were also available to patients enrolled in this trial on demand, this may have tempted some of them to switch to another method being praised by the other women. However, the fact that 60% of the women did not discontinue the study indicates that at least half of those who used either the low or the high dose were genuinely pleased with the method and inclined to continue using it.

The present finding that the combination of a natural estrogen with the simplest progesterone derivative available is as effective and acceptable as the previously available high-dosage combination will certainly come as good news to users of this product.

References

1. Toppozada MK. Existing once-a-month combined injectable contraceptives. *Contraception* 1994;49: 293–301
2. World Health Organization. *Annual Technical Report 1997*. Geneva: World Health Organization, 1998
3. Coutinho EM, de Souza JC. Conception control by monthly injections of medroxyprogesterone suspension and a long-acting estrogen. *J Reprod Fertil* 1968;15:209–14
4. Newton JR, Darcangues C, Hall PE. Once-a-month combined injectable contraceptives. *J Obstet Gynaecol* 1994;14(Suppl 1):1–34
5. Siegel I. Conception control by long-acting progestogens: preliminary report. *Obstet Gynecol* 1963;21:666–8
6. Lande RE. Injectables and implants. *Population Reports* 1995; Series K, No. 5
7. Moore LL, Valuck R, McDougall C, *et al.* A comparative study of 1-year weight gain among users of medroxyprogesterone acetate, levonorgestrel implants, and oral contraceptives. *Contraception* 1995;52:215–20
8. Coutinho EM, Spinola P, Barbosa I, *et al.* Multicenter, double-blind, comparative clinical study on the efficacy and acceptability of a monthly injectable contraceptive combination of 150 mg dihydroxyprogesterone acetophenide and 10 mg estradiol enanthate compared to a monthly injectable comparative combination of 90 mg dihydroxyprogesterone acetophenide and 6 mg estradiol enanthate. *Contraception* 1997;55:175–81

Barriers to contraceptive use in developing countries

10

O. A. Ladipo and J. C. Konje

Introduction

Population explosion poses one of the greatest challenges to reproductive healthcare providers, governments and voluntary agencies as we approach the next millennium. This challenge is greatest in the developing countries where poverty, ignorance and disease prevail. The current world population estimate of 5.8 billion is double the estimate of 1957[1]. It is estimated that every year at the current growth rate, 81 million people will be added to this figure. Of these, 93% will be from the developing countries. By the year 2000, the projected world population will be 5.96 billion, and by 2050 it will be 9.4 billion – an addition of 3.6 billion which is currently the population of Asia[1–4]. Although the use of modern methods of contraception to regulate fertility have to a large extent been widely adopted in the developed countries, uptake remains poor in the developing countries. This is mainly due to the existence of cultural, economic and political barriers[5,6]. While there has been concerted international, regional and national effort to address these unmet needs for fertility control in the developing countries, there must be parallel effort to address these barriers, or access to modern methods of contraception will remain poor.

Socio-economic, cultural and geo-political barriers

Culture and tradition are acknowledged to be major barriers to contraceptive acceptance and practice in developing countries, and in particular in Africa[6]. The ineffectiveness of many family planning programs which exist in many developing countries can be attributed to failure to understand and therefore overcome the cultural barriers of the traditional communities.

Poverty and illiteracy

In developing countries over 50% of the population are poor, illiterate, monolingual and live in rural areas. These are significant handicaps to their knowledge of modern contraceptive methods, and hence utilization is generally poorer than that of their urban counterparts who are better educated and informed. In fact, rural women are not only poor, they are powerless, and always pregnant.

Family size

Large families are the norm in some developing countries because of the high premium placed on childbearing and parenthood, the need to have extra 'insurance' births (fuelled by high perinatal, infant and child mortality) and the status it confers on a man who is economically disadvantaged. In large rural farming communities, children provide manpower for the farms and security in old age – especially as there are no universal pensions or care for the elderly.

Security and safety

In rural communities, grown-up children provide military might and political strength, ensure marriage alliances that create large networks for safety and security of lineage and in many cultural settings (in some regions) are expected to protect the land and fight intruders.

Particular sex preference

In some cultures, sons are preferred over females as they help on the farm, act as insurance for old age, are agents of continuity for the family name and can if required fulfill the priestly duty of pouring libation, without which the ancestral spirits will begin to fade as they are forgotten. In such cultures, therefore, many women who have only daughters continue to try for a son until they are menopausal or die due to complications of high parity. In many Asian countries where cremation is the norm, it is the son that lights the crematorium fire. Infanticide or abortion of prenatally diagnosed females is therefore not uncommon. In many cultures men dominate familial and social relations, including production and reproduction[7].

Filial piety

Culturally, children have an acknowledged duty of filial piety to their parents. The more children parents have, the greater this duty is. This is evidenced by unalloyed honor and respect of parents, support in old age, and the performance of the funeral ceremonies for the parents by the sons. The consequence of failing to have adequate children to perform these traditional rites is the incurrence of the everlasting wrath of the ancestors – something which most parents prefer to avoid.

Distrust of outsiders and political unrest

Many communities remain distrustful of donor family planning providers (agencies, countries or organizations). The programs are generally viewed as a ploy to reduce or eliminate a particular race or tribe. Political and social unrest coupled with insecurity also hinder the logistics of setting up family planning clincs (particularly in parts of Latin America and Africa).

Religious barriers

Most traditional religions value sustained fertility. Children are regarded as the gift of God or as a blessing from heaven, and many traditionalists see no rationale in limiting fertility. Islamic and Roman Catholic leaders oppose contraception in many developing countries and strong moralists link contraception with moral degradation, indiscriminate sexual behavior, early sexual debut, and freedom for illicit extramarital affairs[8,9]. Some fundamentalist groups discourage education and employment outside the home for women, thereby hindering their access to family planning information and services. The majority of these women are in purdah (seclusion of women from public observation). For these women, the decision to seek medical help, including family planning, is only made by the husband, mother, mother-in-law, village elders or other senior family members.

A large number of healthcare providers in some communities are males. Some religions prohibit women from seeking any healthcare services from male providers. They are therefore deprived of opportunities for family planning services and not uncommonly have to resort to poor, if existing, services[10]. Even when some seek contraceptives, they avoid those associated with increased or irregular vaginal bleeding as some religions abhore participation in religious rites during vaginal bleeding.

Barriers due to route of administration and side-effects of contraceptives

In certain cultures it is taboo to handle one's genitals. Contraceptives such as the condom, diaphragm, foam, tablet or jelly are therefore unacceptable, while injected products or long-acting implants and oral contraceptives are preferred. Contraceptives which cause amenorrhea may also be unacceptable in some cultures as this complication is perceived to be evil. In Cambodia, for example, failure to bleed is thought to be associated with darkening of the skin which would make women less healthy and attractive. In others, these contraceptives will be rejected because of concerns about pregnancy.

In traditional and predominantly Islamic regions childhood marriages (usually at menarche or shortly after) are common to ensure virginity and credibility to the family. Contraception is discouraged as it is perceived as promoting promiscuity. In many developing countries, for example, at least 20% of women, and in some about 50%, have had their first child by the age of 18 years. Girls therefore tend to marry older men, are likely to have many children in rapid succession and, because of lack of gender equity, are unable to participate in decisions about child-bearing or negotiate the use of contraceptives.

In most developing countries, marriage is a contract between families in which the wife is expected to contribute to the continuity or viability of the extended family by bearing many children. Where a high bride price is paid, children are regarded as the wealth of the poor, and infertile women are usually rejected by African cultures where polygamy is common and a woman's social status and authority are determined by how many children she has. Large families are therefore common.

Limited access and choice

In many developing countries, family planning services are characterized by obstacles such as poor access and a narrow range of available methods of contraception. In Africa, for example, although availability has increased, couples still have poorer access to fewer methods of contraception, on average, than did couples in either Latin America or Asia more than a decade ago.

Access to contraception is defined as the degree to which family planning services and supplies may be obtained at a level of effort and trust that is both acceptable to, and within the means of, a large majority of the population. In a ranking of contraceptive availability and access based on the work of Maulder and Ross[11], the Population Action International organization found limited access in most parts of developing countries. In addition, the pattern of availability varied widely. In the African region only Tunisia, Botswana and Mauritius had a high accessibility to all five methods. Access was either good or fair for most reversible methods (condoms, pills and intrauterine devices) and very restricted for permanent methods such as sterilization and vasectomy. In India, Iran, Guatemala and Paraguay, on the other hand,

the pattern of access was reversed, with access to oral contraceptives and intrauterine devices lagging behind access to sterilization. Of the 19 countries in the 'poor' category, 13 were in sub-Saharan Africa and most of these had very low access scores for intrauterine devices and sterilization, reflecting the lack of access to clinical health services of any kind. In the 'very poor' category, eight low-income African countries were joined by wealthy but socially conservative Saudi Arabia and Argentina, and by two countries – Laos and Cambodia – where the availability of most social services has been hurt by years of war and civil strife.

The key elements of access to contraceptives as defined by Bertrand and colleagues[12] include geographical or physical accessibility, economic accessibility, administrative accessibility, cognitive accessibility and psychological accessibility. In many developing countries, each of these key elements or a combination are major barriers to contraceptive use.

Quality of care

Bruce[13] identified six categories in this area which are necessary to define adequate quality of care in relation to the provison of contraceptive services. These view clients in a holistic manner and try to identify and meet their needs. Only a few developing countries fulfil these criteria:

(1) Available choice of methods;

(2) Technical competence of service providers;

(3) Information given to clients;

(4) Interpersonal relations;

(5) Mechanism to ensure follow-up and continuity; and

(6) Appropriate constellation of services.

Medical barriers

Medical barriers are defined as 'practices, derived at least partly from a medical rationale, that result in a scientifically unjustifiable impediment to, or denial of, contraception'[14,15]. The most common ones prevailing in developing countries are described here.

Inappropriate contraindications

Some outdated and anachronistic contraindications are still over-zealously applied, thus restricting the use of some forms of contraception[16]. Examples considered as contraindications to oral contraceptive use in some settings, especially where providers are non-physicians, include varicose veins, epilepsy, tuberculosis and diabetes. Headache, for example, is an exclusionary item on a community-based distribution women's oral contraceptive checklist. Migraine headaches are actually a relative rather than an absolute contraindication.

Extremely restrictive eligibility criteria

These may be related to a woman's age, her parity or the consent of her spouse. The oral contraceptive pill, for example, is still restricted to women below the age of 35 years, while in some regions breastfeeding is a contra-indication for any hormonal preparation. In Indonesia, Wells and Sherris[17] found that 90% of women who were given the method they requested continued using it at 1 year, as compared to 28% who had been denied their original choice.

Unnecessary process or scheduling hurdles

These make it difficult for the user to obtain a contraceptive. Such hurdles include physical examinations and laboratory tests. Many procedures have intrinsic merits but are unjustifiable as a pre-requisite to initiation or continuation of contraceptive use. For example, limitations on when a woman may initiate use of injectables or an intrauterine device, or severe restrictions on the number of pill cycles that oral contraceptive users may be given. In some West African countries, for example, it is standard practice to conduct blood tests as a pre-requisite to the prescription of oral contraceptives, in order to rule out diseases of the liver or cardiovascular

system. Family Health International showed that 78% of 139 family planning professionals in 32 African countries considered blood tests necessary, even though they recognized that such tests restricted women's access to these methods through costs and inconvenience, and were an extra burden on overloaded health services. The test results identified very few women to be at medical risk from oral contraceptives[15].

Provider limitations

In some countries, only physicians can perform intrauterine device insertion, when it is recognized that trained nurses, midwives and paramedical staff can be equally proficient. Since there are few physicians in most of these countries, such restrictions undoubtedly deny some women access.

Provider bias

This practice favors some methods and discourages others in the absence of a sound medical rationale, as well as failing to ascertain and to respect the clients' preferences[18].

Inappropriate management of side-effects

Family planning providers sometimes recommend that a client who is experiencing minor side-effects that may or may not be related to the method she is using simply discontinue use of her chosen method, rather than offer adequate counselling and help manage the side-effects.

Regulatory barriers

These are official mechanisms which slow contraceptive development, impede national approval of existing methods or hinder the promotion and advertising of contraceptives in some countries. Failure of the United States Food and Drug Administration to approve the use of Depo Provera until 1992 despite years of international data from the World Health Organization (WHO), for example, influenced the reluctance of several developing countries to offer this method of contraception. Similarly, the Japanese government failed to grant regulatory approval for the use of the oral contraceptive pill despite widespread use for over three decades, and more recently, continued research on quinacrine pellets for chemical sterilization was banned in India.

Underfunding of family planning programs

Family planning programs in many developing countries receive little funding, as economic crises have often led to a substantial fall below the WHO recommendations in funding for health. In 1996, Mauritius had the highest spending on family planning services or supplies of about US $1.65 per person amongst developing countries. Apart from Costa Rica, El Salvador, Mauritius and Zimbabwe, who spend US $1.00 or more annually per person on family planning[19], most developing countries spend less than $1.00 per person. These countries therefore depend on donor countries and organizations for the funding of family planning programs. Recent government policies in major funding countries, such as that of the USA Congress in 1996 to reduce funds for population assistance by 35%, therefore have a very significant impact on the other factors affecting access to contraceptive services. As a result of such policies, there has been a precipitous fall in funding. The predicted consequences of the USA decision, for example, are that 7 million couples in developing countries will lose access to modern contraceptives, resulting in 4 million unplanned pregnancies. Of these pregnancies, 1.6 million would end in abortions. In addition, 8000 more women would die from these pregnancies and 134 000 more infants would die as a result of an increase in high-risk births.

Recommendations

Contraceptive use has increased dramatically over the past three decades. Many couples in developing countries, however, who want to limit or delay births, continue to have no access to modern contraceptives even when services exist in their community. They are therefore denied the numerous benefits of family planning, such as better maternal and child health, reproductive freedom, empowerment of women, economic enhancement and the secondary health benefits of contraception[20,21]. Major obstacles to accessibility of family planning services are the barriers described above. These are complicated, interrelated and international. To eliminate these barriers, national and international efforts should focus on the following:

(1) Removal of policy and medical barriers through dissemination of information and research findings to medical and non-medical staff, policy makers, community leaders and the media;

(2) Dynamic educational events, mass communication, technical assistance, and study forums aimed at the public and those who are privileged to influence government policy;

(3) Introduction of a national curriculum for training medical students, nurses, midwives and all health workers which accommodates more time for didactic and practical training on family planning and related issues.

Continuous updating of medical eligibility criteria

Concerted efforts like the 1994 Cairo International Conference on Population and Development which resulted in the production of two complementary documents intended to update medical eligibility criteria[21] and the required procedures for the use of particular contraceptive methods[22] must be welcomed. An approach to assessing eligibility to use different contraceptive methods, based on the relative health risks and benefits of using a particular method for a woman with a given illness or condition, as adopted in 1994, is a welcome departure from the traditional approach of identifying contraindications to or precautions against method use. We advocate the incorporation of the classification of a woman's eligibility for use of each contraceptive method into the training of family planning providers. Such an approach will provide recommendations to be adopted in more diverse situations and settings in which contraceptives are provided.

Increased funding for family planning programs

Funding for family planning from both national governments and international agencies should be increased. These funds should be directed at the development of a holistic reproductive health program geared towards national needs and backed by a supportive policy environment. In view of limited resources and increasing demand for family planning, other sources of revenue generation should be explored, such as client fees, private sector services, integration of services and reduction of excess spending in the delivery system, minimizing and reducing unnecessary procedures, and increasing government subsidy. We recognize that some of these initiatives may be counter-productive, but tailoring them according to determined need will no doubt meet with success.

Communication strategies

The media is a very important source of information about contraception in developing countries[18]. The electronic, print and traditional methods of communication should therefore be used constructively to inform and educate the public about available family planning methods and their advantages. In addition to educating the public about the existence of modern methods of contraception, the media must expunge the incorrect notion that contraception is alien by discussing the existence of traditional methods of contraception. The media should avoid presenting research results in a sensational way, but should rather provide a rational and balanced view highlighting the risks and benefits of any contraceptive method compared with non-use, and complications from unplanned pregnancy and illegal abortion.

Communications strategies should focus on three main target populations: leaders and health professionals, political and religious leaders, and family planning providers. The communication strategy must aim to facilitate a stronger commitment to high-quality service on the part of leaders and health professionals (in the public and private sectors), and also to enhance their public self-image through media promotion and training. Political leaders, religious leaders and traditional leaders should be informed and encouraged to act as role models in their reproductive aspirations and behavior. The concept of having as many children as God can provide should be discouraged. Family planning service providers should be adequately trained and equipped with up-to-date educational material for counselling in appropriate languages suitable for particular cultures. As providers develop a commitment to high-quality service and learn to focus on the needs of their clients rather than their own needs, medical barriers will be reduced.

Current and potential family planning users

Interpersonal communication and counselling skills of the provider are crucial for decision-making in any family planning services. These often reinforce information about family planning in current and potential clients in many ways. The provision of accurate, complete, simple and clear information reduces one of the most basic medical barriers – withholding important information[22]. Responsive providers can furnish unbiased information, help clarify feelings and, most of all, empower clients to make their own family planning decisions. The special needs of the adolescent should be a priority in view of the large number that will be reaching reproductive age by the beginning of the next millenium.

Research

Finally, scientists in developing countries should be encouraged to participate in a multidisciplinary research effort on current and new methods of contraceptives. In addition to biomedical research, there is a need for:

(1) More social science and epidemiological research and modeling to assess better the risk/benefit ratios of the methods in use;

(2) Operations research to evaluate ways of reducing medical restrictions and to measure the impact of their reduction; and

(3) Market research to understand better the perceptions about contraceptives in the public and professional mind and the fertility aspirations of men and women.

The resulting information would ensure improved product development, emergence of new materials that are more consumer-controlled, improvement of program design and quality of care, and increased contraceptive prevalence[23].

The 1994 Cairo International Conference on Population and Development put forward a plan of action which epitomized the pivotal role of research in improving access to contraception. It concluded that 'governments, with the support of the international community, donors, the private sector, the academic community and non-governmental organizations, should increase support for research to improve and develop new methods for regulation of fertility that meet users needs, and are acceptable, easy to use, safe, free of side-effects, effective, affordable, and suitable for different cultural groups and different phases of reproductive life'. Regional organizations need to co-operate in the areas of funding, training and sharing of experience with countries which have successful family planning programs. Lessons learnt from successful program design, implementation and continued surveillance will ensure that community needs are met[24].

CONCLUSION

As we approach the next millenium, there is an urgent need to address the unmet contraceptive needs of the developing nations. Various barriers contribute to the high prevalence of these unmet needs. To address these effectively, family planning and contraceptive use must be offered as an integral part of reproductive health. Without an adequate policy and financial commitment by national governments and international agencies, the unmet needs for contraception will continue to rise with a consequent increase in unwanted pregnancies, induced abortions, maternal deaths and, regrettably, sexually transmitted infections including the human immunodeficiency virus (HIV). Family planning has a significant impact on all the other basic elements of health care. A woman, for example, who is unable to regulate and control her fertility effectively, sadly cannot be considered to be in a state of complete physical, mental and social well-being[25]. As population scientists and healthcare providers, we must redouble efforts to eliminate or significantly reduce barriers to contraceptive use in developing countries and promote an integrated healthcare service which is accessible and acceptable, and which can easily be moulded to suit different social, cultural and religious settings.

References

1. United Nations Population Fund. *The State of World Populations*. New York: United Nations, 1996

2. United Nations Development Programme. *Explosions, Eclipses and Escapes: Charting a Course of Global Populations Issues*. New York: The Population Council, 1993

3. Population Reference Bureau. *The United Nations Long-Range Population Projection: What They Tell Us*. Washington DC: Population Reference Bureau, 1992

4. Population Reference Bureau. *World Population Data Sheet*. Washington DC: Population Reference Bureau, 1996

5. United Nations. *Prospects: The 1994 Revision*. New York, 1995

6. Caldwell JC, Caldwell P. Cultural forces tending to sustain high fertility in tropical Africa. *World Bank PHM Technical Notes*, 1985: 85–6

7. Isiugo-Abanite UL. Reproductive motivation and family size preference among Nigerian men. *Stud Fam Plann* 1994;3:149–161

8. Barnes AC. In Sciarra JJ, Zatuchni GI, Speidel JJ, eds. *Risks, Benefits and Controversies in Fertility Control*. Maryland: Harper and Row, 1987: 7–11

9. Senanayake P. The politics of contraception. In Runnebaum B, *et al.*, eds. *Future Aspects in Contraception. Part 2. Female Contraception*. Lancaster: MTP Press, 1985

10. Krieger L, El Feraly M. Male doctor, female patient. Access to health care in Egypt. Presented at the *18th Annual NCIH International Conference*, Arlington, Virginia, USA, 1991

11. *Contraceptive Choice: Worldwide Access to Family Planning. PAI, Report on Progress Towards World Population Stabilization* Washington D.C.: Population Action International, 1997

12. Bertrand JT, Hardee K, Mannani RJ, *et al.* Access, quality of care and medical barriers in family planning programmes. *Int Fam Plann Perspect* 1995;21:64–74

13. Bruce J. Fundamental elements of the quality of care; a simple framework. *Stud Fam Plann* 1990; 21:61–91

14. Shelton JD, Angle MA, Jacobstein RA. Medical barriers to access to family planning. *Lancet* 1992; 340:1334–5

15. East and Southern African Regional Workshop. Improving quality of care and access to contraception: reducing medical barriers. USAID, HHRAA, SARA and JHIEGO, 1994

16. Reducing medical barriers and improving contraceptive image. Summary report. Family Health International, Johns Hopkins University, and USAID, Washington DC, June 1992

17. Wells E, Sherris J. Contraceptive services: a client's choice. *Population* 1992;19:8–10

18. Konje JC, Oladini F, Otolorin EO, *et al.* Factors determining the choice of contraceptive methods at the family planning clinic, University College Hospital, Ibadan, Nigeria. *Br J Fam Plann* 1998;24:107–10

19. Birdsall N, Chester LA. Contraception and the status of women. What is the link? *Fam Plann Perspect* 1987;19:14–18

20. World Health Organization. *Family and Reproductive Health. Improving Access to Quality Care in Family Planning: Medical Eligibility Criteria for Initiating Use of Contraceptive Methods*. Geneva: World Health Organization, 1995

21. Technical Guidance Working Groups. *Recommendations for Updating Selected Practices in Contraceptive Use, INTRAH Program, University of North Carolina*. Chapel Hill, NL, USA, 1994

22. *Contraceptive Choice: Worldwide Access to Family Planning*. Washington DC: Population Action International, 1997

23. Marshall A, ed. *The Stage of World Population*. New York: United Nations Population Fund, 1997

24. *Monitoring Family Planning Programmes*. Washington DC: Population Reference Bureau, 1996

25. Fathalla MF. Promoting research in human reproduction. Global needs and perspectives. *Hum Reprod* 1988;3:7

Contraceptive medicine: past, present and future

S. J. Segal

Introduction

As the calendar closes on the 20th century, we can list an amazing array of scientific achievements that have changed our lives in ways that could not have been imagined. One thinks about the conversion from gaslight to electricity, from the horse and buggy to the modern automobile and air travel, the telephone, radio and telegraphic communication, and the conquest of many diseases with drugs and vaccines. Consider also the exploration of space and the launching of satellites, the awesome power of nuclear fission and of the minute silicon chip. Modern contraception warrants inclusion on this list of titanic advances in science that have guided the course of human history, particularly for its impact on the lives of women.

Before the contraceptive pill, the intrauterine device (IUD) and other modern methods, couples had a limited choice of contraceptive methods that were dismally ineffective for preventing conception. A 1935 survey revealed that contraceptive use in the United States was equally divided among the condom, douche, rhythm, and 'other' methods, primarily withdrawal. Failure rates must have been huge, forcing women to choose between high fertility or illegal and unsafe abortions in those pre- antibiotic years. With the advent of the new methods beginning shortly after the middle of the century, fertility began to decline as contraceptive use grew.

World-wide, there has been a dramatic increase in contraceptive use over the past 35 years. The number of couples using systems of fertility control has increased more than ten-fold. In the developing countries, the number of contraceptive users has increased from under 30 million before 1960 to almost 400 million in 1996. The prevalence rate, representing the percentage of couples in the reproductive age group using contraception, has increased from 8% to over 50%, and is continuing to rise in most of the developing world[1].

Consequently, fertility has been steadily declining. In developing countries, the number of children a woman will have in her lifetime has decreased from over six in the 1960s to less than four, more than half way to the replacement level[2]. Most industrialized countries are at or even below replacement levels of fertility.

National surveys have provided detailed information on the methods that people choose. Patterns of methods used differ, but around the world contraception is practiced chiefly by women. Surgical sterilization, primarily tubal ligation, ranks first among methods chosen by American couples[3]. Oral contraception is the most widely used reversible method. In other countries the pattern is different. In Sweden and France, the IUD is the preferred reversible method[4]. Modern hormonal methods for women are not openly available in Japan; the predominant method used is the condom. Of couples using contraceptives 75% report that the condom is the method used. Oral contraceptive use has never been sanctioned by Japan's Ministry of Health and Welfare, which claimed most recently that it would lead to the spread of HIV/AIDS. In fact, the issue is linked to medical politics and economics. The government's decision is guided by the advice of a committee of obstetricians/ gynecologists. Japan has the highest ratio of obstetrics and gynecology doctors to total doctors of all countries and many depend for their income on the volume of surgical abortions. Since Japan does not strictly enforce its prescription drug regulations, oral contraception use would be a transaction between user and pharmacy, without involving the obstetrics/gynecology specialist. In practice, the condom is backed up by easy access to legal and safe abortion. Given the high failure rate of condom use, it is not surprising that over one quarter of pregnancies in Japan are voluntarily terminated[5].

In Latin America and Africa, male use of contraception is negligible. In India, on the other hand, where surgical sterilization is the chief method used to prevent pregnancy, there was a period in the recent past when vasectomy was emphasized. Presently, most sterilization operations are tubal ligations. Male methods account for about 15% of the contraceptive prevalence, which has climbed in recent years to about 40% of couples in the reproductive age group[6]. Some provinces of China rely heavily on vasectomy; 10% of contraceptive use is attributed to vasectomy, mainly in Sichuan and other Southern provinces where the simplified procedure of no-scalpel vasectomy was perfected and put into general use[2]. Nevertheless, in the developing world as a whole, as in most industrialized countries, when couples wish to prevent pregnancies, contraception usually involves methods that women use. In some regions and cultures the use of a male method is a rarity.

In countries where abortion is illegal and done under unsafe conditions, when a contraceptive method fails to protect against unwanted pregnancy, the health of the woman is placed at risk. Even with the availability of so-called modern methods, contraceptive failure is not uncommon. Surgical sterilization by tubal ligation, for example, usually assumed to be the 'gold standard' with respect to effectiveness, does not always succeed. During the first year postoperatively, about four cases per thousand will learn by having a pregnancy that the operation was not successful[7]. Among reversible methods, failure rates for 1 year of typical use are lowest with copper-carrying IUDs or progestogen-releasing intrauterine systems, contraceptive implants or injectable progesto-

gens (in each case, less than 1%). The conventional pill, the mini-pill and inert plastic IUDs fail at a rate of 3–5%. Failure rates with use of the condom, vaginal sponges or spermicides, cervical cap, diaphragm, periodic abstinence and withdrawal range from 12 to 21%[8].

It is a simple matter to calculate the number of pregnancies that result from contraceptive failure by multiplying the number of users of each method by its annual failure rate. Based on 1988 figures reported by the Alan Guttmacher Institute's survey of contraceptive use, unplanned pregnancies in the United States resulting from contraceptive failure totalled 1.74 million. In the United States, of the 3.2 million pregnancies that occur annually, one-half occur while a couple is using a method of contraception. Studies show that about one-half of these are carried to term and the other half are terminated by abortion[9,10].

There is no surer way to reduce the number of unplanned pregnancies and abortions in the United States and throughout the world than by improving the effectiveness of contraception. If for no other reason, the less than satisfactory performance of presently available methods, including the so-called modern methods of recent decades, prompts the search for new and improved methods that can meet the varied needs of the world's diverse population[11].

Contraceptive advances: 1960–1999

Since the initial wave of contraceptive innovations in the 1960s (several oral contraceptives and plastic IUDs), some major advances have been made in contraceptive technology. Most notable among the new products introduced have been the copper-bearing IUDs, the levonorgestrel-releasing intrauterine contraceptive system, the 5-year subdermal contraceptive and injectable progestogens.

The copper T-380A, the most effective of copper-bearing IUDs, was developed through research sponsored by the Population Council of New York[12]. It was initially marketed by the G.D. Searle Co. of Skokie, Illinois, along with a slight variation of the original design, known as the Copper 7. Within months after Searle was acquired in 1985 by the giant chemical corporation, Monsanto, both IUD products were removed from the market. Monsanto executives cited as the reason for this decision the mounting cost of defending lawsuits and their unwillingness to expose the entire assets of the corporation for the sake of products which, though medically safe[13], were vulnerable to litigation while adding little to total corporate revenues. There is substantial epidemiological evidence that American women living in stable monogamous relationships have no increased risk of pelvic inflammatory disease (PID) when they use an IUD. Ortho Pharmaceutical of New Jersey, which also distributed a Copper T-IUD, followed Monsanto out of the US market. Consequently, IUDs virtually disappeared from the United States for several years until a single-product company (GynoPharma, Inc.) was formed to market the Copper T-380A under a license from the Population Council. Because distribution has been limited, IUDs were used by relatively few American women. This is changing now that the product has been acquired by Ortho, a company with excellent experience in the marketing of contraceptives and willing, once again, to enter the IUD market.

Intrauterine contraception, using the same products that were withdrawn from women in the United States, is the method of choice in many other countries, representing a range of different cultures. It is used by 30% of women using contraceptives in Sweden and by more than half of all couples using reversible contraception in China and Cuba[14]. Its appeal is based on simplicity of use, ease of reversibility, absence of systemic side-effects, low cost and remarkable effectiveness. A World Health Organization (WHO) study found that the cumulative 7-year pregnancy rate for the Copper T-380A, the device available in the United States, is 1.6. This averages to fewer than two pregnancies per 1000 women per year, an effectiveness rate equal to that of surgical sterilization[15]. Subsequently, the WHO has reported that the TCu-380A maintains its effectiveness for 10 years and the Population Council has extended its observations on effectiveness to 12 years[16].

Another intrauterine contraceptive system gaining popularity in European countries is not yet available to American women, although the research needed for its development was co-ordinated by the New York-based Population Council and the technology (hormone release from synthetic polymers and the T-shaped carrier) originated in the Council's laboratory. This is the levonorgestrel-releasing intrauterine system[17]. It is as effective as the Copper T-380A and in some studies has shown the added advantage of reducing the incidence of sexually transmitted disease. The Copper T-380A has at least a 10-year lifespan; the levonorgestrel-releasing intrauterine system, marketed under the trade name Mirena®, lasts for 5 years.

The Norplant® system, a novel long-acting contraceptive based on the release of a steroid hormone from an elastomer polymer, has been marketed in the United States since 1991. The subdermal Silastic capsules, also a product of Population Council research[18,19], slowly release the synthetic progestogen levonorgestrel, establishing a blood level above the threshold required to inhibit ovulation or to provide an additional contraceptive effect through the secondary mechanism of preventing sperm passage through a thickened cervical mucus. An effective blood level can be maintained for at least 5 years, although a user has the option of removing the capsules at any time. Norplant contraception is another reversible method that is in the range of effectiveness experienced with surgical sterilization. The main side-effect is irregular vaginal bleeding[20]. By 1999, Norplant had been registered in 26 countries and used by over 10 million women in 44 countries.

Shortly after Norplant approval was announced by the Food and Drug Administration (FDA), the potential use of the method for 'social engineering' was widely discussed in the press and in some State legislative bodies. Editorial writers were quick to suggest that women, particularly adolescents, receiving government welfare payments, should be offered incentives to accept Norplant so that they could avoid unwanted pregnancy[21]. Similar legislative proposals were introduced in several States, but none were enacted. A California

State judge offered a woman convicted of child abuse the choice of Norplant insertion or prison. These coercive uses were unequivocally and publicly opposed by researchers[22] who had developed Norplant. Nevertheless, the method became the target of criticism by some consumer, feminist and human rights advocates who perceived with trepidation the potential for abuse of a method that a woman cannot control herself.

Norplant has also become the target of product liability litigation in the United States. Although none of the thousands of claims, ranging from loss of vision to autoimmune diseases, that have been filed against Wyeth–Ayerst Laboratories and/or physicians who have provided the Norplant system have been upheld in court, this avalanche of litigation is a threat to the survival of the product. Only a handful of similar lawsuits have arisen in other countries in which Norplant has been in use for over a decade. Wyeth–Ayerst is mounting a vigorous defense of Norplant, but the legal costs could become staggering and therefore this resolve could be shaken by financial considerations. Medical and scientific findings, which led to FDA approval and WHO consultative group endorsement, are unchanged and have been reaffirmed by both of these agencies[23]. Norplant has also received strong backing from an expert committee of the American Society for Reproductive Health, the nation's largest professional organization of reproduction health professionals[24].

The adverse publicity associated with the lawsuits has had a dramatic effect on Norplant use in the United States and, in addition, has influenced acceptance elsewhere. According to a *New York Times* report, sales in the United States dropped from the peak level of about 5000 per week to less than 500[25]. In the UK, after an initial burst of consumer interest immediately after the introduction of Norplant in 1993, the level of sales has subsequently declined. After seeking and obtaining regulatory agency approval in France, Wyeth–Ayerst International has postponed introduction of the product in that country. Developing country use has not been noticeably affected by the events in the United States.

As American use of Norplant has declined, interest in injectable contraceptives has risen. Contraceptive preparations based on injectable forms of synthetic progestogens are not new, but have experienced a revival of interest in recent years. Depoprovera®, a 3-monthly injection of the progestogen medroxyprogesterone acetate, was approved for use as a contraceptive in the United States in 1993, after having been used in over 40 other countries for decades. It was first proposed as a contraceptive in 1966 when a Brazilian investigator reported that doses of 150 mg administered intramuscularly caused temporary sterility by inhibiting ovulation for at least 3 months[26]. The same investigator, Elsimar Coutinho, reported 2 years later that conception control with less disturbance of menstrual bleeding could be achieved by monthly injections of the same progestogen combined with a long-acting estrogen[27]. The combination-injectable product has been re-introduced in some countries recently under the trade name Cyclofem® after extensive research sponsored by the WHO[28].

New subdermal contraceptives

Even as use of the Norplant system declines in some countries with reports of product liability lawsuits appearing in the news media, research is progressing with other subdermal contraceptives. Several are in the research pipeline. The most advanced is the levonorgestrel 2-rod system. It has two main advantages. The first is that the same contraceptive effect can be achieved with two subdermal inserts instead of the conventional six used in the original Norplant system. The second is the simplicity of manufacture. Both advantages result from a design modification. The insert consists of an inner rod containing a mixture of elastomer and progestogen, covered by a thin flexible tubing. The two-rod system has been studied extensively in comparison to the six-capsule system. In one study, Swedish women used either Norplant or the new system. The two devices performed similarly over 3 years of use[29]. Reducing the number of subdermal inserts results in easier insertion and removal procedures, and reduces the incidence of any complications that might be associated with these techniques. Leiras Oy of Turku, Finland, is prepared to market the levonorgestrel 2-rod system in Scandinavia and other countries. The United States FDA has ratified a modification of the original Norplant new drug approval (NDA) to authorize the sale of the levonorgestrel 2-rod system by Wyeth–Ayerst Laboratories. Unless the legal cost of defending the original product causes a change in current marketing plans, the company will introduce the new product in 1999 or soon after, most likely under a different name. When introduced, the levonorgestrel 2-rod system can be expected to renew interest in the use of subdermal contraception.

There are three subdermal insert systems under development that attempt to simplify the insertion and removal procedure even further, by reducing the insert number to one. One of these is the Uniplant[®] method, a product being tested by the South to South Co-operation in Reproductive Health, of Salvador, Brazil, a non-profit-making group of developing country researchers who work together to develop new health technologies[30]. The active progestogen of Uniplant is nomegestrol acetate. A proprietary compound of Théramex, Monaco, it is used in other Théramex products for various gynecological indications and has an excellent record for safety. Théramex, after reviewing the decline of Norplant sales in the United States and the UK, withdrew from the development partnership, requiring South to South to negotiate an agreement with another commercial partner. Uniplant employs the polymeric matrix used in Norplant. As a subdermal contraceptive, it is used for 1 year before being replaced. A 3-year system is being studied by Organon International, located in Oss, Holland. Named Implanon[®], this product uses the active metabolite of the progestogen used by Organon in its oral contraceptive products[31]. This compound, 3-keto-desogestrel, is effective in inhibiting ovulation and therefore it can be expected that Implanon will offer satisfactory contraceptive protection. Implanon is made of ethyl vinyl acetate, a polymer approved for some medical applications, but not previously used subdermally.

The third single-rod product is the Nesterone[®] system, under development by the Population Council[32]. It is designed to last for 2 years and uses a polymeric system different from the design of Norplant. The synthetic progestogen is similar in structure to nomegestrol. It is not active when taken orally, so that if used by nursing mothers, any of the steroid that reaches the milk would not have a biological effect in the infant.

Hormonal vaginal contraceptives

Another method of contraception is also based on the release of steroid hormones from a polymeric matrix. This is a vaginal ring which a woman can insert and remove herself, eliminating the disadvantage of clinic dependency associated with intrauterine and subdermal contraception. Vaginal ring contraception has been under investigation for over 25 years, primarily by the Population Council[33] and also by a contraceptive research program of the WHO. From time to time there has been commercial interest in bringing a vaginal ring contraceptive to the market, but this has not yet materialized. In 1987, a company in the UK was prepared to introduce a vaginal ring product, but, at the eleventh hour, the manufacturer of the plastic used for the ring discontinued its production because of new testing required by the US Environmental Protection Agency (EPA).

The conventional oral contraceptive is a combination estrogen–progestogen pill. It is also effective when used vaginally. A large international study by the South to South research group has demonstrated that two popular brands of the contraceptive pill, used *per vaginam* on the usual dosage schedule, are just as effective as when taken by mouth[34]. Absorption of contraceptive steroids through the vaginal mucosa is well known, so this result is not unexpected. This procedure has the advantage of bypassing the liver when the drug first enters the bloodstream. Women who experience nausea or gastric upset when using an oral contraceptive can benefit from using the pill vaginally. Nausea is not fully eliminated as a side-effect because it is frequently a systemic effect of estrogen, regardless of the route of administration. A Brazilian company is seeking authorization to market the first vaginal pill and has received preliminary notification of approval from Brazil's Ministry of Health. If approved, the vaginal pill will be marketed under the trade name Amorette and could be on the Brazilian market in 1999.

Morning-after pill

Postcoital contraception that could prevent a pregnancy from becoming established has been possible for several decades. Until recently, there has been no commercial interest in a product development effort and few health-care providers were aware of the effectiveness of 'off-label' use of existing products for this purpose. Now, thanks to the efforts of several women's health advocacy groups, there is an emerging interest in what has come to be called 'emergency contraception'[35] and the first dedicated product has reached the American market.

During the 1960s, orally active estrogenic products were shown to initiate menstrual-like bleeding when taken within a few days of an unprotected intercourse. The sloughing of the uterine lining means that pregnancy cannot take place even if a fertilized egg is present. It would be expelled, as routinely occurs in almost half of the cycles in which fertilization occurs. The product used most frequently was diethylstilbestrol (DES)[36]. One study, carried out at a university student health service, found that no pregnancies occurred among 1000 young women who took DES near mid-cycle within 6 days of unprotected intercourse[37]. The main disadvantage was that the doses used caused severe nausea and vomiting. Other estrogens were tried, but presented the same problem. This was an era when there was great caution over the use of estrogens, so that the few scientific papers that were published did little to elicit professional or commercial interest.

Later, it was demonstrated that a high dose of the conventional pill, a combination of estrogen and progestogen, can prevent pregnancy from becoming established when taken up to 72 h after intercourse[38]. This work prompted greater interest and the method's use was adopted mainly by emergency room physicians treating rape victims and by student health services on university campuses. Companies marketing oral contraceptives in North America have been unwilling to label their products to indicate this activity, although the identical combination pill is approved and marketed as an emergency contraceptive in several European countries[39]. In the United States the FDA has responded to a petition, filed by the Center for Reproductive Law and Policy, by convening a panel of experts who unanimously endorsed the conclusion that the method is safe and effective. Until now, however, none of the companies with appropriate products on the market have initiated steps to include this use in their labelling, but one new company has sponsored a new drug application and now has its product on the market.

The WHO has sponsored studies of an anti-progesterone, mifepristone (discussed below), as an emergency contraceptive, with results that are extremely encouraging[40]. Without an estrogenic component, the compound is equal in effectiveness to the high-dose combination pill method and causes far fewer of the transient side-effects. There is evidence that some progestogens, without estrogen, can have this same advantage[41]. There is a progestogen-only product on the market in some countries and interest in this approach is beginning to intensify.

A pill to terminate early pregnancy

An adequate level of progesterone in a woman's blood is necessary for the establishment and maintenance of pregnancy. Compounds that do not act as progestogens, but occupy progesterone receptor sites on target cells (in the uterus, for example), prevent the natural hormone from carrying out its progestational role and are, therefore, contragestational[42]. The first of these progesterone antagonists is mifepristone (RU-486) and by 1999 it had been registered as an approved drug for medical abortion in

France, China, Sweden and the UK and had been used successfully by over half a million women. By 1999, over 250 000 women in China had used the locally produced mifepristone and prostaglandin combination and distribution of the French product in France and other European countries had exceeded 350 000. Abortion induction has been the first clinical application of this important new class of drugs. The first studies used mifepristone alone. The success rate in women with established pregnancies who had amenorrhea for less than 7 weeks ranged from 64 to 85%[43]. The lack of response in some women was most likely due to inadequate uterine contractility. The combination of mifepristone with a prostaglandin (misoprostol), which induces contractions, given 48 h later by intramuscular injection, by vaginal suppository or orally, has resulted in a rate of complete abortion exceeding 95%[44]. The oral route, using misoprostol, has become the therapy of choice[45]. The combination is highly effective for up to 9 weeks since the last menstrual period.

Political opposition to mifepristone in the United States has prevented its availability as a medical abortifacient several years after it was introduced in Europe and has impeded progress on the investigation of its use for a number of other indications in gynecology and oncology. Unwilling to remain in the eye of the storm of controversy, the Roussel–UCLAF company of Paris (now a part of the Hoechst Marion Roussel group) assigned all North American rights to mifepristone to the Population Council. An American clinical trial has been completed and the Council has submitted an NDA for review by the FDA. The relevant advisory committee has recommended approval and the agency has declared the product approvable. The Council has transferred its rights to a start-up commercial company and final action awaits completion of arrangements for manufacture and distribution.

Meanwhile, another 'abortion pill' procedure has been suggested and results of the early experience highly publicized. Like the use of mifepristone, this method also involves using an abortifacient drug (methotrexate) in combination with misoprostol[46]. Methotrexate is a potent antimetabolite that has a long history of use as a chemotherapeutic agent for the treatment of choriocarcinoma. It interferes with cell division by acting as an inhibitor of folic acid. In recent years, at lower doses than those employed for cancer therapy, the drug has been used for the non-surgical management of some ectopic pregnancies[47] and at even lower doses for alleviating the symptoms of arthritis and for some dermatological disorders. Now the abortifacient use, discussed over 30 years ago but never pursued because of concern over potential toxicity, is being reconsidered and is currently under investigation by clinics of The Planned Parenthood Association of America, with FDA authorization.

The main advantage of this procedure would be that the two drugs employed are already approved and in use for other purposes. They could, therefore, be prescribed for an 'off-label' use without additional FDA authorization. The main disadvantage from a user's perspective is the prolonged time required to initiate and complete a medical abortion by this procedure.

From the perspective of the health-care provider, there may be a reluctance to prescribe a potent antimetabolite with teratogenic potential for an off-label purpose that might be difficult to defend in the event of malpractice litigation.

A contraceptive vaccine for women

The most comprehensive program toward the development of a contraceptive vaccine is based on the use of human chorionic gonadotropin (hCG) as the antibody-stimulating component[48]. The underlying rationale is to develop antibodies that will interfere with or prevent the action of hCG, which is essential for the establishment and maintenance of an early pregnancy. Without the action of hCG, the uterine lining would lose its progestational support and, at the time of the next expected menses, endometrial sloughing and a menstrual flow would occur whether or not the preceding ovulatory cycle had been fertile. The most advanced approach to the development of an hCG-inhibiting vaccine utilizes the principle of coupling a component of the native hCG molecule to a carrier protein that acts as an immunogen stimulator. This is usually tetanus toxoid or diphtheria toxin, substances that have proven to be safe as vaccines in large-scale use in human populations. Work done primarily in India, sponsored by that country's National Institute of Immunology, utilizes a synthetic molecule that resembles the three-dimensional structure of hCG. This is linked to the tetanus or diphtheria macromolecule. A clinical study was completed in India in 1992. Pregnancies did not occur in women who developed antibody titers that exceeded the threshold adequate to neutralize hCG of early pregnancy. A report of this work in 1994 was published in the United States in the *Proceedings of the National Academy of Sciences*[49], but this has failed to stimulate confirmatory scientific work or commercial interest in this line of development.

The Indian vaccine induces a temporary immunization of short duration so that frequent booster shots are required in order to maintain antibody levels above the threshold required for effective hCG neutralization. This feature is sometimes overlooked by critics who are concerned about the potential irreversibility of an hCG vaccine. Work toward developing adjuvants that would permit a feasible and acceptable schedule for temporary but longer periods of immunization is necessary.

Research on the development of contraceptive vaccines has become politically controversial. Some feminist groups and women's health advocates have expressed grave concern about the potential for misuse of an antifertility vaccine. They fear its involuntary or coerced application in order to sterilize women forcibly. Given this perceived potential for abuse, they question the ethics of working on contraceptive vaccines and call for restraint on the part of scientists and organizations that support scientific research[50]. At least one start-up biotechnology company that initially undertook a development program for an anti-hCG vaccine has discontinued its investment in the project.

A male pill

The most extensive clinical experience with a systemic male contraceptive has been accumulated with a pill tested mostly in China, but also investigated in other countries. It consists of gossypol, the yellow pigment found in cottonseed. First tested as a male contraceptive in the 1970s by a team of Chinese investigators, the idea sprung from the serendipitous observation that uncooked cottonseed oil (which contains gossypol) had been responsible for an epidemic of infertility in a rural area in China.

More than 10 000 Chinese men were enrolled in studies employing several dose levels of gossypol. The initial country-wide study reported a success rate of 99.4% for suppressing sperm production to levels believed to be incompatible with fertility. The dosage schedule began with a daily 20-mg pill for approximately 3 months and was then reduced to every other day. The antifertility effect was achieved without lowering plasma testosterone levels so that, unlike other approaches to male contraception, hormone replacement therapy to maintain libido and other secondary sexual characteristics was not required[51]. In this study, hypokalemia (reduction in blood potassium levels) at the dosage of gossypol used was raised as an issue of concern and this matter has clouded subsequent attitudes toward the potential use of gossypol as a male contraceptive[52]. There were several shortcomings in the initial Chinese work. Among other problems, the gossypol used at the participating centers was not standardized and there were no control cases. Without adequate controls, it was not possible to gauge the association of gossypol to this change in blood chemistry. Although several studies have attempted to establish an animal model or a mechanism of action for the imputed hypokalemic effect of gossypol, these have not been definitive. When gossypol has been tested as a contraceptive in countries other than China, no evidence of hypokalemia has been reported[53]. Doses higher than the male contraceptive regimen, used in the United States for the treatment of adrenal cancer, failed to cause hypokalemia[54]. A comparative clinical study determined that plasma potassium levels of Chinese men tend to be lower than the values of men in other countries and that this appears to be related to dietary rather than genetic factors[55].

The usefulness of gossypol as a male contraceptive will be determined by its reversibility. It appears that the chances for reversal decrease with higher doses and longer duration of use. Even though men who use gossypol for 1 year or longer are able to resume spermatogenesis after cessation of treatment, it will not be possible to assure an individual user that fertility can return within a specified time period. The implication of this is that gossypol, if otherwise proven to be safe and effective as a male contraceptive, would have application as a medical alternative for men seeking surgical vasectomy rather than as a guaranteed reversible method. An international, multicenter trial has been carried out by the South to South research group to test the use of gossypol for this purpose and the results will be published in 1999.

A joint development agreement exists between the South to South Organization and a Brazilian company that specializes in the development of pharmaceuticals from natural products, Hebron S/A of Pernambuco, has been signed. The company has succeeded in scaling up to industrial levels the extraction and purification of gossypol from Brazilian cotton plants. Reuters and other news agencies reported this item following an announcement released by the president of the Hebron Company in Brazil in December 1996. The press release contained several inaccuracies that were later retracted in a subsequent statement from Hebron S/A, but the product development plan is proceeding as initially claimed. South to South is undertaking the laboratory and clinical testing of the Hebron product for effectiveness and safety.

A male implant system

In contrast to the serendipitous disclosure of gossypol's contraceptive action in rural China, the discovery of gonadotropin releasing hormone (GnRH), a small peptide molecule from the brain that indirectly controls the function of the human gonads, was the product of sophisticated biotechnology that earned Nobel Prizes for two American scientists. Research teams led by Roger Guillemin and Andrew Schally competed furiously to be the first to announce the structure of the small polypeptide that regulates the release of gonadotropic hormones from the pituitary gland which, in turn, control the function of the testis and the ovary. Both published their results in 1971 and the two scientists were subsequently awarded the Nobel Prize for this important achievement. After many years of frustrating research to utilize this discovery for contraception, the synthesis of peptide antagonists of GnRH, free of undesirable side-effects, is a positive step toward a male contraceptive based on the principle of GnRH inhibition[56]. Developing acceptable delivery forms of this chemical class of compounds for contraception has been a challenge. Unlike the extensive experience with polymeric release of steroids for long-acting delivery systems, there is no similar technology to borrow from to create a delayed-release system for water-soluble peptides. To be practical, several criteria must be met. The delivery system must employ materials that can be used clinically without causing a local or systemic foreign body reaction, the solubility and stability of the peptide must be sufficient to permit storage of an adequate amount to assure a significant period of effectiveness, and the release rate of the peptide from the vehicle must be slow and constant enough to provide a reasonably constant blood level over the period of use. Synthetic polymers similar to the one used for soft lens products (Hydron) may meet these requirements[57]. Used extensively for many years, Hydron only rarely initiates a foreign body reaction when placed in proximity to the epithelium of the cornea. Although the solubility of peptidic compounds in this mucopolysaccharide has been known, the material has not been used clinically as the basis for a long-acting drug delivery system.

A male method based on GnRH will need to meet another requirement. Since the releasing hormone indirectly controls both the sperm-producing and the hormone-producing functions of the testis, men treated with an antagonist to suppress spermatogenesis would require androgen replacement therapy to maintain libido, potency and other secondary male sex characteristics. The development of suitable hormone replacement therapy for men is complicated by the fact that concurrent testosterone treatment can interfere with the inhibitory effect of GnRH analogs on spermatogenesis[58].

Potential toxicity and metabolic issues further complicate the development of appropriate androgen replacement therapy. Unlike estrogens and progestogens, androgens that can be used orally are not available. When androgen therapy is used for the treatment of sexual dysfunction or hypogonadism, frequent intramuscular injections are required. Although studies with delivery systems such as pellets or microspheres suitable for steroids suggest that injectable preparations that would last for 6 months may be feasible, no such preparations are commercially available.

Longer-acting superandrogens may hold even greater promise for overcoming the problem of a suitable sustained release form for androgen replacement therapy. One analog of testosterone can be prepared in a polymeric matrix that has a lifespan of at least 1 year when placed subdermally. Used in conjunction with a GnRH analog-releasing Hydron implant, this product of Population Council research could resolve many of the problems that have confronted researchers striving to develop a practical male contraceptive over the past several decades[59]. In fact, this 19-nortestoterone derivative, Ment™, is sufficiently powerful as a gonadotropin inhibitor and weak as a prostate stimulator that its use alone for contraception seems very promising.

A male injectable contraceptive

Although reports continue to surface from time to time on the use of injections of androgens, progestogens or androgen–progestogen combinations for the prevention of sperm production via the suppression of pituitary gonadotropins, it is unlikely that these research activities will lead to the development of an acceptable and practical system for male contraception. It has been nearly 40 years since steroidal suppression of gonadotropins was proposed as an approach

to male contraception and some of the same basic uncertainties remain today[60]. The daunting challenge when using an androgenic steroid to suppress gonadotropins is to establish a dose that would remain within normal limits for all men, without reaching hyperandrogenic levels in some.

Any method that risks exceeding physiological blood levels would be viewed with skepticism because of the critical role of androgens in cardiovascular events and prostate stimulation. It is hard to visualize the acceptability of a contraceptive product based on the use of the same hormones that disqualify athletes from international competition. One need only observe the controversy aroused by the approval of occasional medical use of marijuana to predict the outcry that would greet the suggested contraceptive use of a controlled substance.

A vaccine for men

As scientists, armed with the powerful tools of molecular biology and dramatic advances in understanding the immune system, attempt to develop an array of new vaccines to combat disease, they have included the exploration of potential immunological means to suppress male fertility.

One line of research is based on the principle of GnRH inhibition, similar to the use of antagonist analogs, mentioned earlier. The decapeptide itself is too small a molecule to be significantly antigenic, but linking it to a carrier protein enhances substantially its ability to stimulate antibody formation[61]. With a vaccine based on this principle, spermatogenesis would be inhibited by GnRH-neutralizing antibodies and androgen replacement therapy would ensure normal male secondary sex characteristics and functions. Some men with prostate cancer have been immunized safely with a GnRH vaccine in order to suppress androgen stimulation of prostatic tissue, but these preliminary studies have not dealt with the issue of androgen replacement, an essential component of a vaccine that would be used to control fertility in normal men.

The action of the pituitary gonadotropic hormone follicle stimulating hormone (FSH) in stimulating the production of sperm by the testis is not fully understood, although it is clear that it plays a role in initiating and maintaining this process. This has led to studies to try to develop an anti-FSH vaccine that would be used in the male and which might avoid the complication of concurrent suppression of testicular hormone production[62].

Percutaneous vasectomy

Simplification of the operative procedure may enhance the popularity of vasectomy. There are short-term complications of the conventional operation which include hematoma, infection, epididymitis and the longer-term problem of spontaneous recanalization of the vas. A technique perfected by surgeons in China has been popularized as the 'no-scalpel' vasectomy. The scrotal skin is punctured at the midline and the vas is visualized through the tiny puncture hole. The advantages are to minimize bleeding and other side-effects. No sutures are required to close the entry site. In China, over 15 million vasectomies have been performed using this procedure and it is now being adopted by American urologists[63].

Vaginal microbicide

Finally, in this era of acquired immunodeficiency syndrome, a review of contraception cannot be complete without emphasizing the need for methods that women can use to protect themselves from sexually transmitted diseases, including human immunodeficiency virus (HIV). Throughout the world women face a growing risk of infection with HIV. Consistent condom use is not always feasible for many women. The vaginal sheath, vaginal virucidal creams or gels, medicated condoms or other means to reduce the potential of transinfection of women by infected men urgently need greater attention than ever before. This is a complicated line of research that cannot depend on laboratory results alone. Ultimately, clinical trials will be required and the design of such trials present daunting challenges of ethics as well as pharmacology. Some explorations are in progress, but this line of research should receive a much higher allocation of resources and the attention of scientists, commercial companies and funding agencies throughout the world[64].

References

1. Segal SJ. Trends in population and contraception. *Ann Med* 1993;25:51–6
2. United Nations Department of Economic and Social Information and Policy Analysis. United Nations, New York, Population Division, 1994
3. Harlop S, Kost K, Forrest JD. *Preventing Pregnancy, Preventing Health: A New Look at the Birth Control Choices in the United States.* New York: The Alan Guttmacher Institute, 1991
4. Segal SJ. Contraceptive development and better family planning. *Bull NY Acad Med* 1996;73: 92–104
5. International Planned Parenthood Federation. East and South East Asia and Oceania Region. *Country Experiences on Abortion: Japan.* 1994: 10–25
6. International Institute for Population Sciences. *National Family Health Survey (MCH and Family Planning). India 1992–93.* Bombay: National Institute for Population Sciences, 1994: 46
7. Hatcher RA, Trussell J, Stewart F, *et al. Contraceptive Technology*, 16th edn. New York: Irvington Publishers, 1994
8. Jones EF, Forrest JD. Contraceptive failure rates based on the 1988 National Survey of Family Growth. *Fam Plann Perspect* 1992;19:12–19
9. Forrest JD. Epidemiology of unintended pregnancy and contraceptive use. *Am J Obstet Gynecol* 1994;170:1485–8
10. Institute of Medicine. Brown SS, Eisenberg L, eds. *The Best Intentions: Unintended Pregnancy and*

the Well-Being of Children and Families. Washington DC: National Academy Press, 1995

11. Institute of Medicine. Harrison PF, Rosenfield A, eds. *Contraceptive Research and Development: Looking to the Future.* Washington: National Academy Press, 1996

12. Sivin I, Tatum HJ. Four years experience with the TCu-380A intrauterine contraceptive device. *Fertil Steril* 1981;36:159–63

13. Lee NC, Rubin GL, Boruck R. The intrauterine device and pelvic inflammatory disease revisited: new results from the women's health study. *Obstet Gynecol* 1988;71:1–6

14. Segal SJ, Mauldin WP. Contraceptive choices. Who, what, why? In Diczfalusy E, Bygdeman M, eds. *Fertility Regulation Today and Tomorrow.* New York: Raven Press, 1987:305–17

15. World Health Organization. Human Reproduction Programme: task force on safety and efficacy of fertility regulating methods. The Tcu 380A, Tcu220, Multiload 250 and Nova T IUDs at 3, 5, and 7 years of use – results from three randomized multicentre trials. *Contraception* 1990;42:141–52

16. World Health Organization. *Special Programme of Research, Development, and Research Training in Human Reproduction. Annual Technical Report: 1992.* Geneva: WHO, 1993:289.

17. Luukkainen T, Toivonen J. Levonorgestrel-releasing IUD as a method of contraception with therapeutic properties. *Contraception* 1995;52:269–76

18. Segal SJ. Contraceptive technology: current and prospective methods. *Milbank Memorial Fund Q* 1971;49:145–71

19. Segal SJ. Future prospects in contraception. *Excerpta Med Int Cong Ser No. 133. Proceedings of the 5th World Congress on Fertility and Sterility,* Stockholm, 1966

20. The Population Council. *Norplant®, Levonorgestrel Implants: A Summary of Scientific Data.* New York: The Population Council, 1990

21. Editorial. Teenage pregnancy and Norplant. *Baltimore Sun,* 12 February 1993

22. Segal SJ. The uses of Norplant. Letter to the editor, *Baltimore Sun,* 18 February 1993

23. World Health Organization. *Post-marketing Surveillance of Norplant®.* Geneva: World Health Organization, 1995

24. American Society for Reproductive Medicine. Committee on methods of fertility regulation. *Statement on Norplant®.* Birmingham, Alabama: American Society on Reproductive Medicine (formerly American Fertility Society), June, 1995

25. New York Times. Will the lawyers kill off Norplant? *New York Times,* Money and Business Section, 28 May 1995

26. Coutinho EM, De Souza JC, Csapo AI. Reversible sterility induced by medroxyprogesterone acetate. *Fertil Steril* 1966;17:261–6

27. Coutinho EM, De Souza JC. Conception control by monthly injections of medroxyprogesterone suspension and a long-acting oestrogen. *J Reprod Fertil* 1968;15:209–14

28. Hall PE, d'Arcangues C. Long-acting methods of fertility regulation. In World Health Organization *Research in Human Reproduction, WHO Special Programme of Research, Development and Research Training in Human Reproduction. Biennial Report, 1986–1987.* Geneva: World Health Organization, 1988

29. Olsson SE. Contraception with Norplant® implants and Norplant-2 implants (2 covered rods.) Results from a comparative study in Sweden. *Contraception* 1988;27:61–73

30. Coutinho EM. One year contraception with a single subdermal implant containing nomegestrol acetate (Uniplant). *Contraception* 1993;47:97–105

31. Olsson SE. Clinical results with subcutaneous implants containing 3-keto-desogestrel. *Contraception* 1990;1–11

32. Diaz S, Croxatto H, Sivin I. Clinical trial with Nesterone subdermal contraceptive implants. *Contraception* 1995;51:33–8

33. Mishell DR, Talas M, Parlow AF, Moyer DL. Contraception by means of a silastic vaginal ring impregnated with medroxyprogesterone acetate. *Am J Obstet Gynecol* 1970;107:100–17

34. Coutinho EM, Alvarez F, Barbieri I, Ladipo O. Comparative study on the efficacy and acceptability of two contraceptive pills administered by the vaginal route: an international multi-center clinical trial. *Clin Pharmacol Ther* 1993;53:65–72

35. Ellertson C. History and efficacy of emergency contraception: beyond Coca-Cola. *Int Fam Plann Perspect* 1996;22:50–7

36. Segal SJ, Atkinson LE. Systemic contragestational agents. In Osofsky HJ, Osofsky JD, eds. *The Abortion Experience.* New York: Harper and Row, 1973: 200–414

37. Kuchera L. Post-coital contraception with diethylstilbestrol. *J Am Med Assoc* 1971;218:562–3

38. Yuzpe A, Lancee WJ. Ethinylestradiol and *dl*-norgestrel as a postcoital contraceptive. *Fertil Steril* 1977;28:932–6

39. Glasier A, Ketting E, Palan VT, *et al.* Case studies in emergency contraception from six countries. *Int Fam Plann Perspect* 1996;22:57–61

40. Glazier A. Mifepristone (RU 486) compared with high dose estrogen and progestogen for emergency postcoital contraception. *N Engl J Med* 1992;327:1041–4

41. Kesseru E. The hormonal and peripheral effects of *d*-norgestrel in postcoital contraception. *Contraception* 1974;10:411–24

42. Segal SJ. Mifepristone (RU486). *N Engl J Med* 1990;322:10

43. Herrmann W, Wyss R, Riondel A, *et al.* Effet d'une steroide antiprogesterone chez la femme. *C R Seances d'Acad Sci (III).* 1985;294:933–8

44. Bygdeman M, Swahn ML. Progesterone receptor blockage: effect on uterine contractility and early pregnancy. *Contraception* 1985;32:45–61

45. Peyron R, Aubeny E, Targosz V, *et al.* Early termination of pregnancy with mifepristone (RU486) and the orally active prostaglandin misoprostol. *N Engl J Med* 1993;328:1509–13

46. Creinin MD, Darney PD. Methotrexate and misoprostol for early abortion. *Contraception* 1993;48:339–48

47. Tanaka T, Hayashi H, Fujimoto S. Treatment of interstitial ectopic pregnancy with methotrexate. *Fertil Steril* 1982;37:851–2

48. Talwar GP, Sharma NC, Dubey SK, *et al.* Isoimmunization against human chorionic gonadotropin with conjugates of processed beta-subunit of the hormone and tetanus toxoid. *Proc Natl Acad Sci USA* 1976;73:218–22

49. Talwar GP, Singh OM, Pal R, *et al.* A vaccine that prevents pregnancy in women. *Proc Natl Acad Sci USA* 1994;91:8532–6

50. Call for a stop of research on antifertility 'vaccines' (immunological contraceptives.) Open letter signed by 232 organizations, sponsored by Women's Global Network for Reproductive Rights, Amsterdam, 3 November 1993

51. National Co-ordinating Group for Male Contraceptives. Gossypol – a new antifertility agent for males. *Chinese Med J* 1978;4:417–28

52. Prasad MRN, Diczfalusy E. Gossypol. Presented at *2nd Congress of Andrology,* Tel Aviv, June 1981

53. Coutinho EM, Melo JF, Barbosa I, Segal SJ. Antispermatogenic action of gossypol in men. *Fertil Steril* 1984;42:425–30

54. Flack MR, Pyle RG, Mullen NM, Reidenberg M. Oral gossypol in the treatment of metastatic adrenal cancer. *J Clin Endocrinol Metab* 1992;76:1019–24

55. Reidenberg MM, Gu ZP, Lorenzo B, *et al.* Regional differences in serum potassium concentrations in normal men. *J Clin Chem* 1993;39:72–5

56. Leal JA, Williams RF, Danforth DR, *et al.* Prolonged duration of gonadotropin inhibition by a third generation GnRH antagonist. *J Clin Endocrinol Metab* 1988;67:1325–7

57. Kuzma P, Moro D, Quant H. US Patent No. 5266325. Washington DC: US Patent Office, 30 November 1993

58. Michel E, Bents H, Bint Akhtar F, *et al.* Failure of high-dose sustained release luteinizing hormone releasing hormone (Buserelin) plus oral testosterone to suppress male fertility. *Clin Endocrinol* 1985;23:663–75

59. Sundaram K, Kumar N, Bardin CW. 7-Methyl nortestosterone (MENT): the optimal androgen for male contraception. *Ann Med* 1993;25:199–295

60. Heller CG, Laidlaw WM, Harvey HT, *et al.* Effects of progestational compounds on the reproductive process of the human male. *Ann NY Acad Sci* 1958;71:649–61

61. Ladd A, Tsong YY, Prabhu G, *et al.* Effects of long-term immunization against LHRH and androgen treatment on gonadal function. *J Reprod Immunol* 1989;15:85–101

62. Moudgal NR, Murthy GS, Rao AJ, *et al.* Development of ovine FSH as a vaccine for the male. In Talwar GP, ed. *Immunological Approaches to Contraception and Promotion of Fertility.* New York: Plenum Press, 1986:103–10

63. Schlegel PN, Goldstein M. Vasectomy. In Shoupe D, Haseltine FP, eds. *Contraception.* Clinical Perspectives in Obstetrics and Gynecology Series. New York: Springer-Verlag, 1993: 181–91

64. Elias CJ, Coggins C. Female-controlled methods to prevent sexual transmission of HIV. *AIDS* 1996;10(Suppl):S43–S51

Elcometrine for long-term contraception and clinical management of endometriosis

12

E. M. Coutinho and M. Montgomery

Introduction

Elcometrine (ST-1435), also referred to in the scientific literature by the trade name Nestorone, is a 19-norprogesterone (16-methylene-17α-acetoxy-19-nor-4-pregnene-3,20-dione), devoid of both androgenic and estrogenic properties. The compound is related structurally to the derivatives of 19-nortestosterone, such as norethindrone and levonorgestrel[1]. It is also chemically related to 17α-hydroxy derivatives of progesterone such as medroxyprogesterone acetate. Elcometrine was registered as a contraceptive in Brazil in 1998 to be used as a subdermal implant for 6 months. During this time interval, a single implant containing 50 mg of the compound inhibits ovulation, providing contraceptive protection comparable only to that afforded by sterilization or long-acting injectables[2]. In the largest published series, a single implant of elcometrine was used by each of a group of 282 women seeking contraception. A total of 1720 woman-months of use were recorded over the first 6-month period. At the end of the second 6 months, 3373 woman- months were recorded. For the first 6 months, Pearl index was 0.36[3].

Long-acting contraception for nursing women

During the early phase of development, it was found that elcometrine was ineffective as a contraceptive when administered orally. This lack of effect by the oral route was in contrast with its high efficacy by parenteral administration. The suggestion of using elcometrine as a contraceptive for lactating women has been evaluated at the Climério de Oliveira Maternity Hospital of the Federal University of Bahia during the last 2 years. In one trial, 66 breast-feeding women receiving elcometrine by the subdermal route were enrolled. These women were compared to 69 women also breast-feeding who elected to use copper T 380 intrauterine devices. The intrauterine device users served as controls. The women and their infants were observed until the end of the first postpartum year[4].

There were no significant differences in growth and development measurements among the infants in the elcometrine and control groups. The percentage of infants continuing to breast-feed at 3 and 6 months was significantly higher in the elcometrine group. There were no significant differences between the concentrations of elcometrine among the infants in the elcometrine and control groups. There were no significant differences between the concentrations of elcometrine in the blood and milk of the mothers. At 75 days, blood levels of elcometrine in the infants were near the non-detectable level and significantly lower than the levels in maternal blood or milk ($p < 0.01$). In 15 out of 25 infants, blood levels of elcometrine were at the limit of assay sensitivity or undetectable. Two pregnancies occurred in women using intrauterine devices, and none in those using implants. There were bleeding irregularities in both groups.

During the first 90 days, the percentage of the women on elcometrine who developed amenorrhea was only 7.7%. This percentage increased during the second 90-day interval to

27%, reaching 36.7% during the third 90-day interval. Amenorrhea in the women using intrauterine devices reached 27% during the first 90-day interval but decreased to 12.9% during the second 90-day interval and to 7.1% during the third 90-day interval (Figure 1).

The combined incidence of prolonged bleeding and frequent, infrequent and irregular bleeding throughout the study is shown in Figure 2. During the first 90-day interval, the percentage of women presenting any type of bleeding with the exception of regular menstrual bleeding was higher in the elcometrine group (51%) as compared to the control group (8%). During the second 90-day interval, while the incidence decreased from 51% to 31% in the elcometrine users, it increased from 8% to 16% in the control group. During the third 90-day interval, while it decreased further to 27% in the elcometrine group, it further

increased to 19% in the intrauterine device users.

Regular bleeding, similar to menstruation, was less than 5% in the elcometrine group throughout the study while it increased from 11% in the first 90-day interval to 35% during the third 90-day interval in the control group (Figure 3). This increase in the number of women in the control group with regular menstruation is in agreement with the re-establishment of regular ovulation in these women. As ovulation did not occur in the elcometrine implant users, regular menstruation was almost absent in this group of subjects.

Clinical management of endometriosis

In view of its ovulation and menstruation suppression properties, elcometrine has been used successfully in the treatment of endometriosis. In one study published in 1995, it was shown in 30 subjects presenting with large endometriomata in the ovaries that a regression of tumor size occurred following the insertion of a single implant of elcometrine[5]. In a larger series of 51 patients with endometriomata in one (19 patients) or both (32 patients) ovaries, one elcometrine implant made of Silastic® tubing (Technical Products, Georgia, USA) containing 50 mg of the compound was inserted in each of the 51 subjects[6]. At the end of every 6-month interval, subjects were offered a new implant. Dysmenorrhea was present in 37 patients (73%) and chronic pelvic pain in 28 (54.9%).

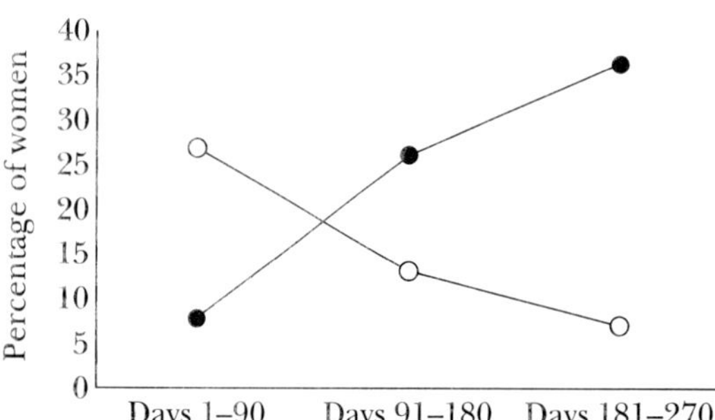

Figure 1 Incidence of amenorrhea throughout the study. Open circles, intrauterine device users; closed circles, elcometrine users

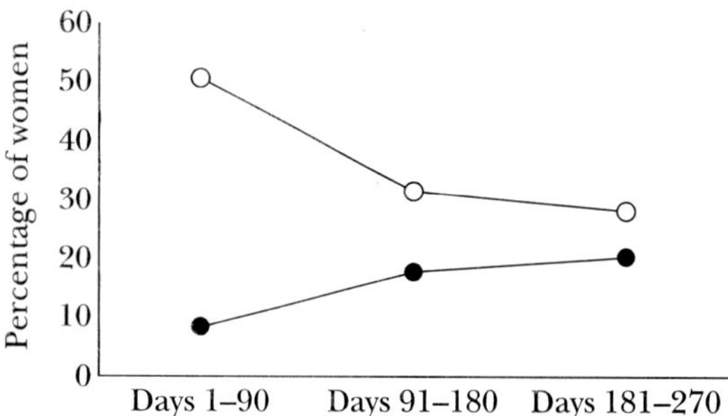

Figure 2 Combined incidence of prolonged bleeding and frequent, infrequent and irregular bleeding throughout the study. Open circles, elcometrine users; closed circles, intrauterine device users

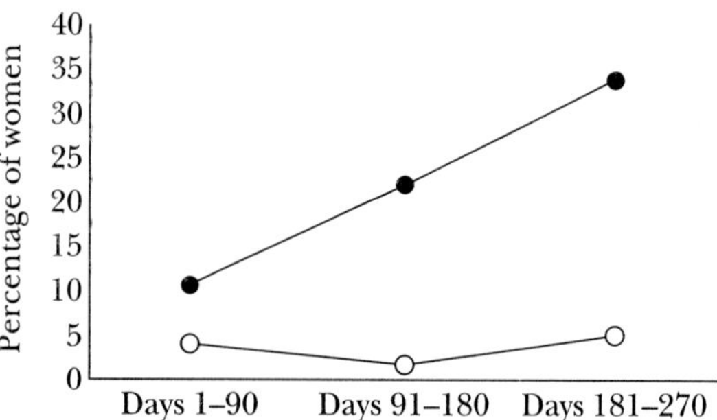

Figure 3 Incidence of normal bleeding throughout the study. Open circles, elcometrine users; closed circles, intrauterine device users

Dyspareunia was reported by 15 (29.4%). The intensity of pain was rated as incapacitating or severe in 82% of subjects, moderate in 12% and weak or absent in 6%. All 51 women completed the first segment of 6 months. Forty-four women had a new implant inserted at the end of the first 6-month interval and completed 1 year of treatment. Fifteen subjects discontinued at the end of 1 year. The remaining 29 received a third implant, completing 18 months of treatment. Thirteen of these discontinued while the remaining 16 received a fourth implant and completed 2 years of treatment. Nine women received a fifth implant and of these three received a sixth implant. Of these three, two received a seventh implant, completing 3.5 years of treatment. Most patients felt relief of pain a few days after insertion of the implant. At the end of the third month of implant use, no patient reported incapacitating or severe pain, 10% of subjects reported moderate pain and 90% reported weak pain or no pain at all.

The volume of endometriomata decreased in 94.1% of patients. In 74.5% of subjects ovarian volume was restored to normal. Figure 4 illustrates one such case. In 19.6% volume reduction was incomplete and in only 5.9% was there no change in volume. In this series the mean weight gain was 2.9 kg. The most common complaint was a reduction in libido, which was reported by 21.5% of patients. The second most common complaint was heaviness in the lower limbs, reported by 13.7% of subjects. Side-effects associated with low estrogen levels, such as hot flushes and sweating, were not reported. Thirty-three per cent of subjects were symptom-free at the end of 1 year following discontinuation of treatment.

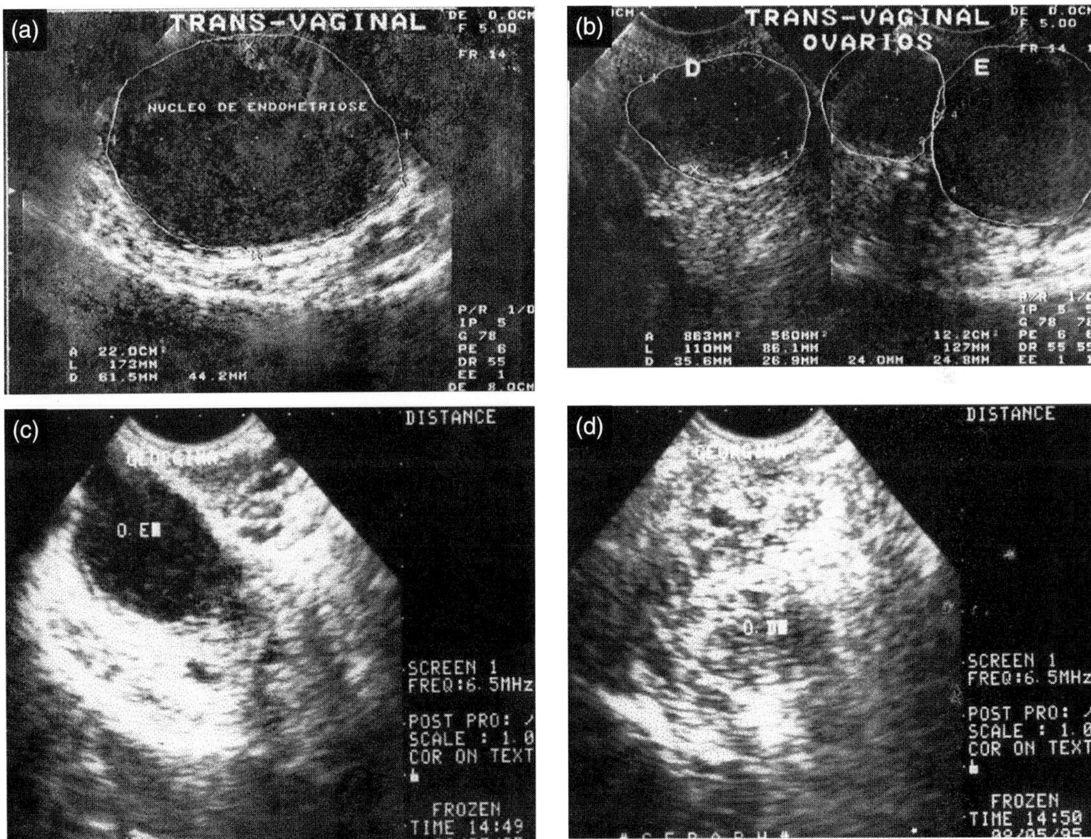

Figure 4 Effect of elcometrine on ovarian endometriomata, shown by transvaginal ultrasound. (a) Left ovary before treatment, volume 95.0 ml; (b) right ovary before treatment, volume 51.0 ml; (c) left ovary after 19 months of treatment, volume 25.5 ml; (d) right ovary after 19 months of treatment, volume 9.1 ml

These studies show that elcometrine implants represent a novel alternative for the treatment of endometriosis, which has proven to be as effective as the leuteinizing hormone-releasing hormone (LHRH) analogs, without the side-effects associated with the use of these peptides.

Elimination of premenstrual syndrome

The physical and psychological changes that occur during the period that precedes menstruation are the result of the retention of salt, water and metabolic products generated under the influence of ovarian hormones in preparation for pregnancy. When pregnancy does not occur, hormones are withdrawn, anabolic phenomena are reverted, and salt, water and organic compounds are released into the extracellular spaces, provoking the symptoms which characterize the premenstrual syndrome (PMS), also known as premenstrual tension (PMT)[7].

Edema, abdominal distention and discomfort, headache and tiredness associated with menstruation are reported by over 40% of all women. PMS may have devastating effects on the lives of these women. It can change behavior, and affect relationships with family members, friends and colleagues, disrupting the marital, social and professional lives of the women. The most extreme cases may require hospitalization. The mental condition of the women may lead to suicide or to the practice of violence. Crimes committed by women suffering from PMS generally occur in the premenstrual phase and this fact has been used to diminish criminal responsibility. Treatment for PMS is based on salt and dietary restrictions, and use of diuretics, hormones and tranquilizers, which provide alleviation of symptoms. The most efficient treatment is based on ovulation inhibition[8].

The use of elcometrine in the treatment of PMS is being investigated at the Centro de Pesquisas e Assistência em Reprodução Humana (CEPARH) in Salvador, Bahia, and at the ABC School of Medicine in São Bernardo, São Paulo, Brazil. In a preliminary report, Coutinho and Montgomery related their experience with 26 women aged 18 to 37 years with PMS who opted for ovulation suppression with elcometrine implants. All women enrolled suffered from severe PMS and had previous experience with traditional medication. One single implant containing 50 mg of elcometrine was inserted in the gluteal region of subjects, preferably between days 3 and 8 of the menstrual cycle, in order to inhibit ovulation in the admission cycle. PMS was absent in the first cycle following insertion in 19 out of 26 women and in 25 out of 26 during the following 5 months of implant use. Twenty-two women requested reinsertion at the end of 6 months. Two women who failed to request a reinsertion had PMS in the first cycle following removal of the implant. One subject became pregnant following discontinuation. One subject who was under psychiatric treatment failed to report back to the clinic.

The most important complaint was irregular bleeding or spotting, which was reported by approximately half of the women during the use of the first implant. For those women who had a second implant, the incidence of irregular bleeding or spotting was reduced to 30%. The second most frequent complaint was reduced libido, which was reported by 15% of subjects.

Elcometrine implants seem, therefore, to be an alternative for the medical control of PMS with the advantage over traditional medication of their long-acting effect combined with few adverse side-effects.

References

1. Coutinho EM, da Silva AR, Kraft HG. Fertility control with subdermal silastic capsules containing a new progestin (ST-1435). *Int J Fertil* 1976;21:103–8

2. Coutinho EM, da Silva AR, Carreira CMV, Sivin I. Long-term contraception with a single implant of the progestin ST-1435. *Fertil Steril* 1981;36:737–40

3. Coutinho EM, da Silva AR, Carreira C, *et al.* Contraception with a single implant and mini-implants of ST-1435. In Zatuchni G, Goldsmith A, Shelton JD, Sciarra JJ, eds. *Long-Acting Contraceptive Delivery Systems.* Philadelphia: Harper & Row, 1984:450–5

4. Coutinho EM, Athayde C, Dantas C, *et al.* Use of a single implant of elcometrine (ST-1435), a non-orally active progestin, as a long-acting contraceptive for postpartum nursing women. *Contraception* 1999; in press

5. Coutinho EM, Carreira C, Bastos GJO. ST-1435: a new alternative for medical therapy of endometriosis. In Coutinho EM, Spinola P, Hanson de Moura L, eds. *Progress in the Management of Endometriosis.* New York, London: Parthenon Publishing, 1995:277–80

6. Coutinho EM, Bastos GO, Carreira C, *et al.* Tratamento da endometriose com implantes subcutâneos de elcometrina. *Rev Brasil Ginecol Obstet* 1999; in press

7. Keye WR. *The Premenstrual Syndrome.* Philadelphia: WB Saunders, 1988

8. Goldenstein S, Halbreich V. Psychotropic medications as treatment of dysphoric premenstrual syndrome. In Smith S, Schiff I, eds. *Modern Management of Premenstrual Syndrome.* New York: Norton & Co., 1993

Overview: contraceptive research accomplishments in the 20th century and present use of contraceptives

13

E. D. B. Johansson

Introduction

Over a period of less than 50 years, women and men have witnessed a revolution in their ability to take command of their reproductive lives with the development of modern contraceptives. These methods enable women to choose when to become pregnant – a truly unique change in the condition of women in the world. New methods are gradually being added, but equally important is the gradual improvement of oral contraceptives: over time, more is learned about their safety and interaction with the body to produce health effects. Most of the positive effects can only be detected by extensive epidemiological studies when the use of a given method has reached a substantial level. These studies have found existing methods to be efficient and safe; most are health-promoting in some ways and some are even user-friendly[1–3].

However, development has not only been marked by an improvement in the products available – the attitude of the user has also changed. In some countries, these changes have been dramatic. In Sweden, efficacy was the most important issue early on, in the 1950s and 1960s. In the late 1960s and the 1970s, safety was the major concern owing to the finding of thromboembolic risk with oral contraceptives and the possible association between intrauterine devices (IUDs) and pelvic inflammatory disease (PID). The decreased dosage of ethinylestradiol in oral formulations, together with proper screening of patients, has drastically reduced the thromboembolic risk[3]. In the case of the IUD, the PID problem was mainly associated with the Dalkon Shield product. Again, proper evaluation of the patient's risk – in this case for PID – and greater attention applied to the insertion technique has changed the attitudes of many users[2]. Efficacy and safety are taken for granted. User-friendliness and ancillary health benefits have become, for women, the most important factors in choosing a method of contraception. The attitudes of the providers have also changed. As many of the medical risks disappear, it is logical to let women choose their method of contraception.

Current use of modern contraceptives

The term 'modern' implies (for contraceptives) a scientific development, quality-controlled production and monitored clinical trials. This includes oral contraceptives, IUDs, injectables, implants and barrier methods. However, even if development and evaluation of the methods are well anchored within evidence-based medicine, the use of the methods is based less on biological facts than on religious, cultural or legal bias. Also, economic realities for providers, hospitals, family planning organizations and foreign aid organizations have a very strong influence on the choice of method as well as the relative merits of the different methods. These are, of course, depressing facts for those involved in the development and evaluation of contraceptive methods. However, in countries with a wide choice of methods and a non-oppressive religious and/or political system, the customer is the decision-maker. This is a very encouraging development that will hopefully spread around the globe.

Owing to the biased nature of choice and the difficulty that most women have in choosing a method that fits their circumstances, the use of different methods varies enormously between countries. However, global figures give the magnitude of use. As women are the main users of modern contraceptives (probably because of the dearth of male methods), this chapter will focus on methods for women.

According to the World Health Organization (WHO), tubal sterilization is the most widely used method globally (17%), followed by IUDs (12%) and oral contraceptives (8%). These figures are the numerations for global use; individual countries differ. The higher figure for tubal sterilization is derived from its dominant use in large countries such as India and China, but also from many users in developed countries such as the USA (Table 1). The copper IUD is a very low-cost product and is favored for this reason by many family planning service providers. A copper IUD can be purchased for less than one US dollar by family planning organizations in developing countries. As a Copper T 380A gives excellent pregnancy protection for 12 years without resupply or medical support, it is by far the most economic contraceptive method. The present author is willing to predict that, for the foreseeable future, no new methods will be developed to outperform the copper IUD on the economic front. By this measure, if affordability is the main reason for the development of new contraceptives, then development should cease. Hopefully though, as with other essential products, the development of contraceptives will never stop. Even if the Copper T 380A is regarded by many as the gold standard

of IUDs and is the most used model, development still continues with the aim of reducing side-effects[4].

Oral contraceptive pills are the most used reversible method in the USA (Table 1)[5]. Currently, 54 different brands are available, but the difference between brands is decreasing. All use ethinylestradiol as estrogen in a dosage of $20–50\,\mu g$[6]. The most commonly used estrogen dose is $30\,\mu g$. The real choice for women is very limited despite the large number of different brands. In Europe, oral contraceptives also dominate, but IUDs are used and are available in several forms. The use of IUDs varies greatly from country to country. France, Finland and Sweden in particular have many women using IUDs. The 'infection backlash' in the mid-1970s affected countries in Europe in various ways. In some countries (such as Denmark), use virtually stopped and physicians were no longer instructed in the insertion and use of IUDs during training. In other countries such as Sweden, use picked up again when it was shown that life-style was the most important factor for PID infection. Greater care with insertion also dramatically reduced the incidence of PID[7].

The early 1990s saw regulatory breakthroughs for long-term, reversible hormonal contraceptives. The Food and Drug Administration (FDA) approved Norplant® (Wyeth-Ayerst) in 1990 and Depo Provera® (Pharmacia-Upjohn) in 1992. Approval in the USA has global consequences, as FDA approval is needed for the purchase of contraceptives by USAID for distribution in developing countries. The Copper T 380A (Paragard®; Ortho) was reintroduced in the USA in 1988, after copper IUDs had been taken off the market because of litigation; it is currently the only copper IUD on the market in the USA. Given the influence of fundamentalist religious groups and the litigation culture in the USA, every new contraceptive has gone through this 'purgatory' of litigation. The oral contraceptives were put on trial in the late 1960s to the early 1970s and endured, as the major companies defended their products. The attacks on IUDs were more successful (and the products less profitable), so they were taken off the market entirely.

Table 1 Use of contraceptive methods in Western Europe and USA (%), 1996. Market value for oral contraceptives 1995: USA $US1160 million; Western Europe $US1050 million. From reference 22

Method	Western Europe	USA
Oral contraceptives	41	28
Intrauterine device	15	1
Sterilization	13	42
Condom	8	18
Barrier (female)	1	3
Natural/other	22	8

Norplant is currently under attack by litigation. At the end of 1998, some 60 000 claims had been filed, but so far the courts have not found any fault with Norplant. The side-effects were well established in the clinical trials and clearly described in the labelling of the product. However, as a result of the adverse publicity, sales of Norplant have decreased markedly in the USA, and in the United Kingdom where similar litigation attacks have occurred. For a summary of the current situation on Norplant, see the Norplant consensus statement and background review[8].

The levonorgestrel intrauterine system (Mirena®; Leiras–Schering) releases 20 µg of levonorgestrel directly into the uterine cavity. Its contraceptive effect is local, with profound changes in the uterine environment making a hostile climate for passing sperm. The endometrium is thin and resistant to estrogen stimulants. This makes menstrual bleedings scant or absent, and pain-free. Mirena offers carefree contraception for at least 5 years with many health benefits. It is the first contraceptive developed with health benefits as important objectives, in addition to high contraceptive efficacy and a good safety profile. Mirena was launched in Finland, the country of manufacture, in 1990. It is now in all European markets and many others, including China. Mirena is likely to be approved by the FDA in the early years of the next millennium.

The current use of these four long-term methods and the changes from 1996 to 1997 in the manufactured value are indicated in Table 2. These methods are as effective as tubal ligation in preventing pregnancies. The large range of estimated users is because of different estimates of average use (and the difficulty in obtaining figures from China). To exemplify, the Copper T 380A has been shown to be effective for 12 years, although the label in the USA shows effectiveness for 10 years. On the other hand, clinical practice in many countries is to change the IUD after a few years of use.

Subcutaneous implants

The developmental history of subcutaneous implants goes back to the mid-1960s with the demonstration that Silastic® polymers could release steroids at a constant rate. An implant placed under the skin with years of action, eliminating user-failures and gynecological attention, was at that time considered to be an ideal contraceptive for mass distribution. When the International Committee for Contraception Research (ICCR) was formed in 1971, implants were a top priority area. Many steroids were investigated.

An implant system using megestrol acetate was in phase 3 clinical trials but was withdrawn owing to findings of increased incidence of breast cancer in beagles treated with progesterone derivatives. Later on, it was realized that all progestins (and progesterone) increase the rate of breast cancer in beagles, but by then all progesterone derivatives had been taken off the market. Only medroxyprogesterone acetate (MPA) was saved. Nowadays, MPA is widely used in hormone replacement therapy (HRT), as an injectable contraceptive (Depo Provera) and in the treatment of cancer of the endometrium. In 1973, levonorgestrel was chosen as the steroid in the development of the implant system that was to become Norplant. Two clinical centers stand out in the development of implants: Professor Elsimar Coutinho's clinic in Salvador, Brazil and Professor Horacio Croxatto's clinic in Santiago, Chile.

Development took time. Many obstacles had to be overcome, to standardize the system for pharmaceutical manufacture. It is important to note that a clinical trial to prove 5 years of efficacy will, with recruitment and follow-up, require 8 years. Norplant was approved in Finland (it was manufactured and distributed by Leiras in Turku, Finland) in 1983. The Population Council played a very active role in the introduction of Norplant in the developing

Table 2 World-wide use of long-term contraceptives and change of sales: 1997 vs. 1996

	Estimated users (millions)	Change vs. 1996 in sales (%)
Depo Provera®	12	–6
TCu 380	50–80	+15
NORPLANT®	5–7	+15
Mirena®	1	+67

world. Indonesia became the country of most widespread use. It was not until 1990 that Norplant received FDA approval in the USA. This was not as a result of any lengthy approval process but the time required to find an American company (Wyeth–Ayerst) interested in the product. Wyeth–Ayerst managed a very successful launch of Norplant, which caused initial problems as training in removals did not keep up with the widespread use of the method. In addition, Norplant became popular with young women. As circumstances change more rapidly for young people, this added to the demand for removal. Then, in 1994, Norplant was attacked by organized litigators just as oral contraceptives and IUDs had been previously.

Norplant consists of six capsules. It was realized early on in development that a reduction in the number of implants would improve acceptability from the perspectives of the provider and the user. Parallel with the development of Norplant, therefore, efforts were made to develop a more effective implant delivery system. The aim of this project was to develop an implant system with the same efficacy and active life as Norplant but with fewer implants. The two-levonorgestrel-rod system (Jadelle[®]; Schering–Leiras) was the outcome of this effort. Pregnancy rates, bleeding patterns and continuation rates at 5 years are essentially identical to those with Norplant, but insertion and removals are less time- consuming. The two-rod system was initially approved for 3 years, but recently the 5-year data were published[9], again matching the performance of Norplant. However, it is also evident from this comparative multicenter study that the two-levonorgestrel-rod system will not give high protection beyond 5 years, while Norplant is good for 7 years.

Subcutaneous implants have, with some exceptions, had a slow start on the global market. Development continues, however, with other organizations also entering the field (Table 3). A new concept needs more than one actor to be successful. Implanon[®] (Organon), a single implant releasing ketodesorgestrel and active for at least 3 years, has been approved for sale in Europe[10]. Uniplant[®], developed by South-to-South with headquarters in Salvador, works for 1 year[11].

Nestorone[®]-one is a single implant effective for 2 years and developed for lactating women. Nestorone, a progesterone derivative, is not orally active, so even if the steroids enter the breast milk – as other steroids do – it will not affect the nursing infant[12].

Norplant is the only subcutaneous implant for contraception with widespread use. It is approved in 60 countries and about 10 million women have experience with it. Norplant consists of six small (34 mm in length and 2.4 mm in diameter) Silastic capsules each containing 36 mg levonorgestrel. The 5-year pregnancy rate is one per 100 women.

Intrauterine levonorgestrel-releasing system Mirena[®]

The development of Mirena (Leiras–Schering) was initiated by Professor Tapani Luukkainen in 1970. After a few years, it was one of the projects within the ICCR of the Population Council. From the start, the aim was to achieve reduction of menstrual blood loss in addition to high

Table 3 Current global development status of subcutaneous implants for contraception. Clinical studies have shown high contraceptive efficacy up to 7 years for Norplant[®], 5 years for two-levonorgestrel rods and 3 years for Implanon[®]

Name	Number of implants	Use experience	Approval status	Contraceptive effectiveness (years)	Sponsor
Norplant[®]	six	10 million	60 countries	5 → 7	Schering AG, Wyeth
Two-levonorgestrel rods	two	studies	USA, Finland	3 → 5	Schering AG, Wyeth
Implanon[®]	one	studies	W. Europe	2 → 3	Organon
Uniplant[®]	one	studies	phase 3	1	South-to-South
Nestorone[®]-one	one	studies	phase 3	2	Population Council

contraceptive efficacy. The delivery system, however, had to be developed further, to achieve long action. The goal was a 5-year method. The development of a suitable delivery system was carried out in parallel with the development of the levonorgestrel-rod system. The next crucial step was to find a dose that would not suppress ovarian function and estrogen production in particular. A study of daily oral doses of 30 µg levonorgestrel had shown minimal effects on ovarian function, including ovulation[11]. Release rates of 10, 20 and 30 µg per day were tested. All doses gave excellent reduction of menstrual blood loss and the 30 µg dose had a slightly higher initial effect on ovarian function[13]. The 20 µg dose was chosen, and the delivery system was calculated to provide contraceptive protection well beyond 5 years. The release rate was remarkably stable and decreased slowly from a minimal release of 30 µg to 14 µg 5 years later[14]. Two large multicenter studies, one Nordic study by Leiras[15], the manufacturer, and one study by the Population Council[16], showed remarkably good contraceptive efficacy of below one at 5 years of use. Early on, it was clear that it was very important to counsel the women on the unique bleeding pattern of Mirena: the initially increased number of spotting days decreases along with the number of bleeding days and the amount of blood lost during the first 3 months, to reach scanty or absent bleeds. The initial studies were randomized against copper IUDs, so the women did not know what to expect. Also for the doctors, it was a new situation, with hormone-induced uterine amenorrhea: well- informed women who were assured that the contraceptive efficacy was so high that they did not need menstrual bleedings to demonstrate that they were not pregnant had very good continuation rates.

The reduction in menstrual blood loss was so dramatic that it was evident that this device could be used in the treatment of menorrhagia. Andersson and Rybo[17] showed in a well-controlled study of 20 women that blood loss could be reduced by more than 90% at 12 months. Several studies have confirmed these results. With the widespread use of Mirena in Scandinavia, many more invasive treatment procedures such as hysterectomy and endometrial resection are avoided. In a Finnish study, women on a waiting list for hysterectomies owing to menorrhagia were randomized to receive a levonorgestrel-releasing intrauterine system or continue with their current medication while waiting for hysterectomy. After 6 months, 64% of the women in the levonorgestrel-releasing intrauterine system group had cancelled surgery, while only 14% in the control group had done so[18].

The market introduction of Mirena was delayed by 5 years because of withdrawals from the market of an enzyme needed in the production of the Silastic polymer. However, after the initial launch in Scandinavia in the early 1990s, Mirena will by the end of 1999 be available in all European countries and also in many developing countries. Mirena is an emerging product that will not only be a major contraceptive method, but will also benefit women with heavy menstrual bleedings and menstrual pain, and those who are in need of estrogen substitution. Its role in the prevention of uterine fibromas, endometriosis, adenomyosis and other uterine diseases has only started to be investigated[18]. When Mirena attains a high percentage of users, the demand for gynecological surgery will decrease, and women wanting tubal ligation will be a rarity. However, the present author predicts that the most revolutionary change will be in women's attitudes to menstrual bleedings[19]. Who will want to have them if you can avoid them and increase your well-being?

Future of contraceptives

The future of contraceptives for the third millennium is very bright. First of all, the number of customers is increasing very rapidly for two major reasons:

(1) The world is only at mid-point in its rapid population growth. In the next 25 years, two billion people will be added. Owing to the young age structure in the developing world, a record number of young, sexually active people will need contraceptives in the coming years. The

world already has more than one billion teenagers.

(2) The total fertility rate has decreased to below 2.1 in most industrial countries. In some regions in Europe the total fertility rate is just above one. As the age of menarche is early (9–13) in well-fed populations and as the average age of menopause still appears to be increasing as it approaches 52, a woman with only one child may need contraceptives for up to 40 years. As the transition from high to low fertility now proceeds rapidly, particularly in Asia and Latin America, the number of women who need contraceptives is increasing rapidly. The speed of the transition to low fertility is so rapid that, within a generation, most women will need contraceptives for up to 40 years. This will mean a customer base of 2.5 billion women by 2025. This is indeed a very impressive market for the pharmaceutical industry to serve.

Another important reason for the bright future is that the safety questions that have been troubling both providers and users of oral contraceptives (OCs) and IUDs have been resolved or well defined in order that women with high risk of side-effects (for example women with previous thromboembolic disease) should not use OCs[3], and women with repeated PIDs should not be fitted with an IUD[2].

Furthermore, the health benefits of avoiding unwanted pregnancies have been well established, and are additional to the prevention of the ill effects on the mother, the father and the child. Also, several available products add health benefits by their hormonal actions. Oral contraceptives and Norplant reduce menstrual blood loss by about 50%. These products have also been shown to improve both hemoglobin and ferritin levels in anemic women in developing countries[20]. The levonorgestrel intrauterine system reduces blood loss by more than 90%, and has been established as a very effective treatment of menorrhagia[21]. This effect is so predictable that Mirena competes with hysterectomy[18]. The use of OCs to reduce menstrual pain and blood loss is a very common

introduction to OCs for young girls even before they need protection from pregnancy. The use of OCs by young women significantly reduces their costs for sanitary protection products, and soiled underwear and bed linen (J. Kristjansdottir and colleagues, manuscript in preparation). It also significantly reduces absence from school, compared to young women with natural menstrual periods. The liberation of young women from the tyranny of religion and family will have a dramatic effect on the demand for contraceptives that have minimal or no vaginal bleedings. As the modern long-term contraceptives have efficacy rates that are equal to or even better than female sterilization, the need of menstrual bleeding as a pregnancy test has disappeared.

What are the new methods still needed?

(1) A variety of methods to satisfy changing requirements during the fertile life of women: this will include new delivery forms such as vaginal rings and transdermal patches that will increase compliance and be under the control of women. Several such methods are under development. The need for contraceptives will also change during the fertile life of a woman. For instance, a woman over 40 has different needs than a woman who simply wants to space her children. A woman over 40 is likely to need a contraceptive of high efficacy as she is less likely to want more children. She is likely to be tired of her menstrual bleedings as they will probably have increased both in amount and duration. She is also approaching the age when she will benefit from estrogen supplementation. Ovarian estrogen production decreases gradually over many years prior to the last menstrual period. The levonorgestrel intrauterine system is the answer to all these demands. The local levonorgestrel concentration in the uterus will protect the endometrium from any estrogenic stimulation, and the woman can surf through menopause with the device in her uterus.

(2) Vaginal microbicides/contraceptives: protection against sexually transmitted diseases including human immunodeficiency virus (HIV) is very important. Many laboratories and organizations are working to develop vaginal microbicides. It is a very difficult task owing to the lack of surrogate endpoints. Large efficacy trials are required to prove the effect. The Population Council is trying to develop a microbicide without contraceptive effects to give a choice to women who want to become pregnant.

(3) Emergency contraceptives: this is an important niche, as it is human nature to utilize hindsight rather than foresight. Currently, the top priority is to spread the awareness of existing methods. However, it is clear that women need specially designed products that are easy to use and have few side-effects.

(4) As many as 70 000 young women die every year as a result of botched abortions, and many more suffer infections and bleedings that impair their future health and fertility. There is a clear need to increase the safety of surgical abortions and introduce quality-control for this procedure. Medical abortion, particularly the mifepristone/misoprostol combination, has been proved to be very safe and effective in different environments[22]. When no instruments are introduced into the uterine cavity, infections are extremely rare! The global introduction of medical abortion would drastically reduce mortality and morbidity among young women.

(5) Men have a limited choice of methods. Condoms have their problems, vasectomies are virtually final, and most men are poor at abstinence or withdrawal. Recently, however, several new approaches to male contraception involving combinations of androgens and progestins have been shown to suppress spermatogenesis. A new potent androgen, 7α-methyltestosterone, has been shown not to undergo 5α reduction, thus avoiding the specific stimulation of the prostate gland that the conversion of testosterone to dihydrotestosterone creates. This raises the hope that men, too, may get a hormonal contraceptive that will have health benefits[23].

References

1. Diczfalusy E. *The Contraceptive Revolution: an Era of Scientific and Social Development.* Carnforth, UK: Parthenon Publishing, 1997
2. Mishell DR. Intrauterine devices: mechanisms of action, safety and efficacy. *Contraception* 1998;58: 455–535
3. Ory HW. Cardiovascular safety of oral contraceptives – what has changed in the last decade? *Contraception* 1998;58:95–135
4. Wildermeersch D, Van Kets H, Vjijens M, *et al.* The Gynefix intrauterine implant. *Ann NY Acad Sci* 1997;816:440–50
5. Johansson EDB. Comparison of the availability of contraceptive methods in selected European countries and the United States. In *Review of Law and Social Change.* New York: New York University, 1997;23:471–6
6. Kannitz AM. Oral contraceptive estrogen dose. *Contraception* 1998;58:95–135
7. Grimes DA, Chaney EJ, Connell EB, *et al.* Modern IUDs. *Contracept Rep* 1998;9:1–15
8. Fraser IS, Tiitinen A, Affandi B, *et al.* Norplant® consensus statement and background review. *Contraception* 1998;57:1–9
9. Sivin I, Campodonico I, Kiriwat O, *et al.* The performance of levonorgestrel rod and Norplant® contraceptive implants: a five year randomized study. *Hum Reprod* 1998;13:3371–8
10. Implanon®, a new single-rod contraceptive implant. Presentation of clinical data. *Contraception* 1998;58(Suppl 6)
11. Coutinho EM, de Souza TC, Barbosa IC, *et al.* Multicenter clinical trial on the efficacy and acceptability of a single contraceptive implant of

nomegestrol acetate, Uniplant. *Contraception* 1996;53:121–5
12. Diaz S, Lähteenmäki P, Croxatto HB, *et al.* Clinical trial with Nestorone® subdermal contraceptive implants. *Contraception* 1995;51:33–8
13. Larsson-Colin U, Johansson EDB, Gemzell C. Effects of continuous daily administration of 0.03 mg of *d*-norgestrel on the plasma levels of progesterone and the urinary excretion of estrogens. *Acta Endocrinol* 1971;66:702–10
14. Luukkainen T. Levonorgestrel intrauterine device. *Ann NY Acad Sci* 1991;626:46–9
15. Andersson K, Odlind V, Rybo G. Levonorgestrel-releasing and copper-releasing (Nova-T) IUDs during five years of use: a randomized comparative trial. *Contraception* 1994;49:56–72
16. Sivin I, Mahgoubs EI, McCarthy T, *et al.* Long-term contraception with the levonorgestrel 20 μg/day (LNg 20) and Copper T 380Ag intrauterine devices: a five-year randomized study. *Contraception* 1990;42:361–78
17. Andersson JK, Rybo G. Levonorgestrel-releasing intrauterine device in the treatment of menorrhagia. *Br J Obstet Gynaecol* 1990;97:690–4
18. Lähteenmäki P, Haukkamaa M, Puolakka J, *et al.* Open randomized study of use of levonorgestrel releasing intrauterine system as alternative to hysterectomy. *Br Med J* 1998;316:1122–6
19. Johansson EDB. Future aspects of the levonorgestrel-releasing intrauterine system. *Gynecol Forum* 1998;3:31–2
20. Task Force for Epidemiological Research on Reproductive Health. *Effects of Contraceptives on Hemoglobin and Ferritin.* Geneva: WHO, 1998;58: 261–73
21. Levels and trends in contraceptive use. In *United Nations World Contraceptive Use.* New York, 1996
22. Winikoff B, Sivin I, Kurus MA, *et al.* Safety, efficacy and acceptability of medical abortion in China, Cuba and India: a comparative trial of mifepristone–misoprostol versus surgical abortion. *Am J Obstet Gynecol* 1997;176:431–7
23. Sundaram K, Kumar N, Bardin CW. 7α-methyl-nortestosterone (MENT): the optimal androgen for male contraception. *Ann Med* 1993;25: 199–205

Contraception for the 21st century: challenges and prospects   14

J. Guillebaud

Introduction

I predict that the supremacy of the combined steroid hormone pill will be increasingly challenged through the arrival of the following new choices: new female-directed methods not requiring a clinician (new vaginal caps, female condoms, spermicides and virucides); loose-fit internally-lubricated (therefore much more user-friendly) plastic condoms for men; new intrauterine methods (intrauterine devices and intrauterine systems); new steroid hormone delivery systems for women and for men (implants, patches, injectables); more acceptable high technology fertility-awareness-based methods, such as the new Persona®; methods based on antiprogestogens (including 'contragestion', which is highly controversial, but also improved postcoital 'emergency' methods and the use of small oral doses to interfere with ovulation on a regular basis); luteinizing hormone releasing hormone (LHRH) analogs and antagonists, either to ablate the menstrual cycle or in men to block spermatogenesis (in either sex there would be the need for add-back gonadal steroid treatment, with estradiol in the woman or testosterone in the man); the possibility of human chorionic gonadotropin (hCG)-receptor chemical blockers to prevent follicular development or implantation or to stop the action of peptides important in the complex process of sperm–oocyte fusion; and, perhaps one day, after many 'false dawns', the long-awaited immune methods operating variously in the male and female genital tracts.

This review focuses on the reversible methods; detailed references are to be found in my chapter in a recent book[1]. Lacking a 'crystal ball', it can only be one researcher's overview. It cannot be comprehensive, nor does it allow for sudden unforeseeable breakthroughs.

Negative publicity about contraceptives ever since the 1970s has meant that contraceptive research and development have been seen as unprofitable; hence, as was predicted by Djerassi[2], no entirely new birth control technologies have emerged in recent years. Rising each year by around 90 million, we will start the next millennium with over 6000 million, mostly utterly destitute, human beings. We will never meet human needs without stabilizing human numbers on a finite planet.

It is estimated that up to 64% of pregnancies world-wide are either mistimed or totally unwanted. Therefore, a large proportion of the 580 000 maternal deaths occurring annually represent deaths not only from unsafe abortions, but also full-term deliveries which resulted from pregnancies the women never wanted.

The combined oral contraceptive

The pill will, I am sure, remain popular in the 21st century, regardless of the uncertainty triggered on 18 October 1995 by the letter from the Committee on Safety of Medicines (CSM) in the UK[3]. This was based on studies suggesting a doubling of the risk of venous thromboembolism with desogestrel- or gestodene-containing pills as compared with those containing levonorgestrel or norethisterone and its pro-drugs. The extra annual risk was estimated as 15 per 100 000, equating to a tiny excess mortality risk of around two per million, from the one condition of venous thromboembolism.

The differential risk has not been confirmed in more recent studies, but, even if real, it is a very tiny risk in comparison with those that are accepted in life generally.

Regardless of loss of confidence through 'pill scares', its supremacy in the contraceptive field is being increasingly challenged. A useful criterion for new methods is that their 'default state' should be contraception (rather than conception, as when the pill user defaults!). Older parous women have had such methods (e.g. copper intrauterine devices (IUDs)) as first-line choices for some time: there is a great need for such 'forgettable' contraceptives for much younger women.

Mifepristone and other progesterone antagonists

At the time of writing, aside from research, products of this type are used solely for medical termination of pregnancy. However, mifepristone is close to 100% effective for postcoital contraception when used according to the same criteria as the existing combined estrogen–progestogen approach, with far fewer women reporting side effects. The only problem so far seems to be delay in the next menses and re-establishment of cycling, particularly among women treated before ovulation. Use of much lower doses may overcome the problem of menstrual delay, and the effectiveness of the method may be extended to beyond 72 h after coital exposure.

Studies are also in progress in Edinburgh and elsewhere which may lead to methods of regular birth control. This could be by regular 'contragestion', which would interfere with implantation during the final days of the cycle and would therefore be rejected by some as abortifacient. But mifepristone and its clones also show promise in small oral doses used early in the cycle in such a way as to interfere with ovulation on a regular basis. The problems with bringing progesterone antagonists to the market, even for uncontroversial pre-fertilization applications, are not so much medical as legal and ethical.

Female-directed methods

There are two interesting vaginal caps, both simpler to use than the diaphragm, neither requiring any form of clinical fitting procedure, although both are used with spermicides. It is claimed that their efficacy is of the order of that a well-fitting diaphragm. The vaginal caps are entering the market in some countries, although we await more efficacy data. Their names are 'Lea's Shield' and 'Femcap'.

Female condoms

On the market there is 'Femidom' ('Reality' in the USA). The 'bikini condom' failed dismally on esthetic grounds. But the 'pantycondom' – with a replaceable lubricated vaginal pouch secured to some lacy and not unerotic undies – shows promise, empowering the woman whose man should but will not use a condom of the male variety.

Virucides/spermicides

This approach has been ludicrously underfunded to date, despite its huge potential benefit. The testing of numerous candidate compounds is at last under way, in the hope of identifying a substance which in a suitable delivery system would reduce, if not eliminate, virus transmission. It is relevant to consider user-friendly microbicides in the context of contraception, even if a successful product was not able to be recommended itself as an adequately effective contraceptive. This is chiefly because using it would then enable potentially human immunodeficiency virus (HIV)-exposed couples to employ one of the more effective 'medical' methods of contraception, which would otherwise not be an option. At present, male condoms are often used badly for both contraception and HIV protection, so leading to many unwanted conceptions.

This research must pay great attention to the vehicle: the base could be suitably scented and the product marketed as a 'sex aid'. There is even the potential for vaginal rings to release the active ingredient over days or weeks, thereby vastly improving compliance.

New loose-fit internally lubricated male condoms

There is a renewed interest in male condoms, partly through the observation that many men prefer the 'freedom' of coital movement within the female condom. Using both latex and polyurethane materials, various agencies are actively researching lubricated loose-fit male condoms in which the shaft and glans penis are allowed free movement. 'Ez-On' is the first marketed product, available in the Netherlands.

New hormone delivery systems for women

Injectables

Already widely used world-wide is depot medroxyprogesterone acetate (DMPA), given at a dose of 150 mg every 12 weeks, and norethisterone enanthate, 200 mg every 2 months. More recently, monthly combined injectables have been devised through the World Health Organization (WHO) working chiefly in South America and have proved very popular. They lead to a bleeding episode approximately monthly and are highly effective.

The most promising is Cyclofem® (25 mg DMPA with 5 mg estradiol cypionate). This can be delivered efficiently in programs: a special self-injector helps to overcome the problem of frequent injections. Advantages include the more regular bleeding pattern, lack of hypoestrogenic symptoms and potential risks, and the fact that patients who develop symptoms do not have to wait so long for reversal to be achieved.

Subdermal progestogen implants

Norplant® is likely to be supplanted by the single ethylene vinyl acetate rod releasing 3-keto-desogestrel (over 3 years) (Implanon®), and similar single capsules or others which are biodegradable are expected. Compared with Norplant, Implanon is far quicker and simpler to insert and remove (removal time averages 2.6 min). So far, no failures have been reported in 2300 insertions. Its main remaining problem is, as with all other progestogen-only methods, irregular bleeding.

Vaginal rings

One version was close to being marketed in 1993, releasing levonorgestrel over a period of 3 months; unfortunately, however, in a study at the Margaret Pyke Centre, some erythematous vaginal patches were detected which, on histology, showed evidence of inflammation. It is not certain whether this was due solely to mechanical pressure or whether there was a component of chemical reaction or allergy to either the levonorgestrel or the polymer. The vaginal ring concept remains viable. The combined 3-keto-desogestrel plus ethinylestradiol ring, which is softer and more flexible than the levonorgestrel ring, appears most promising at present. Rings might also be possible vectors for microbicides (see above).

Transdermal patches

At present, these are marketed primarily for administering hormones for estrogen replacement therapy and in the very near future will be marketed as an alternative to the pill.

Luteinizing hormone releasing hormone (LHRH) analogs and antagonists

These show potential for use both to ablate the menstrual cycle and, in men, to block spermatogenesis. In both sexes there would be the need for add-back gonadal steroid treatment, with estradiol in the woman or testosterone in the man. This would prevent the unacceptable side-effects of loss of libido (and hot flushes in the woman); however, in women, it would also be necessary to protect the endometrium from overstimulation and this could be done by the levonorgestrel-releasing intrauterine system (see below).

Other peptide-based approaches

There is the potential to produce long-acting follicle stimulating hormone (FSH)-receptor or human chorionic gonadotropin (hCG)-receptor blockers to prevent follicular development or to block implantation, respectively. The same technology might also be used to block the action of peptides important in the complex process of sperm–oocyte fusion.

Other approaches to systemic contraception for men

Research is currently in progress through WHO using testosterone esters. These can either be used alone or in smaller doses in combination with progestogens. All can be given as long-acting injections or, in due course, potentially by other routes such as subcutaneous implants. There is a risk that the testosterone-based methods might create an increased risk of arterial disease, prostatic hypertrophy or aggression, but careful titration of the doses should minimize such hazards.

There would be an advantage for compliance if any marketed product were not, in fact, a 'male pill': an injection or implant could be given or at least supervised by his likely more reliable partner!

Immune approaches in both sexes

The most advanced immune approach in Phase II trials is the method based on active immunity to hCG using the appropriate antigen plus adjuvants. However, this method has already been under development for 25 years without a reliable product emerging. Another approach being considered is immunity to the zona pellucida or to various sperm antigens. In the latter case, the intention is to simulate natural conditions in which a man is entirely healthy, but his sperm fail to fertilize. However, the approach appears likely to be more successful within the woman, rather than raising auto-antibodies to the man's sperm.

With all the potential immune methods, the problem of individual variation is acute, in that some are poor responders, so that conception results despite oft-repeated booster doses, whereas others are hypersensitive with the risk of immunosterilization. The avoidance of the

risk of (auto)immune disorders is also a high priority.

Fertility awareness-based methods

In developed countries, these are likely to be more widely used through the development of better technology, both to predict and to detect ovulation. Already marketed is Persona®, the small hand-held electronic computer and urine-testing device. This predicts ovulation through measurement of the first significant rise of estrone-3-glucuronide in a dipstick placed in the woman's urine and instructs her through a red light that she is entering her fertile period. The end of this is detected through measurement of the LH surge followed by computer calculations of the time necessary in that woman's case for any ovulated egg to become non-fertilizable. In ongoing use, the system adapts to the individual woman by referring to her stored data for the previous six cycles.

From the main European trial (Keith May of Unipath, personal communication), the best estimate for the first-year failure rate among consistent users is six per 100 woman-years. This makes it inappropriate for women who need greater efficacy, unless they are prepared to use barriers or abstain during the first 'green' phase (pre-ovulatory phase, always less effective due to the capriciousness of sperm survival) as well as the red one. It is also likely to prove prohibitively expensive for most Third World countries.

Intrauterine contraception

Copper IUDs

Wildemeersch and co-workers[4] have produced a banded copper delivery system (GyneFix®) (Figure 1) based on a single polypropylene thread bearing a knot, which is pushed by a special inserting stilette 1 cm into the fundal myometrium. Studies show that when the devices are properly inserted, this approach retains the excellent efficacy of the copper T-380 and its clones, yet minimizes the risk of both expulsion and uterine pain. It also shows potential (with the knots enhanced in various ways) for immediate postabortal and postplacental insertion.

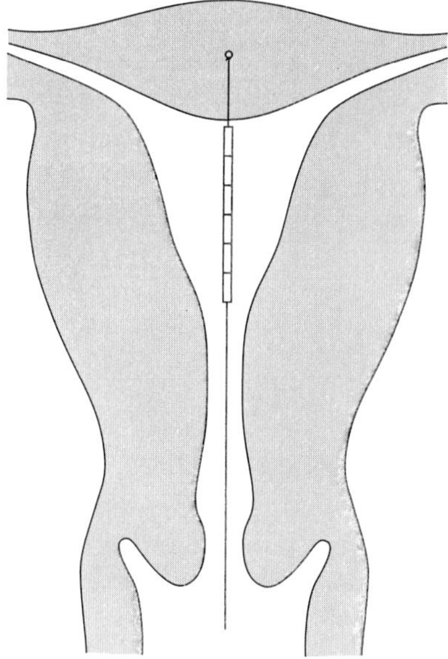

Figure 1   The GyneFix

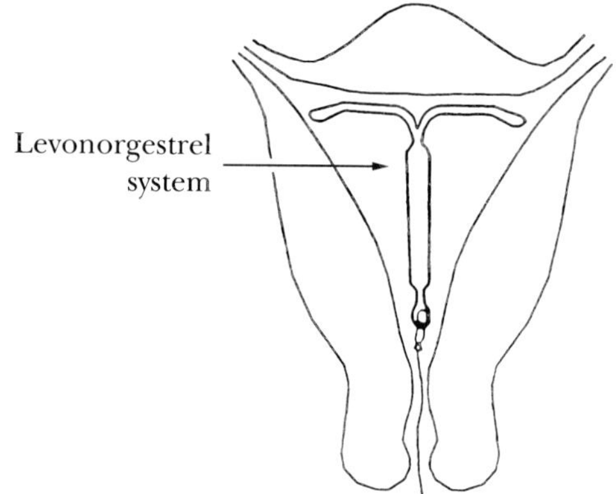

Figure 2   The Mirena levonorgestrel-releasing intrauterine system

It is hoped that this technology might in due course be applied also to Silastic cylinders or threads releasing progestogenic hormones, since in the form already marketed (as Mirena®, the levonorgestrel-releasing intrauterine system), intrauterine progestogen already conveys so many other advantages. I predict that this uterine implant technology will be a crucial ingredient of the contraceptive 'mix' of the 21st century!

The levonorgestrel-releasing intrauterine system (Mirena)

This releases 20 µg/24 h of levonorgestrel from its polydimethylsiloxane reservoir through a rate-limiting membrane (Figure 2). Its main contraceptive effects are local, by endometrial suppression and changes to the cervical mucus and uterotubal fluid which impair sperm migration. The blood levels of levonorgestrel are about one-quarter of the peak levels in users of the progestogen-only pill and therefore ovarian function is altered less. Most women continue to ovulate and in the remainder sufficient estrogen for health is produced from the ovary, even if they become amenorrheic as many do: this is primarily a local end-organ effect and should be seen as a benefit. Postmenopausal estradiol levels have not been detected, even in those who have no uterine bleeding.

Clinical advantages and indications

I maintain that for most parous women this represents the future already here, yet this is still not recognized by many providers, even where the system is on the market. It has unsurpassed efficacy, less than 0.2 per 100 woman-years in the first year. Return of fertility is rapid and appears to be complete. Combining most of the best features of hormonal and intrauterine contraception without most of the problems of either, it fundamentally 'rewrites the textbooks' about IUDs. The user of this system can expect a dramatic reduction in the amount and, after the first few months (discussed below), the duration of blood loss. Dysmenorrhea is also generally improved.

The levonorgestrel-releasing intrauterine system is certainly the contraceptive method of choice for most women with heavy menses or who are prone to iron deficiency anemia – a specially relevant bonus one would wish to offer freely to our sisters in the Third World. It also shows promise for a number of gynecological indications: as a first-line treatment for frank menorrhagia; as part of the management of severe premenstrual syndrome (PMS) with high-dose (100–200 µg) estradiol skin patches; possibly also to prevent fibroid growth; in the management of uterine pain from adenomyosis; and in the treatment of endometrial hyperplasia.

Perimenopausal use

Here it provides progestogenic protection of the uterus during estrogen replacement therapy by any chosen route. Our studies at the Margaret Pyke Centre confirm those elsewhere, that this is a fully contraceptive regimen, most women achieve amenorrhea whether the intra-uterine system be inserted before or after final ovarian failure and progestogenic (PMS-type) side-effects are very rare.

Main adverse effects

Like any IUD it can be expelled, and there is the usual small risk of perforation, minimized by its 'withdrawal' technique of insertion. The infection risk may be reduced, but not entirely eliminated, by its marked progestogenic effect on genital tract fluid. A more important problem is the high incidence in the first post-insertion months of uterine bleeding which, though small in quantity, may be very frequent or continuous and can cause considerable inconvenience. There is a also small incidence of steroidal side-effects such as acne and breast tenderness.

Conclusions

This method – particularly once the thread-borne variant mentioned earlier is available –

Table 1 Main features of the 'ideal' contraceptive

100% reversible
100% effective (with the 'default state' = contraception)
100% convenient (discreet, and non-coitally-related)
100% free of adverse side-effects (neither risk nor nuisance)
100% protective against sexually transmitted infections
Possessed of other non-contraceptive benefits
Non-medical, maintenance-free (needing no on-going medical intervention)

fulfils many of the criteria for an 'ideal' contraceptive (Table 1). Adverse side-effects are few and in general they are in the category 'nuisance' rather than hazardous.

Given the urgency of the human numbers problem, it is to be hoped that new contraceptives fulfilling even more completely the ideal criteria of Table 1, particularly methods requiring no special skill to be applied/distributed, without nuisance side-effects and protective against sexually transmitted infections, be developed for widespread use in the 21st century. In the meantime, the levonorgestrel-releasing intrauterine system sets a high standard, and hopefully a cheap public sector price can soon be set in order to obtain both its contraceptive and health benefits for the maximum possible number of women on the planet.

References

1. Guillebaud J. Contraception for the 21st century. In Johansson EDB, ed. *The Levonorgestrel Intra-uterine System – The New Contraceptive Option for Parous Women.* Carnforth, UK: Parthenon Publishing, 1998:11–32
2. Djerassi C. *The Politics of Contraception.* New York: WW Norton, 1979
3. Committee on Safety of Medicines. Combined oral contraceptives and thromboembolism [Letter]. London: Committee on Safety of Medicines, 1995
4. Wildemeersch D, Batar I, Webb A, *et al.* Gynefix. The frameless intrauterine contraceptive implant – an update. For interval, emergency and post-abortal contraception. *Br J Fam Plann* 1999;24:149–59

The contraceptive efficacy of low-dose gossypol in Brazilian men

15

E. M. Coutinho, C. Athayde, C. Hirsch, M. da Paixão Campos, G. Atta, M. Reidenberg and S. J. Segal

Introduction

Gossypol, a yellow pigment isolated from cottonseed oil, suppresses spermatogenesis, can be taken once a day, and maintains normal testosterone levels and libido. Its safety, however, is controversial. The outcome of the Chinese clinical trials involving 8806 men[1] uncovered the incidence of irreversible infertility (10%) and the appearance of hypokalemic-induced paralysis in a small number of treated men (0.75%). These facts damped the enthusiasm of investigators. On the other hand, hypokalemia is relatively common in Chinese men who are healthy and not taking any drugs[2,3]. In view of the poor prospects available for the development of an alternative male contraceptive, and given the importance of the subject, we decided to carry out a clinical trial in Brazil, using a lower gossypol dose than that used previously in China, to evaluate its effectiveness and safety.

Materials and methods

Thirty-two subjects voluntarily seeking vas ligation were enrolled in Brazil (Salvador, Bahia). The study inclusion criteria were the following: sperm density > 20 million/ml with more than 50% normal forms, progressive sperm motility > 30%, blood serum potassium > 3.8 mmol/l, female partner not known to be infertile, completed family, normal electrocardiogram, age between 26 and 42 years, age of female partner < 40 years. The subjects accepted the possibilities of lack of efficacy and reversibility or irreversibility occurring. The protocol was approved by the institution's clinical review board (IRB).

Two oral regimens of gossypol acetate produced in China were evaluated for efficacy, acceptability and side-effects as a male contraceptive. Gossypol was given orally at a dose of 15 mg/day for 12 weeks or for 16 weeks, if needed, to reach spermatogenesis suppression. This was followed by random allocation of the subjects to the doses of 7.5 mg/day or 10 mg/day for 40 weeks. If spermatogenesis suppression was not attained at the end of 12 weeks, subjects continued at 15 mg/day for an additional 4 weeks. If suppression was not reached at the end of 16 weeks, subjects were discontinued from the study. A third group of 23 healthy men who did not receive any drug were enrolled as a control group. Gossypol was prepared from the seeds of *Gossypium barbadense* by the Shanghai Pharmaceutical Company (Shanghai, China). A single batch of gossypol acetic acid was used for the entire study. Urinalysis, semen analysis, hematology, SMA12, determination of levels of potassium, testosterone, follicle stimulating hormone (FSH), and luteinizing hormone (LH), and clinical examination, including testicular volume, were carried out twice before starting treatment. Plasma gossypol was measured once as a pretreatment control. Subjects visited the clinic monthly for follow-up. Men were clinically examined in weeks 12, 24, 36 and 52. Testicular volume was determined with the use of Prader's orchidometer. During weeks 8, 12, 16, 24, 36, 44 and 52, urine samples were collected and examined for leukocyte counts, proteins, hemoglobin and glucose. Semen analysis was carried out in weeks 4, 8, 12, 16, 24, 36, 44, and 52.

Semen collection and analysis were carried out according to the World Health Organization Laboratory Manual for the Examination of Human Semen and Semen–Cervical Mucus Interaction. Samples were collected after 72 h of sexual abstinence. Blood cell counts and clinical chemistry were performed in weeks 8, 12, 24, 36, 48 and 52. Potassium was measured every month from week 8. Testosterone and LH levels were measured in weeks 12, 24, 36 and 52. FSH was determined every month from week 12. Blood was collected for plasma gossypol in weeks 12, 36 and 52. The blood was centrifuged in a refrigerated centrifuge after adding reduced glutathione as an antioxidant to stabilize the gossypol. The plasma was removed, frozen and sent to New York in the frozen state. Gossypol concentration determinations were carried out by high-performance liquid chromatography using an electroconductivity detector at the Department of Pharmacology at the Weill Medical School of Cornell University, New York. The method has been presented in detail[4]. Men in the control group did not receive gossypol, but were willing to provide blood samples for evaluation of potassium levels and SMA12 measurements on the same schedule as treated subjects. Post-treatment recovery was evaluated at 6 and 12 months after the treatment period (weeks 72 and 104 of the study). Couples were instructed to use other means of contraception following the treatment phase. The contraceptive methods of the couple's choice were provided as part of the study. If by 1 year after stopping treatment sperm counts were not within the subject's normal pre-treatment range, but were > 20 million/ml with > 30% forward motility, the subject was considered as having semen quality within the range of normal healthy men and therefore to have recovered. Data were statistically analyzed using the Wilcoxon test. Student's t test was used for comparisons of gossypol concentration.

Results

The mean age and other subject characteristics at admission are shown in Table 1. Varicocele was clinically diagnosed in 47% (15/32) of

Table 1 Characteristics at admission of subjects in the treatment group ($n = 32$)

Characteristic	Number of subjects (mean ± SD)
Age (years)	31.2 ± 7.1
Weight (kg)	63.9 ± 9.1
Systolic blood pressure (mmHg)	118.4 ± 10.5
Diastolic blood pressure (mmHg)	81.2 ± 7.1
Height (cm)	168.4 ± 5.9
Right testicular volume (ml)	25.0 ± 5.4
Left testicular volume (ml)	24.4 ± 6.4

subjects. The median reported frequency of intercourse among subjects at admission was ten times per month (range 4–28). A prostate of normal size without inflammatory signs was observed in 72% (23/32) of subjects during rectal examination at admission, whilst 28% (9/32) presented a prostate of normal size with signs of congestion. Seventeen of the 32 men (53%) who entered into the study discontinued before completing 1 year of treatment for the following reasons:

(1) Weakness and tiredness (1);

(2) Did not reach spermatogenesis suppression (4);

(3) Non-compliance (3);

(4) Failure to maintain sperm suppression (1);

(5) Other non-medical reasons (8).

Twenty-six of the 32 men (81%) who entered into the study completed the loading phase. Of these, 22 men (85%) attained spermatogenesis suppression (19 at 12 weeks and 3 at 16 weeks of treatment) and in four men (15%) there was no spermatogenesis suppression. In the four subjects who failed to meet the criteria to continue the study, there was an increase in the total number of immotile spermatozoa in the sample from 20% at admission to 62% at week 16. The 22 subjects in whom spermatogenesis was suppressed were allocated at random to one of the two treatment groups: Group 1 – 7.5 mg/day (11 subjects) or Group 2 – 10.0 mg/day (11 subjects). Body weight increased at week 52 only in the 10.0 mg group. Blood pressure was unchanged during treatment. Testicular volume decreased consistently with both drug regimens. The reported frequency of intercourse per month did not vary significantly. There were no changes in urine analysis, except for one subject who presented with a positive hemoglobin test between weeks 12 and 36 of treatment and a positive protein test at weeks 24 and 36. The blood cell counts were unchanged during treatment. Once sperm density fell to values around 1 million/ml, it was maintained in both groups, except in one subject in the 7.5 mg/day group, who was discontinued from the study at week 52 of treatment for failing to maintain sperm suppression. Serum potassium values fluctuated inconsistently at a few times in both treated and control subjects (Table 2). No subject developed hypokalemia.

Serum glutamic-oxaloacetic transaminase, serum glutamate pyruvate transaminase, bilirubin and alkaline phosphatase fluctuated inconsistently at a few sampling times. All individual values were found within the normal range. Sodium, phosphorus, glucose and total protein varied inconsistently at a few sampling times in both treated and control subjects. The concentration values of urea, creatinine, albumin, uric acid and calcium were unchanged throughout the treatment period. Testosterone and LH were unchanged, while FSH increased consistently (Table 3). Plasma gossypol levels measured at 12 weeks were 160 ± 71 ng/ml (mean $\pm$ SD) in the patients who had sperm suppression ($n = 14$) and 201 ± 108 in those in whom there was no suppression ($n = 4$).

Table 2 Potassium levels in Brazilian men taking gossypol. Values are mean $\pm$ SE

| | *Potassium level* (mmol/l) (*n*) | | | |
	15 mg/day gossypol	*7.5 mg/day gossypol*	*10 mg/day gossypol*	*Control group*
Admission	4.12 ± 0.05 (32)	—	—	4.12 ± 0.06 (23)
Week 8	3.94 ± 0.08 (25)	—	—	4.05 ± 0.10 (23)
Week 12	$3.95 \pm 0.08^{\dagger}$ (26)	—	—	4.17 ± 0.07 (23)
Week 16	—	$3.90 \pm 0.06*$ (14)	3.96 ± 0.10 (11)	4.03 ± 0.09 (23)
Week 20	—	$4.00 \pm 0.09*$ (11)	$3.75 \pm 0.08*^{\ddagger}$ (8)	4.09 ± 0.06 (22)
Week 24	—	$3.86 \pm 0.11*$ (11)	3.81 ± 0.12 (8)	$3.98 \pm 0.07*$ (23)
Week 28	—	4.10 ± 0.12 (11)	3.81 ± 0.07 (8)	3.98 ± 0.10 (22)
Week 32	—	4.06 ± 0.13 (11)	$3.68 \pm 0.09^{\dagger}$ (8)	4.00 ± 0.09 (23)
Week 36	—	4.01 ± 0.13 (11)	3.83 ± 0.16 (8)	$3.90 \pm 0.07**$ (23)
Week 40	—	4.19 ± 0.17 (10)	3.80 ± 0.16 (8)	4.07 ± 0.10 (23)
Week 44	—	4.00 ± 0.16 (9)	3.80 ± 0.09 (8)	4.01 ± 0.08 (21)
Week 48	—	4.06 ± 0.11 (9)	4.00 ± 0.18 (8)	4.07 ± 0.07 (23)
Week 52	—	$3.91 \pm 0.11^{\dagger}$ (8)	4.02 ± 0.16 (8)	4.27 ± 0.07 (23)
Week 72	—	4.00 ± 0.18 (7)	4.07 ± 0.15 (7)	4.15 ± 0.07 (19)
Week 104	—	$3.94 \pm 0.06^{\dagger}$ (5)	3.83 ± 0.11 (7)	$3.58 \pm 0.09*$ (6)

Follow-up visits versus admission: $*p < 0.05$, $**p < 0.01$; potassium levels of treated versus control subjects at sampling points: $^{\dagger}p < 0.05$, $^{\ddagger}p < 0.01$

Table 3 FSH levels in men taking gossypol. Values are mean ± SE

	FSH *level* (IU/l) (*n*)		
	15 mg/day gossypol	*7.5 mg/day gossypol*	*10 mg/day gossypol*
Admission	2.47 ± 0.25 (26)	—	—
Week 12	2.76 ± 0.27 (26)	—	—
Week 16	—	3.09 ± 0.52 (14)	3.09 ± 0.47 (11)
Week 20	—	3.93 ± 0.86 (11)	4.34 ± 0.96 (8)
Week 24	—	4.76 ± 1.30 (11)	4.64 ± 1.16 (8)
Week 28	—	5.91 ± 1.67* (11)	5.94 ± 0.98* (8)
Week 32	—	6.52 ± 1.63* (10)	7.63 ± 1.57* (8)
Week 36	—	6.41 ± 1.57* (11)	8.21 ± 1.38* (8)
Week 40	—	6.82 ± 1.83* (9)	9.07 ± 1.44* (8)
Week 44	—	7.71 ± 1.66* (9)	8.36 ± 1.63* (8)
Week 48	—	8.80 ± 2.42** (9)	8.59 ± 1.18* (7)
Week 52	—	9.05 ± 2.71* (8)	10.0 ± 1.34* (8)
Week 72	—	10.20 ± 2.45* (7)	11.10 ± 2.23* (7)
Week 104	—	10.40 ± 2.55* (4)	7.93 ± 0.87 (3)

Follow-up visits versus admission: *$p > 0.05$, **$p > 0.01$

Post-treatment recovery was evaluated at 6 and 12 months after gossypol discontinuation. Testicular volume returned to values not statistically different from those at admission by 12 months postsuspension in both groups. In the 7.5 mg/day group, three out of seven subjects (43%) recovered spermatogenesis (20, 51 and 77 million/ml), two subjects within 6 months and one within 12 months post-treatment suspension; three of seven remained azoospermic and one of seven reached a sperm count of 12 million/ml. In the 10.0 mg/day group, only one of seven subjects (14%) recovered (20 million/ml), three of seven remained azoospermic and three of seven remained oligospermic (1, 1 and 4 million/ml). Mean levels of FSH at 6 and 12 months post-treatment were still increased when compared to admission in both groups.

Discussion

The present study shows that 22 men out of the 26 who completed loading phase (12–16 weeks on 15 mg/day) were rendered infertile. Four men failed to reach azoospermia at 16 weeks. In these men an insufficient reduction in sperm density from a mean of 53 million/ml to a mean of 13 million/ml occurred, but a simultaneous increase in the number of immotile spermatozoa from a mean of 20% to a mean of 62% could have rendered them subfertile.

Only one man failed to maintain sperm suppression during the maintenance phase (7.5 mg/day group). This subject presented with a sperm density increase from week 36 to week 52, from 4 to 38 million/ml. Our gossypol concentration measurements indicate that, within the range of doses and levels studied, the occurrence of sperm suppression does not appear to be concentration-dependent. Apparently, some men are responsive and others are not. However, recovery seems to be dose-dependent in this small study population, since more subjects recovered in the group with the lower dose intake (7.5mg; three out of seven subjects) than in the group taking 10.0 mg/day (one out of seven subjects). Moreover, a higher incidence of azoospermia or severe oligospermia at 1 year postsuspension was observed in the 10.0 mg/day group (six out of seven subjects). A reduction in testicular volume resulting from a decrease in mass of the germinal epithelium was found to be reversible. Nevertheless, full reversibility of spermatogenesis failed to occur in nearly 71% of the men. We have shown in a previous study that long-lasting azoospermia was more likely to occur in men with subclinical varicocele, which was diagnosed in 47% of our volunteers[5]. The present study also shows that hypokalemia, which was observed in Chinese men in earlier trials of gossypol, did not occur in our subjects. We think this is because we included only men with serum potassium values above 3.8 mmol/l at entry to the study and perhaps because our dose of gossypol was lower than that used in prior studies. In addition, hypokalemia is relatively common in Chinese men who are healthy and not taking any drugs[2].

Gossypol has the potential of being a medical alternative to surgical vasectomy when the delay in onset of infertility is acceptable. The possibility of reversal, occurring in 29% of the men on this regimen within 1 year after stopping gossypol, is an advantage for this compound. When taken for 1 year, gossypol causes no reduction in sexual desire or frequency of intercourse. There were no drug-attributable adverse events. Making gossypol available would give men an additional alternative to vasectomy or barrier methods.

Acknowledgements

This study was supported in part by grants from The Rockefeller Foundation, The Gloria Conn Fund, and the CONRAD subproject agreement CSA–94–160.

References

1. Liu ZQ, Liu GZ, Hei LS, *et al.* Clinical trial of gossypol as a male antifertility agent. In Chang CF, Griffin D, Woolman A, eds. *Recent Advances in Fertility Regulation.* Geneva: Attar, 1981:160–3
2. Reidenberg MM, Gu ZP, Lorenzo BJ, *et al.* Differences in serum potassium concentrations in normal men in different geographic locations. *Clin Chem* 1993;39:72–5
3. Gu Z-P, Segal S, Reidenberg MM. Serum potassium values in normal men in Shanghai compared with men from Shanghai living abroad. *Clin Chem* 1994;40:340
4. Bushunow P, Reidenberg MM, Wasenko J, *et al.* Gossypol treatment of recurrent adult malignant gliomas. *J Neuro-Oncol* 1999; in press
5. Coutinho EM, Melo JF, Barbosa I, *et al.* Antispermatogenic action of gossypol in men. *Fertil Steril* 1984;42:424–30

Immunocontraception: past, present and future — 16

G. P. Talwar

Introduction

The possibility of regulating fertility by immunological approaches was indicated by experiments of two illustrious pioneers, Karl Landsteiner[1] and Eli Metchinikoff[2], 100 years ago. Both independently generated antibodies cytotoxic to sperm. The idea lay dormant for nearly 30 years, when a French scientist reported immunizing women against human sperm for temporary sterility[3]. This démarche could not, however, be converted into a practical modality, as sperm, along with the coated seminal plasma components, carried a large number of constituents which cross-reacted with other tissues of the body. It was necessary to refine purification techniques to a stage of obtaining single homogeneous molecules, which could be tested and confirmed as being unique to sperm. The identification of an isozyme of lactate dehydrogenase (LDH-C$_4$) by Goldberg[4] was the first such molecule, which was demonstrated to be specific to sperm and not present in other tissues. A serious limitation, still, was in obtaining such molecules in adequate amounts from natural sources. It was only after the dawn of DNA recombinant technology that alternative ways of obtaining such antigens became possible. Advances in better understanding of the immune system, emergence of hybridoma technology, analytical delineation of binding epitopes and synthetic protein chemistry have contributed enormously to the current research on development of immunological approaches for regulating fertility.

Past

Animal experiments

In years gone by, fertility regulation was demonstrated either in laboratory animals or in veterinary species. The antigens used were crude extracts and a strong adjuvant, such as Freund's complete adjuvant (FCA), was invariably employed. It did achieve castration in males and block of fertility in females, but no attention was paid to the side-effects. FCA produced noxious granuloma and abcess. Observations were limited to short periods and no serious attention was given to reversibility and systemic side-effects, nor was necropsy carried out to see immunopathological damage to various tissues.

Clinical observations

A large number of clinical reports have appeared over years assigning unexplained infertility to immunological factors[5–13]. In many patients, this was ascribed to the presence of antisperm antibodies in the circulation; titers above a threshold (depending on the method employed) were considered to be the basis of infertility. Treatment with immunosuppressing agents, such as corticosteroids, helped a percentage of such patients to conceive[12]. Cases have been reported[14] where both husband and wife carry antibodies directed at the same sperm constituents. Sera from infertile patients have served to sift out the putative antigens as potential contraceptive antigens. No clinical abnormalities other than inability to bear progeny have been reported in the numerous cases examined, giving support to the hypothesis that fertility control can be exercised by immunological approaches without systemic side-effects. What is not known in most cases is the mode by which people got immunized in these 'Nature's' experiments. The only clear association is of vasovasectomy with circulating antisperm antibodies[15]. Nearly two-thirds of subjects undergoing this operation form antibodies reactive with sperm. The titers are not universally high and a large variation exists in the extent and duration of the response. This variation may be due in part to the differences in surgical handling and manipulation, over and above individual constitutional factors. What is indicated, however, is the presence of auto-antigens on the sperm to which the body is not tolerant and which can evoke an immune response in the individual.

The present status of immunocontraception

Research has progressed world-wide to identify antigens to make vaccines that can evoke humoral and/or cell-mediated immune responses for the regulation of fertility. The interception of fertility can take place at several steps. Human (and mammalian) reproduction results from the penetration of the sperm into the egg and the initiation of a series of events leading to the multiplication of embryonic cells. Both the sperm and the egg carry numerous antigens; an immune response against any of these antigens can prevent fertilization. Factors are being identified by scientists engaged in *in vitro* fertilization (IVF) and assisted reproduction which are important for normal cleavage and initial embryonic development[6]. The early human embryo starts making human chorionic gonadotropin (hCG)[17], which has now been identified to play a crucial role in the nidation of the embryo onto the uterus. Antibodies against hCG prevent implantation in marmosets[18]. This is also the case in humans. Hyperfertile women who are immunized with the anti-hCG vaccine and protected from becoming pregnant do not manifest any elongation of the luteal phase or experience heavy bleeding[19], implying therefore that the vaccine does not act as an abortifacient and, in fact, prevents the onset of pregnancy by blocking implantation.

A cascade of hormones play a critical role in the generation of gametes and in the production of sex steroids required to prepare the uterus to receive the embryo and to sustain pregnancy until such time as the fetoplacental unit makes by itself the requisite hormones, including paracrine hormones and growth factors. Normal supply of these is necessary to avoid abortion and carry the pregnancy to term. Figure 1 gives a schematic overview.

In view of the many steps vulnerable to blockage, a number of vaccines are under development. These are summarized in Table 1. They are at different stages of experimental work and evaluation.

Pertinent developments with potential for immunocontraception

The targets selected for immuno-interception fall broadly into two categories: the gamete antigens and the reproductive hormones. Six vaccines (Table 2), all directed at reproductive hormones, have reached the stage of phase I clinical trials after extensive demonstration of their ability to control fertility in experimental animals (including subhuman primates) and their lack of toxicity, which was shown in standard preclinical toxicology studies in two species. They received approval of the Drugs Regulatory and Ethics Committees in nine countries: India, USA, Finland, Chile, Sweden, Brazil, Dominican Republic, Austria and Australia. The trials were conducted under the supervision of renowned clinicians. The findings have shown universally that these vaccines are safe and devoid of any notable side-effects. Furthermore, they are all reversible. Phase II efficacy studies have so far been carried out on only one vaccine, the HSD-TT/DT directed at hCG. The hCG vaccines are thus discussed as an entity separately in the following text.

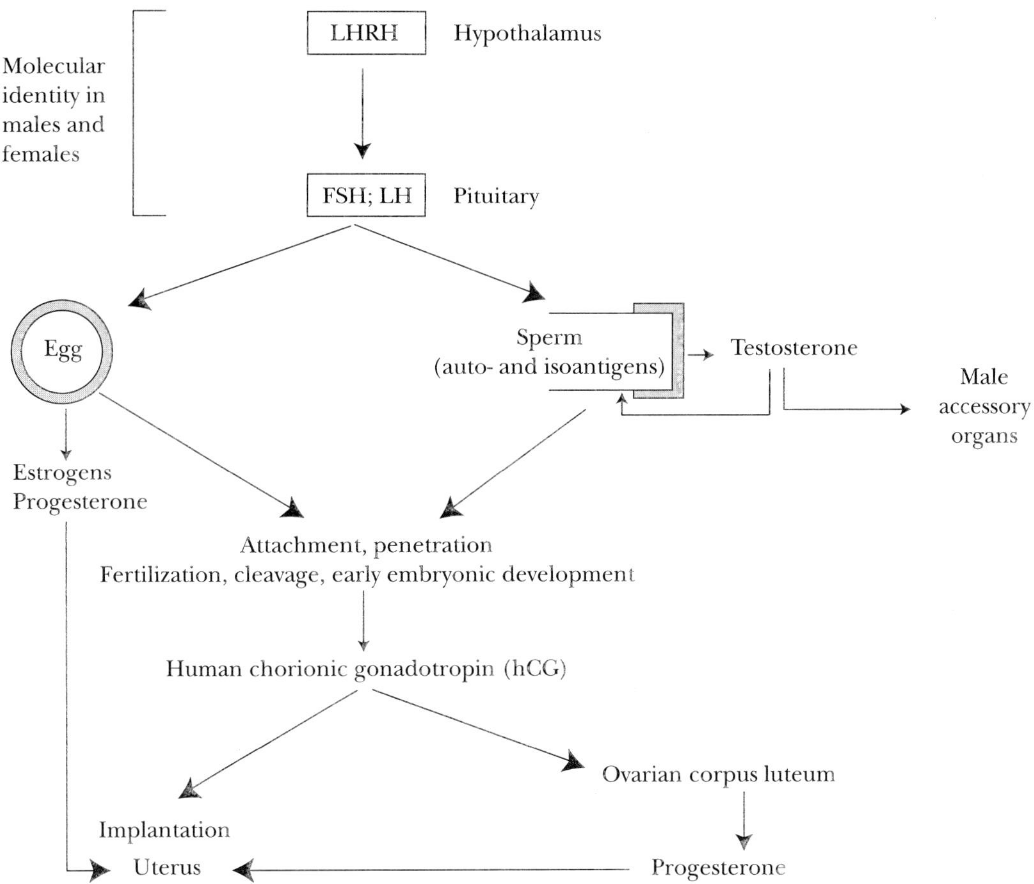

Figure 1 Schematic overview of the hormones involved in preparing the uterus to receive the egg and sustain pregnancy

The vaccines against luteinizing hormone releasing hormone (LHRH) have potential primarily for the control of animal fertility, since its molecular structure is essentially conserved through evolution and is the same from mouse to man. Moreover, it is common to both males and females and hence the vaccines would have application in both sexes. The LHRH vaccine was fully safe in women and reduced the high levels of follicle stimulating hormone (FHS) and luteinizing hormone (LH) in post-menopausal women[20]. Monoclonal antibodies against LHRH arrest the onset of estrus in bitches[21].

Since inactivation of LHRH blocks not only the generation of gametes, but also the production of sex steroids, major human applications of the LHRH vaccine would be in hormone-dependent cancers, endometriosis and pre-cocious puberty, although with androgen supplements it may also be useful for male fertility control. A semi-synthetic LHRH vaccine was devised several years ago[22]. It causes a dramatic atrophy of the prostate in rodents[23] and in monkeys[24]. This vaccine has undergone Phase I/II clinical trials in 28 patients with advanced-stage carcinoma of the prostate in India and Austria[25]. Patients generating anti-LHRH antibodies had a reduction in testosterone to castration levels. There was a concomitant fall in prostate specific antigen and acid phosphatase levels and several patients experienced an improvement in clinical well-being with evidence of a decrease in prostatic mass as seen by ultrasound scans and nephrostograms. Surprisingly, the vaccine also has some but not total inhibitory action on the growth of an androgen-independent Duning tumor clone

Table 1 Birth-control vaccines under development at the experimental stage

Target	Vaccine	Destined use	Status	Principal investigator(s)
Sperm	LDH-C$_4$	female fertility control	immunodominant epitopes identified; protection studies in baboons with chimeric peptide of LDH-C$_4$ with T-epitope of tetanus toxoid was 63–75% successful	E. Goldberg
Sperm	RSA	male fertility control	inhibition of sperm–egg interaction by monoclonal antibodies	M.G. O'Rand
Sperm	PH-20	males and females	fully effective in guinea pigs	P. Primakoff
Sperm	SP-10	females	intra-acrosomal protein. Vaccine trials in baboons caused reduction of fertility	J.C. Herr
Sperm	HSA-63	females	antibodies inhibit human sperm penetration. Cross-reactive with SP-10	M.S. Liu
Sperm	FA-1	females	conserved across species. Antibodies prevent human sperm penetration, also inhibit acrosome reaction. Present in infertile patients; recombinant protein made	R.K. Naz
Sperm	NZ-1 NZ-2	females	antibodies block human sperm penetration; sperm-specific	R.K. Naz
Sperm	CS-1	females	antibodies inhibit first cleavage of pronuclear stage zygotes; antibodies present in infertile patients	R.K. Naz
Sperm	glutathione S-transferases	females	antibodies inhibit fertilization	C. Shaha
Sperm	71-kDa	females/males	antibodies present in infertile couples; cause heavy agglutination of sperm	A. Suri
Sperm	BCG; Talsur	male animals	intratesticular/epididymal administration causes aspermatogenesis without loss of libido	G.P. Talwar R.K. Naz A. Suri
Oocyte	rabbit recombinant 55-kDa and 75-kDa	females	immunization of cynomolgus monkey with 55-kDa protein leads to infertility without affecting ovarian function; 75-kDa protein causes ovarian dysgenesis	B.S. Dunbar
Oocyte	human/ cynomolgus Macaque ZP3 peptide	females	immunization of cynomolgus Macaques leads to infertility with normal ovarian function	C.A. Mahi-Brown
Oocyte	recombinant human ZP3/ porcine ZPE	females	immunization of marmoset monkey leads to infertility associated with ovarian dysfunction, characterized by suppression of folliculogenesis and depletion of the primordial follicle pool	R.J. Aitken
Oocyte	pig zona pellucida	females	demonstrated effect of immunization for control of wildlife population	J.F. Kirkpatrick
Oocyte	synthetic peptide corresponding to mouse ZP3	females	efficacy to block fertility in female mice without concomitant auto-immune oophoritis	K.S.K. Tung

Table 1 *continued*

Target	Vaccine	Destined use	Status	Principal investigator(s)
Oocyte	recombinant pig ZP1 and synthetic peptides	females	mapped the epitope for a monoclonal antibody inhibiting binding and penetration of pig and human sperm in homologous eggs	K. Koyama
Oocyte	porcine ZP3	females	immunization of bonnet monkey with porcine ZP3 along with permissible adjuvants leads to reversible block of fertility	S.K. Gupta
Oocyte	bonnet monkey ZP1/ZP2/ZP3; synthetic peptides	females	cloning, sequencing and expression of bonnet monkey ZP1, ZP2 and ZP3; synthetic peptide epitopes corresponding to monoclonal antibody identified	S.K. Gupta
Oocyte	mouse ZP3 synthetic peptide KLH conjugate	females	immunization of Swiss mice leads to reversible block of fertility; cloning and sequencing of zonae pellucidae	J. Dean
Oocyte	dog, cat, cow, pig cynomologus monkey and human ZPA/ZPB/ZPC	females	cloning, sequencing and expression of the various zona proteins. Testing efficacy to block fertility	Zonagen Inc.
Oocyte	porcine ZP3 cynomolgus deglycosylated form	females	demonstrated contraceptive efficacy in squirrel monkeys and rabbits	A.G. Sacco
Riboflavin carrier protein (RCP)	chicken RCP CTP and RCP-DT	pregnancy interception in females; renders males subfertile	tested in rodents and primates. Immunodominant epitopes determined	R.P. Adiga

LDH-C$_4$, isoenzyme of lactate dehydrogenase; BCG, Bacillus Calmette Guerin; ZP, zona pellucida; KLH, keyhole limpet hemocyanin; RCP, riboflavin carrier protein; CTP, carboxyl terminal peptide; DT, diphtheria toxoid

in rats[25,26]. At present we are making a DNA-recombinant vaccine for LHRH, which could be cheap and amenable to industrial production.

The third hormone against which a vaccine has been developed is FSH. Moudgal and associates[27] have employed ovine FSH to generate antibodies which cross-react with monkey and human FSH. These cause oligospermia in monkeys and, furthermore, the fertilizing ability of the residual sperm is diminished. No decline in testosterone levels occurs. The vaccine is designed for male fertility control. It has entered Phase I clinical trials in men to determine safety and reversibility.

Research on gamete antigens

Immunotargeting of sperm, egg and or their interaction is an attractive approach and, if successful, would achieve a prefertilization block. It is therefore not surprising that a large number of investigators are following this line of research. However, no vaccine or passive immunological approach against the gamete antigens has yet progressed to the human trials stage. The most advanced research is on an isoenzyme of lactate dehydrogenase (LDH-C$_4$). O'Hern and co-workers[28] have made a chimeric conjugate of a B-cell epitope (5–19) of LDH-C$_4$ linked to a promiscuous T-cell determinant of

Table 2 Birth-control vaccines reaching clinical trials

Target	Vaccine	Destined use	Status	Principal investigator(s) and published work
hCG	HSD-TT/DT	women for reversible fertility control	phase I safety and Phase II efficacy trials completed; prevents pregnancy at titers of > 50 ng/ml; no significant side-effects; ovulation maintained with regularity of menstrual cycles	G.P. Talwar and colleagues[19]
hCG	β-hCG-TT	women for reversible fertility control	phase I trials completed in India, Sweden, Finland, Brazil and Chile	ICCR of the Population Council and G.P. Talwar and colleagues[41,43]
hCG	β-hCG-TT	women for reversible fertility control	phase I trials in Chile, Dominican Republic and Finland for determining hormone profiles, which remained normal	H. Croxatto; V. Brache; P. Lehtenmäki; R.M. Thau
hCG	CTP-DT	women for reversible fertility control	phase I clinical trials conducted in Australia	V. Stevens; W. Jones and colleagues[53]
hCG	Vaccinia β-hCG membrane-anchored	men and women, lung cancer-secreting hCG	experimental efficacy *in vitro* and *in vivo* in nude mice using Chago cells; preliminary clinical trials in three lung cancer patients in Mexico	G.P. Talwar; D. Biswas and colleagues[52]; C. Gual *et al.*
LHRH	LHRH-6 DLys-DT	men, carcinoma of prostate	phase I/Phase II trials conducted in India and Austria in patients with advanced-stage carcinoma of the prostate	G.P. Talwar and colleagues[25]; S.N. Wadhwa; S. Sharma; J. Frick
LHRH	LHRH-6 DLys-DT	postmenopausal women	decline in FSH and LH levels; reversible effect with waning of antibodies	G. Carlos and colleagues[20]; G.P. Talwar
LHRH	LHRH-1-TT	men, for fertility control with androgen supplementation and for carcinoma of the prostate	experimental studies completed; Phase I trials initiated in the USA	R.M. Thau; Y. Tsong and colleagues at The Population Council
FSH	FSH (ovine)	men, for fertility regulation without loss of libido and decline in testosterone	phase I trials initiated in India	N.R. Moudgal and colleagues

hCG, human chorionic gonadotropin; HSD, heterospecies dimer; TT, tetanus toxoid; DT, diphtheria toxoid; CTP, carboxyl terminal peptide ; LHRH, luteinizing hormone releasing hormone; FSH, follicle stimulating hormone; Lys, lysine; ICCR, International Committee on Contraception Research

tetanus toxoid. Baboons were immunized with this chimeric peptide, along with a strong adjuvant (squalene–Arlacel A emulsion containing muramyl dipeptide). Optimal immunization lowered the pregnancies by 63–75%. These included three conceptions which ended in miscarriage during the first trimester, which calls for more studies to determine the stage at which pregnancy is interrupted by immunization with this antigen. The effect was reversible and fertility was regained in course of time.

A large number of leads have come from infertile couples. Suri and colleagues[14] identified a 71-kDa antigen from the serum of an infertile woman which reacted with her husband's sperm as well as with sperm from normal donors. Antibodies against this antigen were also present in the husband's serum and caused heavy agglutination of the sperm. The antigen has cross-species reactivity and antibodies inhibit sperm attachment to mouse oocytes *in vitro*.

Naz and co-workers[29] have focussed their attention on the identification of those sperm surface proteins that bind to pertinent zona pellucida proteins involved in sperm–egg interactions. One of these, the FA-1 antigen, has been cloned and sequenced. It has an auto-phosphorylating activity for tyrosine residues, which have a vital role in sperm capacitation and acrosome reactions. FA-1 antigen is testes-specific and is not present in other tissues. Immunization of female mice with recombinant FA-1 reduced the number of babies born by about 75%. FA-1 is a conserved antigen and is cross-reactive in several species. It is believed to be a human sperm receptor (ligand) for binding to the zona pellucida and may also have a role in sperm capacitation and/or acrosome reactions[30]. It is thus a promising antigen. Naz has also described three other antigens on which his group is doing seminal work (Table 1). It is not unlikely that a mixture of several meritorious sperm antigens may be necessary to achieve near to 95% fertility control, which at present has not been achieved with any antigen by active immunization, except for a solitary observation by Primakoff[31] employing the PH-20 antigen in guinea pigs. Table 1 refers to the major work in progress in different laboratories on sperm antigens.

Zona pellucida antigens

Table 1 lists 11 major laboratories working on the zona pellucida antigens, with the aim of identifying one or more antigens that may be specific to the zona, an immune response against which could block the sperm–egg interaction and thereby fertility. Earlier studies with solubilized zona pellucida, or even with one of the purified zona pellucida glycoproteins, caused oophoritis, with permanent loss of ovarian follicles. Molecular cloning of mouse zona pellucida by Dean and allied studies of Tung identified the coexistence of epitopes for B and T cells in the protein sequence[32]. T-cell response was the cause of undesirable autoimmune reactions[33] and this has to be avoided to prevent ovarian damage. Thus, B-cell epitopes are being sifted from zona pellucida proteins and linked to promiscuous T-cell epitopes of extraneous origin to make them immunogenic.

Monoclonal antibodies have been generated by Gupta and co-workers[34] against porcine zona pellucida cross-reactive with monkey and by Koyama and colleagues[35] against the human zona pellucida. It is their reactivity with deglycosylated zona pellucida that is of most interest. Epitope mapping has revealed linear sequences of immunoreactivity. Monoclonal antibodies used for this purpose were screened beforehand for the desirable bioactivity of blocking sperm attachment to hemizonae. Gupta and associates[36] have discussed their strategy of using more than one B-cell epitope of zona pellucida for a contraceptive vaccine. Gupta and colleagues have also cloned and expressed monkey zona pellucida in *Escherichia coli* with good yield[37].

Koyama and co-workers[35] have carried out elegant studies in which they have mapped the binding epitope of a monoclonal antibody which completely inhibited the binding and penetration of human sperm in human eggs *in vitro*. The sequence of an 18-mer region in human zonae containing this epitope was determined. This was rendered immunogenic by linking with diphtheria toxoid. The polyvalent antibodies raised in mice and rabbits against this conjugate retained full efficacy of inhibiting the human sperm–egg interaction.

Summary

From the above, it is evident that the stage is not set for clinical trials on a vaccine against zona pellucida. However, some basic rules for handling zona antigens have been learnt to dissociate the domains generating antibodies for the inhibition of sperm penetration from those generating cytotoxic T-cell response causing an autoimmune reaction, resulting in follicular atresia. Use would have to be made of only B-cell epitopes, avoiding the T-cell determinants in the zona pellucida proteins. More than one B-cell epitope may be necessary in a future contraceptive vaccine for an adequate immune response. At present, zonae pellucidae, especially those prepared by the DNA recombinant route, may be suitable for the sterilization of wild animals. Their potential was explored, for the sterilization of bitches, by Mahi-Brown and co-workers[38]. There were, however, complications of unnatural bleeding, rendering this approach unsuitable for companion animals. In Australia, anti-zona pellucida immunization by live vector-engineered vaccines is being investigated for control of multiplication of wild pest animals.

Induction of aspermatogenesis without decline of testosterone

Immunization with none of the sperm antigens (except PH-20 in guinea pigs) resulted in full fertility control, in spite of employing very strong adjuvants such as FCA, an adjuvant which would be not permitted for use in humans. Could there be an alternate strategy? Sperm are known to carry auto-antigens. These normally remain sequestered within the reproductive tract. Besides, there are other active mechanisms suppressing the generation of an immune response in the testes. We hypothesized that, if the barrier became labile and local suppressive influences were overcome, the immune system should by itself stop spermatogenesis by reacting with sperm antigens to which the body is not tolerant. Leydig cells making testosterone would be spared, as they are present and functional in the fetus and recognized as 'self' components by the immune cells. Spermatogenesis does not occur in fetal life, but begins in puberty, with the result that some proteins on sperm not present in other tissues of the body are potential auto-antigens. We experimented with Bacillus Calmette Guerin (BCG), a vaccine with strong adjuvant and inflammatory properties. An intratesticular injection of BCG caused complete aspermatogenesis in rats, dogs and monkeys[39]. Care had to be exercised to disperse the bacilli and avoid deposits. The animals retained libido and could mate, but the matings were infertile. Semen obtained by electro-ejaculation was totally devoid of sperm. Testosterone levels remained normal. The approach was applicable in all species investigated, including bulls. The hypothesis was, indeed, workable. The effect was highly localized. If injection was given in one testis, the other testis was not affected. No systemic side-effects were noted. No antisperm antibodies were detectable in the circulation. The effect was presumably caused by cell-mediated immune responses. Used in moderate doses, the effect was reversible and the animals regained fertility in the course of time[40]. A major limitation of this otherwise highly effective approach is the local site of immunization. It would further be necessary to isolate the active components in place of using the bacillary suspension.

hCG – the first vaccine providing evidence for prevention of pregnancy in women

The hCG hormone was chosen by our laboratory, the World Health Organization Task Force and the International Committee on Contraception Research of the Population Council to be investigated. It is made in appreciable biologically meaningful amounts only in pregnancy and in some cancers. It is an early signal of conception and is essential for implantation as well as for sustenance of early pregnancy (Figure 1). Women excrete large quantities of hCG in the urine during the first trimester and thus it is obtainable from natural sources. More recently, efficient expression systems have been developed for obtaining subunits of hCG by DNA recombinant methods[37]. Its molecular structure is known, enabling submolecular designs for an eventual vaccine.

The hCG hormone consists of two subunits, α and β, linked to each other covalently to generate the bioactive hormone. The α-subunit is common to three other hormones, thyroid stimulating hormone (TSH), LH and FSH, the β-subunit in each case conferring hormone-specific activity. Thus, the β-subunit of hCG was employed as a potential antigen in the first prototype vaccine designed by us. In order to make it immunogenic in humans, it was linked covalently to tetanus toxoid (TT). β-hCG-TT did induce anti-hCG antibodies in women[41]. The response was reversible and no side-effects of immunization were observed[42]. The main limitation of this vaccine was its low immunogenicity, with only 30% of women responding with high titers. The safety, reversibility and lack of any side-effects of the β-hCG-TT vaccine were confirmed by multicenter Phase I trials conducted by the ICCR of the Population Council[43]. In follow-up studies of the ICCR in Chile, Finland and the Dominican Republic, normal FSH, LH, estradiol and progesterone levels were found in women investigated pre-immunization and at various time intervals after immunization with β-hCG-TT.

The next task was to enhance the immunogenicity of the vaccine. Initially, the vaccine was used absorbed on alum. Inclusion of a sodium phthalyl derivative of lipopolysaccharides, along with alum, on average doubled the antibody titers without any adverse effects on safety. To further improve the intrinsic immunogenicity, two alternative conjugates were employed, in one case linking β-hCG with β-OLH (β-subunit of ovine luteinizing hormone) and in the other using a heterospecies dimer (HSD) of β-hCG associated non-covalently with α-OLH. Both constructs generated increased antibody titers[44]. However, the heterospecies dimer was preferred. It exploited the evolutionarily conserved trait of

the two subunits from two different species to materialize into a 'super'-hormone conformation, which induced an enhanced steroidogenic response compared to the homospecies dimer hCG[45]. Furthermore, the antibodies produced by HSD-TT/DT had higher bioneutralization capacity per unit immunoreactivity[46].

After the standard preclinical toxicology studies, drugs regulatory and ethical approvals, comparative immunogenicity and Phase I clinical trials were undertaken with the HSD-TT, β-hCG–β-OLH/TT and β-hCG-TT vaccines. All of them were safe and no aberrant reaction was noted on metabolic, endocrine or other functions of the body[47]. Ovulation was not impaired, nor was menstrual regularity. HSD-TT produced the highest antibody titers and was selected for Phase II efficacy studies.

During these trials, it was noted that some women became refractory to the immune response against hCG on repeated immunization with the vaccine using TT as the carrier. The carrier-induced immunosuppression could be overcome by using an alternative carrier, such as diphtheria toxoid (DT)[48].

Phase II efficacy trials

Phase II efficacy trials were conducted in three centers in women of reproductive age, of proven fertility, who were sexually active and who were regularly attending the family planning centers of these institutions[19]. The protocol demanded two visits every month, one immediately following menstruation in the first week and the other in the third week for a blood test to determine luteal progesterone and antibody titers. In cases where menstruation was delayed, a pregnancy test was mandatory. Patients maintained a menstrual diary and intercourse record. In cases where antibody titers were tending to decline below 50 ng/ml hCG bioneutralizing capacity, the patient was given a booster injection of the vaccine. Women had the option to leave the trial and not receive the booster immunization. The majority of women, however, continued with the vaccine and were followed up for periods ranging from 6 to 36 months. Only one pregnancy was recorded in 1224 cycles at titers above 50 ng/ml[19]. The ability of the anti-hCG antibodies to prevent pregnancy was further confirmed by postcoital tests conducted in mid-cycle in eight volunteers. In spite of a high mucus score and a high number of motile sperm in the partner, none of them became pregnant[49], whereas at titers below 35 ng/ml, conceptions occurred readily[19].

Immunization did not disturb menstrual regularity, nor was ovulation impaired, as indicated by luteal progesterone levels[19]. The method was fully reversible and fertility was regained by the women when antibody titers declined below the protective threshold in the absence of booster injections. Medical termination of pregnancy was provided according to the protocol. Four women, however, decided to have another baby. Their pregnancies continued to term and the women gave birth to children who have normal physical and cognitive development, as judged with respect to their siblings[50].

In summary, the HSD-hCG vaccine was safe and reversible. It protected hyperfertile, sexually active women from becoming pregnant, as long as the antibody titers were at or above 50 ng/ml hCG bioneutralization capacity. Ovulation was not impaired, nor was the menstrual regularity deranged. No change occurred in bleeding profiles, nor in the amount of blood loss. No systemic contraindications were observed. A follow-up after 10 years of immunization has not indicated any long-term side-effects in vaccinated women (Gopalan and colleagues, unpublished data).

Limitations of the vaccine

While the feasibility of immunocontraception is clearly indicated by the Phase I/Phase II trials with the HSD-hCG vaccine, further optimization and product development is required to make it a practical proposition. The vaccine attained protective threshold titers in only 80% of the recipients and these were sustained for periods of 3 months or more in only 60% of women. Heterogeneity of the immune response is recognized for all vaccines, but in contrast to vaccines for communicable diseases where everyone may not get the infection, the birth-control vaccine will be given to women who are fertile and who must have assurance of protection. Two options emerge. First, limit the use of the presently developed vaccine to high responders. This would call for an initial test. Those who generate high titers could use the vaccine and poor responders could use an alternative method. No method suits all, nor is the same method suitable for a given individual at different stages of reproductive life. Interestingly, the vaccine is usable at all stages of reproductive life, in nulliparous women or in those above 30 years of age, and it may therefore have a place amongst other options.

The second strategy would be to wait until the vaccine can be optimized. Enhancement of immunogenicity could be achieved by inclusion of better adjuvants. Potent adjuvants approved for human use are today available and the mere inclusion of an adjuvant rendered a malaria vaccine which had otherwise no protection, highly protective[51]. We have discussed elsewhere various other strategies which can enhance the antibody response, such as the use of live recombinant vaccine and biodegradable microspheres for single contact point delivery of multiple injections of the vaccine[19,49].

Side benefits

An unexpected property of anti-hCG antibodies is in the inhibition *in vitro* and *in vivo* of lung cancers producing hCG[52]. A large number of cancers which make and secrete hCG are reported in the literature. It remains to be seen whether anti-hCG immunization is beneficial in these diverse hCG-synthesizing cancers.

Current and future positive prospects

It has been demonstrated without ambiguity that the HSD-hCG vaccine is capable of controlling fertility by antibodies which can inactivate hCG. This is achieved without any notable systemic side-effects. The antibodies must be of high affinity, with $K_a \geq 10^9$ M^{-1}. All vaccines (i.e.

the carboxyl terminal peptide of β-hCG[53]) do not generate such high- affinity antibodies. The main drawback in employing vaccines is the uncertainty of the degree and type of immune response. These vary from individual to individual. As antibody is the effective agent (and not the vaccine), a logical alternative is to use preformed antibodies of defined characteristics with respect to affinity, specificity and class of antibody. These could be given at a dose adequate to ensure efficacy. Phase II trials on the hCG vaccine have established the titers of antibodies that are protective (e.g. 50 ng/ml). Another amazing observation was the dominant response to a conformational epitope located in the core part of the molecule[54].

Many years ago, we developed a mouse hybrid cell clone which made monoclonal antibodies against hCG of high affinity ($K_a = 3 \times 10^{10}$ M^{-1}) and high specificity (no cross-reaction with any extraneous organ of the body or with FSH or TSH; < 5% cross-reaction with hLH). The determinant recognized by this antibody happens to be competitive with the major population of antibodies made by the vaccinated women protected from becoming pregnant. This is a bioeffective monoclonal antibody in all experimental test systems. While it may be usable as such for a single time intervention (mouse monoclonal antibodies are in clinical use in cancer patients), a better alternative would be to humanize this monoclonal antibody. Technology has enabled this to be done[55]. It is possible to make engineered therapeutic antibodies in plants[56] and in yeast.

At the time of submission of this manuscript, some progress had been made in the project on 'humanizing' and sifting for 'human' analog antibodies to our meritorious mouse mono-clonal antibody. The genes coding for the variable part of the heavy and light chains of this antibody have been cloned and sequenced. The base sequences of the domains binding with hCG in both heavy and light chains have been delineated.

The aim and the purpose of future work

The aim is to make, in a cost-effective way, 'human' antibodies inactivating hCG by a DNA recombinant route. By virtue of their target specificity, these will be totally safe and free of side-effects. Previous work on the hCG vaccine has outlined the desirable characteristics of a bioeffective antibody and also the amount in which it has to be used to achieve efficacy. Our initial purpose would be to evaluate the passive use of the antibody for emergency contraception. Since hCG is essential for implantation, administration of anti-hCG antibodies any time up to a week after unprotected sex would prevent the onset of pregnancy. Thus there would be a wider time window for intervention than that presently available for Yuzpe's regime (48–72 h). hCG antibodies would be effective for even longer, until the expected day of menstruation, as hCG provides the corpus luteum with support for making progesterone during this period, which is critical for the continuity of gestation.

Acknowledgements

Current work on passive immunization approaches is supported by the Rockefeller Foundation, the Talwar Research Foundation and Indo-German Bilateral Co-operation in Science and Technology.

References

1. Landsteiner K. Zur Kenntnis der specifish auf biutkorperchen wirkenden sera. *Zentralblatt Bacteriol* 1899;25:546

2. Metchinikoff E. Etudes sur la resorption des cellules. *Ann Inst Pasteur (Paris)* 1899;13:737

3. Baskin MJ. Temporary sterilization by injection of human spermatozoa: a preliminary report. *Am J Obstet Gynecol* 1932;24:892–7

4. Goldberg E. Immunochemical specificity of lactate dehydrogenase-X. *Proc Natl Acad Sci* 1971; 68:349–52

5. Behrman SJ. The immune response and infertility. In Behrman SJ, Kistner RW, eds. *Progress in Infertility*. Boston: Little Brown, 1975:793–815

6. Boettcher B, Hjort T, Rümke P, *et al.* Auto and isoantibodies to antigens of the human reproduction systems. *Acta Pathol Microbiol Scand* 1977; 30:173–80

7. Isojima S, Li TS, Ashitaka Y. Immunological analysis of sperm immobilizing factor found in sera of women with unexplained infertiliy. *Am J Obstet Gynecol* 1968;101:677–83

8. Talwar GP. *Immunology of Contraception*. London: Edward Arnold, 1980

9. Katsch S. Immunology, fertility and infertility: a historical survey. *Am J Obstet Gynecol* 1959;77: 946–56

10. Menge AC, Medley NE, Schwarz ML, *et al.* Sperm antibodies in serum and cervical mucus of infertile women. In Bratanov K, Vulchanov VH, Dikov V, *et al.*, eds. *Immunology of Reproduction*. Sofia: Bulgarian Academy of Science Press, 1979: 336–40

11. Rümke P. Sperm agglutinating auto-antibodies in relation to male infertility. *Proc R Soc Med* 1968;61:275–8

12. Shulman S. Agglutinating and immobilising antibodies to spermatozoa. In Cohen J, Hendry WF, eds. *Spermatozoa, Antibodies and Infertility*. Oxford: Blackwell Scientific Publications, 1978:81–99

13. Voisin GA, Toullet F, D'Almeida M. Characterization of spermatozoal auto, iso and alloantigens. In Diczfalusy E, ed. *Immunological Approaches to Fertility Control*. Stockholm: Karolinska Institute, 1974:173–98

14. Suri A, Chhabra S, Upadhyay S. Identification of human sperm antigen recognized by serum of an infertile woman: a candidate for immuno contraception. *Am J Reprod Immunol* 1996;36:317–26

15. Liskin L, Pile JM, Quillan WF. Vasectomy safe and simple. *Populat Rep* 1983;4:61–100

16. Naz RK, Sacco A, Singh O, *et al.* Development of contraceptive vaccines for humans using antigens derived from gametes and hormones: current status. *Hum Reprod Update* 1995;1:1–18

17. Fishel SB, Edwards RG, Evans CJ. Human chorionic gonadotropin secreted by preimplantation embryos cultured *in vitro*. *Science* 1984;223: 816–18

18. Hearn JP, Gidley-Baird AA, Hodges JK, *et al.* Embryonic signals during the pre-implantation period in primates. *J Reprod Fertil* 1988; 36(Suppl):49–58

19. Talwar GP, Singh O, Pal R, *et al.* A vaccine that prevents pregnancy in women. *Proc Natl Acad Sci USA* 1994;91:8532–6

20. Carloss G, Garza-Flores J, Menjivar M, *et al.* Ability of an anti-luteinizing hormone-releasing hormone vaccine to inhibit gonadotropins in postmenopausal women. *Fertil Steril* 1997;67:404–7

21. Talwar GP, Gupta SK, Singh V, *et al.* Bioeffective monoclonal antibody against the decapeptide gonadotropin releasing hormone: reacting determinant and action on ovulation and estrus suppression. *Proc Natl Acad Sci USA* 1985;82: 1228–31

22. Talwar GP, Chaudhuri MK, Jayshankar R. Antigenic derivative of LHRH. *UK Patent* 1992: 2228262

23. Jayshankar R, Chaudhari M, Singh O, *et al.* Semisynthetic anti LHRH vaccine causing atrophy of the prostate. *Prostate* 1989;14:3–11

24. Giri DK, Jayraman S, Neelaram GS, *et al.* Prostatic hypoplasia in Bonnet monkeys following active immunization with semi synthetic anti-LHRH vaccine. *Exp Mol Pathol* 1991;54:255–64

25. Talwar GP, Diwan M, Davar H, *et al.* Counter GnRH vaccine. In Rajalkshmi M, Griffin PD, eds. *Male Contraception – Present and Future*. New Delhi: New Age International, 1998:309–18

26. Furest J, Fiebiger E, Jungwirth A, *et al.* Effect of active immunization against luteinizing hormone releasing hormone on the androgen sensitive Duning R 3327-PAP and androgen independent Duning R 3327-AT2 prostate cancer cell lines. *Prostate* 1997;32:77–84

27. Moudgal NR, Suresh R. FSH and FSH derived vaccines. In Talwar GP, Raghupathy R, eds. *Birth Control Vaccines*. Austin: RG Landes Company, 1995:89–100

28. O'Hern PA, Bambra CS, Isahakia M, *et al.* Reversible contraception in female baboons immunized with a synthetic epitope of sperm specific lactate dehydrogenase. *Biol Reprod* 1995;52: 331–9

29. Naz RK, Ahmad K. Molecular identities of human sperm proteins that bind human zona pellucida: nature of sperm–zona interaction, tyrosine kinase activity and involvement of FA-1. *Mol Reprod Dev* 1994;39:397–408

30. Kadam Al, Fatek M, Naz RK. Fertilization antigen (FA-1) completely blocks human sperm binding to human zona pellucida: FA-1 may be a sperm receptor for zona pellucida in humans. *J Reprod Immunol* 1995;29:239–63

31. Primakoff P, Lathrop W, Wollman L, *et al.* Fully effective contraception in male and female guinea pigs immunized with the sperm protein PH-20. *Nature (London)* 1988;355:543–7

32. Rhim SH, Millar SE, Robey F, *et al.* Autoimmune disease of the ovary induced by a ZP$_3$ peptide

from the mouse zona pellucida. *J Clin Invest* 1992; 89:28–35

33. Lou Y-H, McElveen MF, Garza KM, *et al.* Rapid induction of auto antibodies by endogenous ovarian antigens and activated T cells: implication in autoimmune disease pathogenesis and B cell tolerance. *J Immunol* 1996;156:3535–40

34. Gupta SK, Chadha K, Harris JD, *et al.* Mapping of epitopes on porcine zona pellucida-3α by monoclonal antibodies inhibiting oocyte–sperm interaction. *Biol Reprod* 1996;55:410–15

35. Koyama K, Hasegawa A, Inoue M, *et al.* Blocking of human sperm–zona interaction by monoclonal antibodies to a glycoprotein family ZP$_4$ of porcine zona pellucida. *Biol Reprod* 1991;45:727–35

36. Gupta SK, Jethanandani P, Afzalpurkar A, *et al.* Prospects of zona pellucida glycoproteins as immunogens for contraceptive vaccine. *Hum Reprod Update* 1997;3:311–23

37. Talwar GP, Rao KVS, Chauhan VS, eds. *Recombinant and Synthetic Vaccines.* New Delhi: Narosa Publishing House, 1994:1–512

38. Mahi-Brown CA, Yanagimachi R, Nelson ML, *et al.* Ovarian histopathology of bitches immunized with porcine zonae pellucidae. *Am J Reprod Immunol* 1988;18:94–103

39. Talwar GP, Naz RK, Das C, *et al.* A practicable immunological approach to block spermatogenesis without loss of androgens. *Proc Natl Acad Sci USA* 1979;76:5882–5

40. Naz RK, Talwar GP. Reversibility of azoospermia induced by Bacillus Calmette Guerin (BCG). *J Androl* 1986;7:264–9

41. Talwar GP, Sharma NC, Dubey SK, *et al.* Iso immunization against human chorionic gonadotropin with conjugates of processed β subunit of the hormone and tetanus toxoid. *Proc Natl Acad Sci USA* 1976;73:218–22

42. Talwar GP, Sharma NC, Dubey SK, *et al.* Fifteen papers on toxicology, safety and immunological responses of βhCG-TT vaccine. *Contraception* 1976;13:129–268

43. Nash H, Talwar GP, Segal S, *et al.* Observations on the antigenicity and clinical effects of a candidate anti-pregnancy vaccine; β subunit of human chorionic gonadotropin linked to tetanus toxoid. *Fertil Steril* 1980;34:328–35

44. Talwar GP, Singh Om, Singh V, *et al.* Enhancement of anti-gonadotropin response to β subunit of ovine luteinizing hormone by carrier conjugation and combination with β subunit of human chorionic gonadotropin. *Fertil Steril* 1986;46:120–6

45. Talwar GP, Singh Om, Rao LV. An improved immunogen for anti hCG vaccine eliciting antibodies reactive with conformation native to the hormone without cross-reaction with human follicle stimulating hormone and human thyroid stimulating hormone. *J Reprod Immunol* 1988;14:203–12

46. Pal R, Singh OM, Rao LV, *et al.* Bioneutralization capacity of antibodies generated in women by the β subunit of hCG and βhCG associated with the α subunit of ovine luteinizing hormone linked to carriers. *Am J Reprod Immunol Microbiol* 1990;22:124–6

47. Talwar GP, Kharat I, Dhall K. Phase I clinical trials with three formulations of anti chorionic gonadotropin vaccine. *Contraception* 1990;41:293–316

48. Gaur A, Arunan K, Singh Om, *et al.* Bypass by an alternate carrier of acquired unresponsiveness to hCG upon repeated immunization with tetanus conjugated vaccine. *Int Immunol* 1990;2:151–63

49. Talwar GP, Singh O, Gupta SK, *et al.* HSD-hCG vaccine prevents pregnancy in women, feasibility study of a reversible safe contraception vaccine. *Am J Reprod Immunol* 1997;37:153–60

50. Singh M, Das SK, Suri S, *et al.* Regain of fertility and normality of progeny born during below protective threshold antibody titres in women immunized with the HSD-hCG vaccine. *Am J Reprod Immunol* 1998;39:35–8

51. Stoute JA, Slaoui M, Heppner G, *et al.* A preliminary evaluation of a recombinant circumsporozoite protein vaccine against plasmodium falciparum malaria. *N Engl J Med* 1997;336:86–91

52. Kumar S, Talwar GP, Biswas DK. Necrosis and inhibition of growth of human lung tumour by anti α hCG antibodies. *J Natl Cancer Inst* 1991;84:42–7

53. Jones WR, Bradley J, Judd SJ, *et al.* Phase I clinical trial of a World Health Organisation birth control vaccine. *Lancet* 1988;1:1295–8

54. Deshmukh U, Pal R, Talwar GP, *et al.* Antibody response against epitopes on hCG mapped by monoclonal antibodies in women immunized with an anti hCG vaccine and its implications for bioneutralization. *J Reprod Immunol* 1993;25:103–17

55. Jespers LS, Roberts A, Mahler SM, *et al.* Guiding the selection of human antibodies from phage display repertoires to a single epitope of an antigen. *Biotechnology* 1994;10:899–903

56. Schumann D, Schillberg S, Zimmermann, *et al.* Engineering and expression of bispecific single chain Fv fragments in transgenic tobacco plants. *Nature Biotechnol* 1999;submitted

Pharmaceutical gossypol from Brazil

17

L. F. Pianowski

Introduction

Cotton is native to the Americas, where it is found both as a shrub and a full-size tree. Among the many varieties of cotton, experts, including Hutchinson, distinguish eight classes. Of these, the most important are the Herbacea and the Hirsuta. The Herbacea include the cultivars of Africa and Asia. It is the Hirsuta which are native to South America.

According to the researcher Napoleão Esberard de M. Beltrão, over 90% of the cotton grown in Brazil is *Gossypium hirsutum*. Annual varieties of it are grown in the North–North-East, in part of central Brazil and in the South. Some *Gossypium barbadense*, the sea-island cotton, is cultivated on a small scale elsewhere.

Gossypol is found in every part of the Brazilian plant: in the stem, leaf, flower, capsule and seed (Figure 1). Gossypol content of the seed accounts for between 0.72 and 1.89% of its weight. According to researcher Wilson Paes de Almeida, who works at the Agronomy Institute of the State of Paraná, higher gossypol content is dependent on genotype. The varieties HG, DD and SM1 show a particularly high concentration in their stalks and leaves and a lower concentration in the fruit. These varieties contain over 3% gossypol. We at Hebron intend to change over to these different genotypes in order to obtain a richer yield.

Foreign varieties include *Gossypium klotzschianum Davidsonii*, native to the Galapagos Islands, whose seeds contain over 9% gossypol.

At present, agronomists and the cotton industry are concerned with developing varieties low in gossypol and so geneticists have been developing cotton varieties with a gossypol content close to zero. But, in the light of research currently under way in Brazil and in other countries, attitudes to gossypol are certain to change.

Objectives have not always been clear cut, as the gossypol content of the plant plays a part in protecting cotton plantations against insect pests. Instances have been found of lower resistance to pests, which has led to a reduced output of cotton in some areas where varieties with a low gossypol content have been cultivated.

In crushing cottonseed for oil, oilcake is produced as a byproduct. This oilcake has a gossypol content of around 2% by weight, but is a resource practically ignored by the industry. Small amounts of gossypol are, however, used as an antioxidant for rubber, as a stabilizer for vinyl polymers and as an experimental insecticide.

Indeed, gossypol, which is phenolic, detracts from the value of the oilcake as animal feed; it restricts it to the ruminants, as ruminants tolerate a high gossypol content.

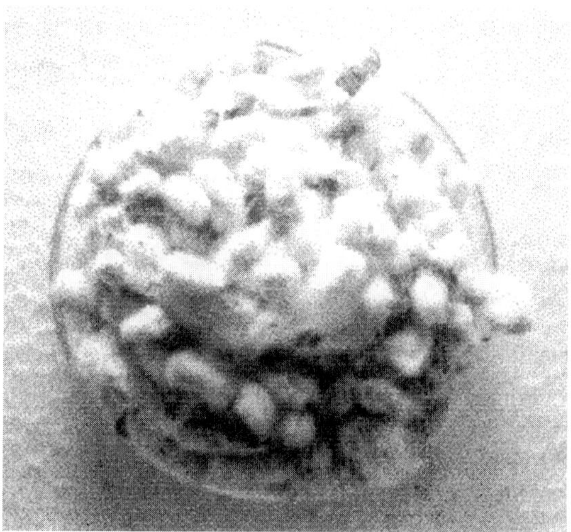

Figure 1 Close-up of cotton

It should be pointed out that the figure of 2% has been supplied to us by the Brazilian Farming Research Company, EMBRAPA, of the city of João Pessoa, capital of the State of Paraíba. My colleagues and I received oilcake supplied by a large company in São Paulo and our analysis does not agree with this figure. Our figure came out at 0.5%. This lower figure could be due to the deleterious effect of heat and light on the gossypol.

We intend to carry out research on fresh oil-cake in comparative studies and extract gossypol from it. We will be making a special effort to maintain freshness and to minimize any degrading effects. We are looking to broaden this research, with a view to developing a partnership between the vegetable oil industry and the fine chemicals industry.

Personally, I would not see it as economically viable for the vegetable oil companies to change their ways so that they can supply the initial demand for gossypol. Preserving the quality of the product would require extraordinary care in extracting it. It is worth emphasizing the importance of research into the strategies of working together, to define a technology symbiosis that would benefit all concerned.

Table 1 shows how much gossypol could be extracted from oilcake, which is itself a by-product of crushing cottonseed for oil. The figures are from 1996.

At the end of the 1970s, Brazil was the world's fifth biggest cotton producer, after the Soviet Union, China, the USA and India. Today Brazil comes twelfth, as shown in Table 2.

Table 3 shows cotton output nationwide, which Table 4 details for some States. The chart shows the drop in output over several years.

Some analysis of these figures will show how much raw material is available. It should be borne in mind that there are other options, as gossypol can be extracted from every part of the cotton plant. Therefore, actually arriving at the gossypol–acetic acid complex is no great difficulty. A monthly output of 300 000 phials, each holding 30 tablets of 20 mg, would call for around 180 kg of the gossypol–acetic acid complex.

Extracting and purifying gossypol

Gossypol was first isolated in 1899, but its structure was not worked out until the 1930s. It is a complex molecule, a binaphthyl compound, occurring naturally in the species *Gossypium*. Although its contraceptive function is related to

Table 1 Potential gossypol extraction ratios

Area	Crude cotton (t)	Oilcake (t)	Available gossypol (t)
All Brazil	1 200 000	480 000	9600
North-east Brazil	200 000	80 000	1600

Table 2 World cotton. Data supplied by EMBRAPA, ICAC 1998, CONAB 1998 and BM&F 1998

Item	1996 ($\times 10^6$ t)	1997 ($\times 10^6$ t)	1998 ($\times 10^6$ t)
Output, raw cotton	57.68	57.59	56.12
Output, cotton	19.61	19.58	19.08
Area under crop	35.20	34.50	33.91
Cotton consumption	19.22	19.47	19.53
Final stock	9.41	9.51	9.06
China, leading producer	4.20	4.20	4.00
Brazil, twelfth major producer	1.21	0.91	1.53

Table 3 Cotton in Brazil. Data supplied by ICAC 1998, CONAB 1998 and BM&F 1998. Research carried out by Napoleão Esberard de M. Beltrão, EMBRAPA, Campina Grande, PB, Brazil

Item	1996 ($\times 10^3$ t)	1997 ($\times 10^3$ t)	1998 ($\times 10^3$ t)
Output, raw cotton	1205.90	911.76	1529.40
Output, cotton	410.00	310.00	520.00
Area under crop	657.50	901.90	1000.00
Cotton consumption	820.00	840.00	850.00
Output, major producing state	119.50, Paraná	69.40, Goiás	130.10, Goiás
Imports of floss	385.00	460.00	300.00

Table 4 Cotton in north-east Brazil. Data supplied by ICAC 1998, CONAB 1998 and BM&F 1998. Research carried out by Napoleão Esberard de M. Beltrão, EMBRAPA, Campina Grande, PB, Brazil

Item	1996 ($\times 10^3$ t)	1997 ($\times 10^3$ t)	1998 ($\times 10^3$ t)
Output, raw cotton	205.90	170.00	166.20
Output, cotton	70.00	57.80	56.50
Cotton consumption	280.00	290.00	300.00
Output, major producing state	159.50, Ceará	160.00, Ceará	160.00, Ceará
Imports of floss	210.00	232.20	243.50

Figure 2 Chemical formula of gossypol

the negative enantiomorph, we use racemic gossypol.

The difficulty in producing gossypol lies in its vulnerability to deterioration before, during and after the extraction process, and in the pharmaceutical procedure followed. Our research has accordingly been carried out with special protective measures. We used different processes on different samples, until we achieved a procedure that yielded consistent results. Samples were drawn from:

(1) Run-off from cotton processing;

(2) Oilcake;

(3) Cottonseed.

Phase 1 We started with the run-off, a by-product of crushing the seed, expecting it to contain a high proportion of gossypol. We tested a range of different solvents following various methods, but the yield was so low that we concluded that the run-off was not an economically viable source (Figure 3).

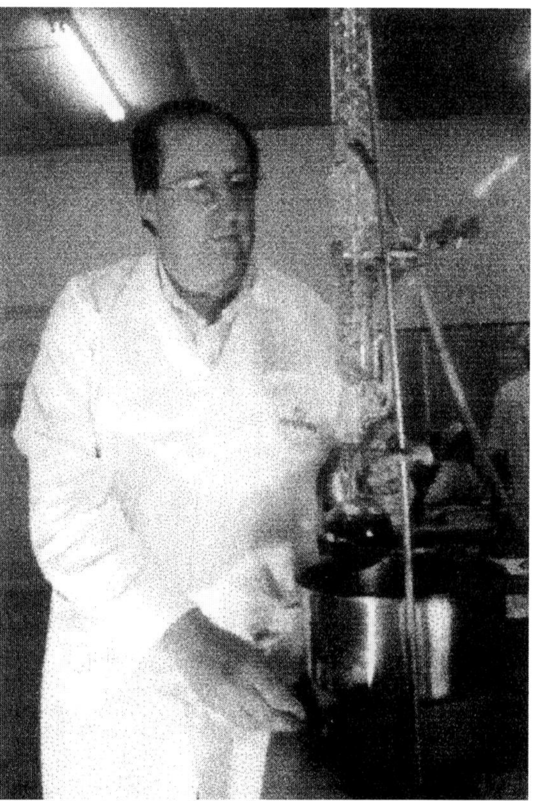

Figure 3 Front view of low-pressure extractor

Phase 2 We then examined the oilcake. Oilcake is a byproduct of crushing cottonseed, made up of seed residue washed in oil solvents. The literature indicated a gossypol content of around 2%. This was not borne out in practice; our highest figure was 0.5%, even with a range of different reagents and procedures.

We have abandoned work with the oilcake for the time being.

Phase 3 We turned to the cottonseed itself, following laboratory routines as set down in the AOCS official methods, and Carruth's procedure.

Our procedure involved washing the seeds with an organic oil solvent and extracting the gossypol and other matter with the use of different solvents, such as acetone, ethyl ether and methanol. Phenylaniline was added to hive off the gossypol, which was then subjected to acid hydrolysis and separated out with acetic acid. Washing and recrystallizing refined the gossypol to a high level of purity.

These procedures gave us a content of 0.3–0.55% of gossypol extract. Aiming at higher concentrations and an industrial scale of operations, we eliminated intermediate steps to optimize processing, which not only saved time, but yielded content of up to 1.42% from the seeds under test.

Some idea might be given here of how unstable the substance is. Treating on different days the seeds that had been crushed together, we found a falling off of 50% in yield over a period of 1 week. This instability forced on us a better understanding of the material we were working with. We controlled the climate and adapted the light of the laboratory until we achieved consistent results.

Stability of the final product

Once the gossypol–acetic acid complex had been separated out, the next step was to ensure stability of the final product. The extreme instability of the salt led to a rapid breakdown of the substance. Figures 4 and 5 show breakdown in the tablets of 40% over the 6 and 12 months, respectively. Instability of this order required keeping the substance in darkness and refrigerated. In the research stage, it is acceptable to have to keep the substance in the refrigerator. However, this restriction affects the marketability of the product, as few consumers would accept it. Concentrations as unpredictable as this would require an increased dosage of the final preparation to ensure adequate medication.

Research was shifted to seeking a means of stabilizing the gossypol–acetic acid complex in tablet form. Methods used were:

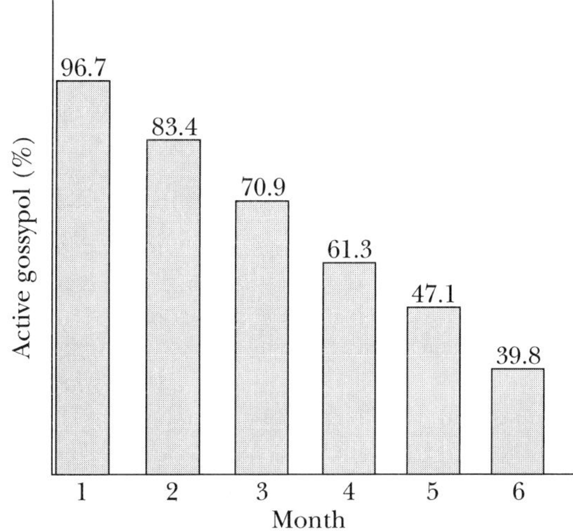

Figure 4 Breakdown of unstabilized tablets over 6 months. Data collected month by month for 1 year

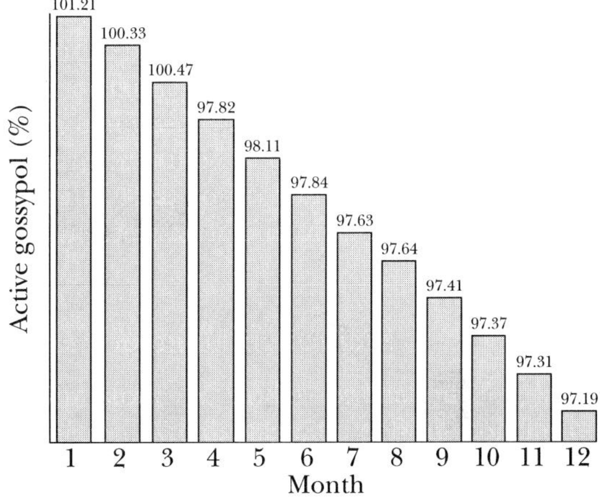

Figure 5 Breakdown of unstabilized tablets over 12 months

(1) Chemical use of chelate-forming substances and antioxidants;

(2) Physical use of a protective coating against ultraviolet light, oxidation and humidity.

Description of end product

(1) White-coated tablets;

(2) Friability of less than 1%;

(3) Disintegration in less than 10 min;

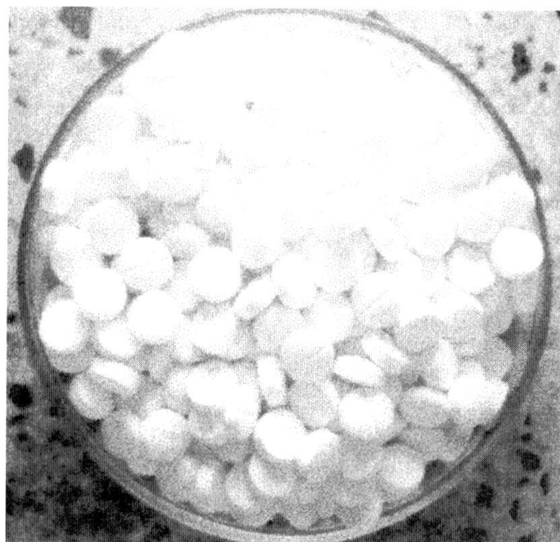

Figure 6 Tablets after coating

(4) Hardness greater than 3 N;

(5) Effective dosage of between 97% and 105% (Figure 6).

Methods of identification and dosage

When all work was concluded, checks were run on identification and dosage by means of high-performance liquid chromatography, thin-layer chromatography, infra-red, mass spectrometry and spectrophotometry.

Bibliography

1. Edwards JD. *Review of the Structure of Gossypol. The Chemistry of Gossypol.* New Orleans: The National Cotton Seed Products Association, 1959
2. Kohel RJ, Lewis CF. *Cotton.* New York: ASA Publications, 1985
3. Kassab AL. *Algodão.* Sao Paulo: Icone Editora, 1986
4. The Merck Index.
5. *Relatório Sobre Algodão da EMBRAPA.* Campina Grande, PB, 1997

Researchers consulted

1. Dr Napoleão Esberard de Macêdo Beltrão, Engenheiro Agrônomo, Doutor pela Universidade Federal de Viçosa. Researcher with EMBRAPA for 25 years
2. Dr Wilson Paes de Almeida, Agonômo, leader of the Cotton Programme of the Instituto Agronômico do Paraná
3. Dr Quezia B Cass, Chair Professor of the Department of Chemistry of the Universidade Federal de São Carlos

Non-hormonal contraception for young adults

18

C. A. Petta

Introduction

One-fifth of the world population is aged between 10 and 19 years. Young people are marrying later, and more are having sex before marriage. As a consequence, they will have an increased risk for unwanted pregnancies and sexually transmitted diseases. In developing countries, 20–60% of young women's pregnancies and births are unwanted or unplanned. Pregnancy puts young women's health at risk, through childbearing or unsafe abortion. In addition, it decreases the chances of education and adequate employment in the future. Half of those infected with the human immunodeficiency virus (HIV) are under 25 years of age[1].

Although contraception and infection prevention are clearly very important issues when talking about young adults, these individuals often have little or no access to reproductive health and sexual services, and lack information and education on the risks of some sexual behavior and its consequences.

Few married youths use contraception before the birth of their first child. In a survey, adolescents said that the main reason they did not use contraception was because they did not expect to have sex at that time[2]. Sexual activity tends to be sporadic and unplanned among young adults. A second common reason is that they lack information about contraceptives. Without adequate information, young people may have unnecessary fears about the effects contraceptive methods can have on their bodies and health. They often know about the more popular methods such as condoms and pills, but do not know how to get them or how to use them correctly[3].

Young adults also have some specific characteristics that may limit the use of contraceptive methods and prevent adequate infection control. They think they are not at risk, and have a feeling of invulnerability that leads them to underestimate the need of prevention for pregnancy and sexually transmitted diseases. They may also lack confidence and motivation to use a method. Adolescents may feel embarrassed to look for a reproductive health service and ask for contraception or orientation. They can fear meeting relatives, neighbors or other adults. Finally, many may not have the power and skill to use contraception or negotiate with a male partner the use of condoms, or are even forced to have sex.

The approach to young adults by health providers is often inadequate. There are no appropriate settings or time schedules to attend them. Services and provision of contraceptive methods should be free of charge. Dialog, instruction and educational materials should be specially designed and tested to reach youngsters. Services should also ideally provide a full range of health services. Peer counsellors can be very effective in providing orientation[4]. A common situation is negative attitudes of the provider towards young adults. Adults generally do not approve of sexual activity among unmarried adolescents. Providers may have personal and religious views about sexuality which can influence their attitudes in a negative manner. Consequently, adolescents may hesitate to tell adult providers that they are sexually active and seek information on contraception and disease prevention.

For all the above reasons, providers need to be trained to have open discussions, and need to have communication skills which enable them to reach the adolescents. Among these points, adequate knowledge and specific training to the contraceptive methods is of paramount importance to the provider. We will now discuss the use of non-hormonal contraceptive methods by young adults.

There is no medical reason to deny the use of any contraceptive method, based on young age alone[5]. However, there are important non-medical issues to be evaluated when considering the use of some methods by young adults.

Abstinence

This is the most effective way to prevent pregnancy and sexually transmitted diseases. There is no ill effect on the health of men or women if they abstain from sex. Young adults can find many ways to express their sexuality without having intercourse. Hugging, holding hands, massage, kissing and masturbation are alternatives. Abstinence can be discussed as an option. However, it requires motivation, self-control, and partner co-operation. It is also necessary to have negotiation skills to deal with social and peer pressure to have sex, elements that frequently make abstinence difficult for many adolescents.

Barrier methods

Barrier methods include both male (condom) and female (condom, diaphragm, spermicides, cervical cap) methods. These methods can be very effective to prevent pregnancy if used consistently and correctly. There is a great user influence on the pregnancy rates. With so-called 'perfect use', which is consistent and correct, the rates can be as low as three pregnancies per 100 women for male condom users. With typical or normal use, the rates can be as high as 21 pregnancies per 100 women for spermicide users[6].

Condoms have gained an important place amongst the contraceptive choices, due to their protection against infection. Condoms can prevent all types of sexually transmitted disease including HIV. Other female-controlled barrier methods can have different degrees of protection. Spermicides containing nonoxynol-9 protect against common bacterial diseases and have been found to inactivate the HIV virus in the laboratory[7,8].

To achieve perfect use and higher protection against pregnancy and sexually transmitted diseases, it is important to explain to youths how barrier methods work, their characteristics and how to use them correctly. For this purpose it is useful to have models, pictures and other instructional materials.

Male and female condoms

Condoms are not the only method proven to be effective against sexually transmitted disease, but they can also have a protective effect against cervical cancer by preventing infection by the human papilloma virus.

The condom has virtually no contraindications for use, except for the rare person who is allergic to latex. It may decrease sensation in the penis because of its thermal insulation properties which can diminish the heat sensation from the vagina, resulting in difficulty for some men in maintaining erection during intercourse. On the other hand, this may help men with premature ejaculation.

Latex condoms can be damaged by exposure to oil lubricants, excessive heat, humidity or light. Plastic condoms are made of a more stable material and can resist these elements without damage. Plastic condoms do not affect sensitivity as latex condoms do, as they can be thinner and stronger. Their use can be ideal for places where storage facilities are not ideal or non-existent and water-based lubricants are not available.

Male condoms can break or slip, and, although the occurrence of this is very rare among experienced users, the rate can be about 5% among the majority of users[9]. Breakage and slippage are basically associated with specific behaviors, such as opening the package with teeth or sharp objects, unrolling the condom before putting it on, having intercourse for more than 20 min or especially intense intercourse. All this information is important for the counseling of new users.

In recent years, a female condom has been developed in response to the need for more female-controlled methods. It is a soft, loose-fitting plastic sheath with a flexible ring at each end. One ring is at the closed end of the sheath and serves as an insertion mechanism and anchor over the cervix. The outer ring forms the external edge of the device and remains outside the vagina after insertion, providing protection to the labia and the base of the penis during intercourse. It is made of plastic which is stronger and more durable than latex. The female condom may be difficult to insert during initial use, and teaching and practice is important before using this method[10].

Since many adolescents are at risk for sexually transmitted diseases, when men are not willing to use a male condom a female condom can be used, giving the woman the ability to decide on this protection.

Spermicides

Spermicides are chemical barriers that prevent the sperm from reaching the superior female tract. They have been described since ancient times, from rags to herbal preparations applied into the vagina to prevent pregnancy. The most commonly used spermicidal chemicals are nonoxynol-9, menfegol and benzalkonium chloride. They are presented in various delivery bases, such as creams, jellies, foams, films, suppositories and tablets.

Since most spermicides are surfactants, they act on the membrane of the sperm and micro-organisms, killing them and consequently preventing pregnancy and some sexually transmitted diseases. Nonoxynol-9 helps to prevent the transmission of gonorrhea and chlamydia, and is suggested to reduce the risk of bacterial vaginosis, trichomoniasis and herpes[7,8]. On the other hand, there is a concern that with the use of spermicides many times each day, vaginal and cervical abrasions may occur, in theory increasing the risk of HIV transmission. Use of spermicide alone is not recommended for preventing HIV infection[11].

Spermicides can be used together or in association with another barrier method such as a condom or diaphragm. Several studies are being conducted with spermicides, using new delivery systems and HIV-preventing compounds.

Diaphragm and cervical cap

The diaphragm and cervical cap are made of soft rubber or silicone and must be fitted by a trained provider for proper sizing. These devices are commonly used with spermicide to increase their efficacy, because they do not make a perfect seal against the cervix and it is possible for them to dislodge during intercourse.

These methods are not recommended for women with cervical or vaginal abnormalities, during the first 6 weeks after childbirth, and for women with a history of toxic shock syndrome. Women with allergies to latex or spermicides do not usually use them[5].

Any trained healthcare provider can fit a woman for a diaphragm or cervical cap. After being taught how to insert and remove them, the woman should practice the technique for about 10 days, with the device in place, for the provider to be sure that she is inserting it correctly. During this practice time she should use a back-up method. The devices should be checked periodically for small holes or material deterioration, and must be fitted again when a woman gains or loses a significant amount of weight, has a baby, or has a second-trimester abortion. A woman with repeated urinary tract infections may be helped by reducing the amount of time she wears a diaphragm, although she must wear it for at least 6 h after intercourse

New barrier methods

There are several new barrier methods at different stages of development, which use new device designs, new materials, new delivery systems, and microbicides and spermicides.

The Femcap® is a new device similar to the cervical cap, which is made of silicone rubber and which can be worn for 48 h. Also made with silicone, Lea's shield is a diaphragm-like device.

Preliminary research has been done on a vaginal ring made of silicone, which releases nonoxynol-9 spermicide at a constant rate for at least 30 days. Various substances are under study, which would protect against sexually transmitted diseases but allow pregnancy. Research into barrier methods is intense, and many new options should be available in the near future[12].

Double protection

As we have seen, the efficacy of barrier methods can vary widely[6], so dual methods can enhance contraceptive efficacy while keeping sexually transmitted disease protection. Barrier methods are not as effective in preventing pregnancy as other methods such as oral contraceptives, injectables and intrauterine devices. If a person is at high risk of infection, providers have a responsibility to help clients decide what method to use, having to decide between emphasizing pregnancy prevention and disease prevention. For this reason, many programs recommend dual methods – one for infection prevention and one for pregnancy prevention. There are many choices of association of a barrier method with a high efficacy method in preventing pregnancy. Adequate counseling can help clients to identify the association which best fits their needs.

Intrauterine devices

Intrauterine devices are very effective methods for preventing pregnancy. The widely used TCu 380, a copper-releasing device, has a 10-year life-span and pregnancy rates lower than one per 100 women using the method for 1 year. Intrauterine device use is independent of coitus, and fertility returns quickly after removal[13].

Intrauterine devices carry with them many myths, mostly resulting from the experience of early larger, non-medicated devices, which were sometimes responsible for serious medical problems, as was the case with the Dalkon Shield and its relationship with infection. Modern devices are usually copper-releasing, but some are hormone-medicated, such as the levonorgestrel intrauterine device or the progesterone-releasing Progestasert®[14].

The mechanism of action of the copper-bearing intrauterine devices is still not completely understood. However, researchers believe that the main mechanism of action is by fertilization prevention[15].

A provider should be trained properly to insert intrauterine devices. The procedure requires a clinic visit and a pelvic examination, that can be a barrier to some young women. In addition, intrauterine devices do not offer any protection against sexually transmitted diseases, including HIV. According to the eligibility criteria of the World Health Organization, intrauterine devices are not recommended for young women with increased risk of sexually transmitted disease. Intrauterine devices may increase the risk of pelvic inflammatory disease and infertility among women who have an untreated sexually transmitted disease at the time of insertion, or if insertion does not follow infection prevention procedures. Careful screening and counselling is necessary, but intrauterine devices may be used by young women in stable, mutually monogamous relationships.

Although the intrauterine device can generally be used safely by women aged under 20 years, expulsion rates can be higher among women at this age who have never borne a child. Expulsion rates also vary with the time of insertion. The lowest expulsion rates are associated with interval insertion, and expulsion rates are higher during the postpartum period[16].

During counselling about intrauterine devices, providers should cover in detail the characteristics of the devices, the client's current and future risks of sexually transmitted diseases, effectiveness and how the device works, insertion and removal procedures, instructions for follow-up visits, possible side-effects and complications, and signs of possible complications. It is also important to emphasize that intrauterine devices should not be used by young women at high risk of infection, including those with multiple partners or those whose partners have multiple partners.

Traditional methods

The traditional contraceptive methods, being the periodic abstinence method and coitus interruptus, are methods always available and frequently used by adolescents, especially as they begin sexual activity, because they may lack knowledge of or access to other methods. In addition, these methods are free.

Unfortunately, these methods have high failure rates and offer no protection against sexually transmitted diseases. The use of them requires a highly motivated couple and knowledge about their bodies and physiology, an understanding of how pregnancy occurs and how to avoid it, and interpretation of the signs of their bodies. These methods can be difficult to practice.

During the first years after menarche, menstrual cycles are often irregular, making it difficult to practice the calendar method of periodic abstinence. Although modern methods can identify fertile periods of the cycle, they can be expensive and also need training for their use.

Sterilization

Sterilization is not an appropriate method for young adults, because they are initiating their reproductive life. They may decide to have children in the future, even those who already have them.

Sterilization performed at a young age may increase the risk of regret. Although reversal may be possible, it is not always successful, is expensive and not available in many locations[17]. For these reasons, sterilization must be clearly understood as a permanent method. Consequently, it is rarely suitable for young adults.

References

1. McCauley AP, Salter C. Meeting the needs of young adults. *Pop Rep* 1995; series J(41)
2. Paira V. Sexuality, condom use and gender norms among Brazilian teenagers. *Reprod Health Matters* 1993;2:98–109
3. Family Health International. *Contraceptive Technology Update Series. Reproductive Health of Young Adults.* North Carolina: Family Health International, 1997
4. Family Health International. *How to Create an Effective Peer Education Project.* Arlington: Family Health International, 1996:9–12
5. World Health Organization. *Improving Access to Quality Care in Family Planning – Medical Eligibility Criteria for Contraceptive Use.* Geneva, Switzerland: World Health Organization, 1996
6. Hatcher RA, Trussel J, Stewart F, *et al.*, eds. *Contraceptive Technology,* 16th edn. New York: Irvington Publishers Inc, 1994
7. Niruthisard S, Roddy RE, Chutivonge S. Use of nonoxynol-9 and reduction in rate of gonococcal and chlamydial infections. *Lancet* 1992;339:1371–5
8. Feldblum PJ, Morrison CS, Roddy RE, *et al.* The effectiveness of barrier methods of contraception in preventing the spread of HIV. *AIDS* 1995; 9(Suppl. A):S85–S93
9. Ritchers J, Donovan B, Gerofi J. How often do condoms break or slip off in use? *Int J STD AIDS* 1993;4:90–4
10. Wisconsin Pharmacal. *Reality Female Condom. A Monograph for Healthcare Professionals: Research Findings and Usage Considerations.* Chicago, IL: Wisconsin Pharmacal, 1994
11. Focus on spermicides. Controversy over HIV protection persists, despite promising studies of nonoxynol-9. *Contracept Tech Update* 1994;15:13–18,23
12. Family Health International. *Contraceptive Technology Update Series. Barrier Methods.* North Carolina: Family Health International, 1996
13. The Population Council and the Program for Appropriate Technology in Health (PATH). *The Copper T 380A IUD (Information Packet).* Seattle, Washington: PATH, 1989
14. Petta CA, Mcpheeters M, Chi IC. Intrauterine devices: learning from the past and looking to the future. *J Biosoc Sci* 1996;28:241–52

15. Ortiz ME, Croxatto HB, Bardin CW. Mechanism of action of intrauterine devices. *Obstet Gynecol Surv* 1996;51(Suppl 12): S42–51
16. Chi IC, Farr G. Review article: postpartum IUD contraception – a review of an international experience. *Adv Contracept* 1989;5:127–46
17. Petta CA, Bahamondes L, Hidalgo M, *et al.* A follow-up of women seeking sterilization reversal. A Brazilian experience. *Adv Contracept* 1995;11:157–63

Section III
Endocrinology of reproduction

adenovirus expressing MMP-9 (AdMMP-9) or a control virus expressing LacZ[9]. Thirty hours after infection, the media surrounding amnions infected with AdMMP-9 contained a prominent proMMP-9 signal detected as a 92-kDa lysis band by zymography and an 83-kDa band beneath it, reflecting processed proenzyme. Amnions infected with AdLacZ stained uniformly for β-galactosidase activity, reflecting efficient gene transfer, whereas amnions infected with AdMMP-9 did not stain for the presence of β-galactosidase.

The AdMMP-9-infected amnions were characterized by a ragged appearance and detachment of cells from the membranes, histological features that are found in amnions collected on days 20 and 21 of pregnancy[3]. AdLacZ-infected amnions were relatively intact, with normal cellularity and without evidence of cytopathic effect. Evidence for increased collagen breakdown in AdMMP-9-infected amnions was obtained from measurement of hydroxyproline in the conditioned media. Media from cultures of amnions infected with AdMMP-9 contained more than four-fold more hydroxyproline than media from cultures of AdLacZ-infected amnions.

AdMMP-9 infection resulted in a marked increase in apoptosis, assessed by immunohistochemical staining for nuclear DNA fragmentation. The AdMMP-9-infected tissues had 5.1 ± 1.9 apoptotic cells per high-power field (high-power field = 400 $\times$, $x \pm$ SD, $n = 3$ cultures per group), a finding that is similar to that which we have observed in amnions collected on day 21 of pregnancy[6]. In contrast, the AdLacZ-infected amnions averaged 0.3 ± 0.2 apoptotic cells per high-power field (significantly different from AdMMP-9-infected amnions, $p < 0.01$ by Student's t test).

The effects of AdMMP-9 infection on amnion structure and amnion cell apoptosis were blocked by the MMP inhibitor, Batimistat®. Batimistat retained amnion membrane integrity, reduced the release of hydroxyproline-containing peptides into the culture fluid and completely prevented amnion cell apoptosis[9].

These findings document that type IV collagen is lost from the rat amnion prior to the onset of labor. The disappearance of type IV collagen coincides with increased expression of two enzymes that degrade type IV collagen, MMP-2 and MMP-9. The increase in MMP-9 is particularly striking as no MMP-9 activity can be detected by zymography prior to the evening of day 20 of pregnancy, whereas MMP-2 activity is detectable on all days of gestation with an increase by day 21. This temporal correlation suggests that the loss of type IV collagen is in fact due, at least in part, to the induction of type IV collagenases.

Our studies demonstrating differential sensitivity of kidney and amnion basement membranes to collagen breakdown by active MMP-9 and bacterial collagenase suggest that the rat amnion type IV collagen chain composition potentially favors collagenase degradation, as compared to the type IV collagen composition of adult renal tubular basement membranes. The relative abundance of cysteine-enriched type IV collagen α-chains in renal basement membranes may impart greater strength to the basement membrane as a result of cross-linking through disulfide bridges. Hence, it is conceivable that type IV collagen composition determines the longevity and integrity of the basement membrane, with basement membranes that are relatively poor in the more cross-linked α-chains, such as amnion, being destined for turnover.

Degradation of the type IV collagen in amnion basement membranes may initiate the process of apoptotic cell death that we have previously described[6]. Indeed, ultrastructural studies of rat amnions documented loss of basement membrane components and delamination of amnion epithelial cells in association with features of cell death[3]. Consistent with this view, our *in vitro* experiments demonstrate that increasing MMP-9 expression promotes collagen breakdown and apoptosis in rat amnions in organ culture. It should be noted that cells remaining anchored to the amnion, in addition to those which had separated from their substrates, were undergoing apoptosis as evidenced by nuclear DNA fragmentation. Hence, apoptosis appears to be initiated prior to complete separation of the amnion cells from their substrate, perhaps as a result of partial detachment or changes in cell shape due to matrix degradation. The MMP inhibitor, Batimistat, prevented the amnion cell apoptosis induced by AdMMP-9.

We corroborated the rat amnion organ culture studies using cultures of human amnion cells (WISH cells) grown in serum-free medium on a combined matrix of type I and type IV collagen. Transfection of the WISH cells with an MMP-9 expression plasmid resulted in cell detachment and apoptosis, whereas transfection of the cells with an empty vector had no effect on cell attachment and cell death. Notably, MMP-9 is also induced in the human amnion with labor[7] and apoptosis has been noted in human amnion[10,11]. Moreover, embryonic membrane matrix metabolism and apoptosis also appear to occur prior to hatching of the chicken, suggesting that the program of matrix degradation and programmed cell death is a common feature of extraembryonic membranes across species[12].

Apoptosis is now recognized to play an important role in fetal and maternal tissues near the end of pregnancy. However, the factors that provoke programmed cell death in preparation for labor and delivery remain to be clarified. Our observations suggest that increased expression of MMPs initiates apoptosis by catalyzing degradation of the basement membranes or pericellular matrix, leading to cell detachment or change in cell shape and subsequently cell demise. This process may reflect a ripening process analogous to changes occurring in the cervix prior to parturition[13]. However, detachment of cells from the amnion is not an immediate death sentence, since viable amniocytes can be collected from amniotic fluid and limited digestion of amnion tissue with bacterial collagenase disperses cells that can be maintained in culture. Thus, the state of the amnion cells, the process leading to their separation from the matrix, or the duration of the separation may be key determinants of cell fate.

References

1. Schmidt W. The amniotic fluid compartment: the fetal habitat. *Anat Embryol Cell Biol* 1992;124: 1–100
2. Parry SD, Strauss JF III. Premature rupture of the fetal membranes. *New Engl J Med* 1998;338: 663–70
3. Paavola LG, Furth EE, Delgado V, *et al.* Striking changes in the structure and organization of rat fetal membranes precede parturition. *Biol Reprod* 1995;53:321–38
4. Malak TM, Bell SC. Structural characteristics of term human fetal membranes: a novel zone of extreme morphological alteration within the rupture site. *Br J Obstet Gynaecol* 1994;101:375–86
5. Bryant-Greenwood GD. The extracellular matrix of the human fetal membranes: structure and function. *Placenta* 1998;19:1–11
6. Lei H, Furth EE, Kalluri R, *et al.* A program of cell death and extracellular matrix degradation is activated in the amnion before the onset of labor. *J Clin Invest* 1997;98:1971–8
7. Vadillo-Ortega F, Gonzalez-Avilla G, Furth EE, *et al.* 92-kDa type IV collagenase (matrix metalloproteinase-9) activity in human amniochorion increases with labor. *Am J Pathol* 1995;146:148–56
8. Lei H, Vadillo-Ortega F, Paavola LG, *et al.* 92-kDa gelatinase (matrix metalloproteinase-9) is induced in rat amnion immediately prior to parturition. *Biol Reprod* 1995;53:339–44
9. Lei H, Kalluri R, Furth EE, *et al.* Rat amnion type IV collagen composition and metabolism: implications for membrane breakdown. *Biol Reprod* 1999;60:176–82
10. Leppert P, Takamoto N, Yu S. Apoptosis in fetal membranes may predispose them to rupture. *J Soc Gynecol Invest* 1996;3:128A
11. Runic R, Lockwood CJ, LaChapelle LL, *et al.* Apoptosis in human fetal membranes: implications in parturition-associated changes in fetal membrane integrity. *J Soc Gynecol Invest* 1996;3: 293A
12. Lei H, Furth EE, Kalluri R, *et al.* Induction of matrix metalloproteinases and collagenolysis in chick embryonic membranes before hatching. *Biol Reprod* 1999;60:183–9
13. Leppert PC, Yu SY. Apoptosis in the cervix of pregnant rats in association with cervical ripening. *Gynecol Obstet Invest* 1994;37:150–4

Reproductive endocrinology towards the next millennium

B. Lunenfeld and E. Lunenfeld

Introduction

The 'conquest of infertility' is an incredible achievement; it is a victory of human will, endurance and technology. However, as we near the millennium, new challenges are arising in relation to scientific, ethical and humanitarian aspects in infertility management. How do we use current and evolving technologies to allow parents to achieve the joy of having children with dignity, to make treatment available to all, to secure universal reimbursement and to increase short- and long-term safety and decrease any adverse impact on the health of both mother and child?

Medicine is racing from triumph to triumph. Somehow, however, the more medicine achieves, the less it satisfies. Medicine does not seem able to fulfil the ever-increasing expectations that have been raised by the promise of new breakthroughs. Until about the mid-1960s, medical research was primarily driven by the desire to cure sick people; today, the shift in research is focusing on the understanding of disease processes and the prevention of disease as well as on improving the quality of life. This is also true for reproductive medicine. According to a position paper by the World Health Organization (WHO)[1], 'Reproductive health is a state of complete physical, mental and social well-being, and not merely the absence of disease or infirmity, in all matters relating to the reproductive system and its functions and processes. Reproductive health therefore implies that people are able to have a satisfying and safe sex life and that they have the capability to reproduce and the freedom to decide if, when and how often to do so'.

In order to attain this ideal state, reproductive medicine must make all possible efforts to enable conception in all couples desiring it, and must also avoid maternal and neonatal complications such as the hyperstimulation syndrome, multiple pregnancy and premature delivery. These are formidable goals, and, in order to reach them, new detailed information regarding physiology of reproduction must be obtained, and new efficient treatment methods must be devised. The ethical, sociopolitical and economic problems related to these goals must not be underestimated. They have to be discussed, taken into consideration and dealt with.

In the near future, we should expect significant advances in reproductive basic and applied research, diagnostic tools, drug development, and the clinical management of infertility.

New developments in the treatment of post-infectious infertility

Post-infectious infertility is obviously a world-wide problem. It is estimated that 11% of patients will be infertile after one episode of pelvic inflammatory disease (PID), 23% after two episodes and 54% after three or more episodes[1]. Up to 64% of African women and 25–35% of patients in other areas of the world have infertility that can be traced to prior infection.

Specifically, an infectious etiology for infertility can be directly related to a history of sexually transmitted disease, pelvic inflammatory disease, male genital tract infections and pregnancy complications of an infectious nature. Clearly, sexually transmitted diseases are a major cause of infertility throughout the world and prevention of pelvic infection should be a high priority both for medical scientists and for governments. Chlamydia is probably the most common sexually transmitted disease today. WHO estimates that the minimal global incidence is 50 million per year[2].

New techniques for the rapid diagnosis of chlamydial infection are therefore essential. There is now some promise that a rapid screening test to indicate the presence of chlamydial salpingitis can be developed. In addition, the development of a vaccine against the major outer membrane protein of chlamydia should be possible, and should be a high priority worldwide. This development alone would have a dramatic effect in every area of the world in reducing female infertility due to tubal disease.

New directions in basic research

In vitro maturation of gametes

Priority areas for basic research should be *in vitro* maturation of gametes, regulation of meiosis, and the ability to control the production of the sperm head decondensation factor by the oocyte and of the oocyte activation factor by the male gametes.

In vitro maturation of spermatocytes or spermatids has to date not been possible. There have been very few reports on children born following intracytoplasmic sperm injection (ICSI) with spermatids[3], and these should be viewed with caution since it is difficult to differentiate between a late spermatid and an early spermatozoan.

It has been proposed that cytoplasmic changes in spermiogenesis mainly concern the Golgi apparatus (acrosome vesicle), centrosomal material (flagellum), mitochondria (periaxonemal ring) and cytoplasm volume (drastic reduction). These changes may not be necessary in ICSI and their absence could be without consequences for post-fertilization development. Spermatid gene transduction produces new proteins which are related to fertilization (acrosomal enzymes, flagellum proteins, protamines, etc.) and which seem no longer useful after gamete fusion. There is no report of genomic imprinting occurring during spermiogenesis in mammals. Moreover,

the important sperm changes during epididymal maturation (formation of disulfur bonds, acquisition of motility and of molecules for oocyte recognition, methylation of certain genes) were found to be unnecessary for embryo development in cases of ICSI with epididymal or testicular spermatozoa[3]. However, nuclear changes affect chromatin with the substitution of histones by protamines and other transitional proteins to insure sperm DNA stability across male and female genital tracts, and may also be important or even essential in the fertilization process.

The *in vitro* maturation of oocytes will become reality and a routine procedure in the not too distant future. Successful pregnancies followed by liveborn children have been reported[4–6]. If these procedures prove themselves and become routine, they will simplify and significantly decrease the costs and risk of assisted reproductive procedures for the mother, but may increase the risks of faulty pre- or post-meiotic development of the gametes with profound consequences for fertilization, embryonic development and expression, even in later generations, due to gene deletions, mutation or amplification of mutations. Examples of such amplification of mutations are the fragile X syndrome, myotonic dystrophy, Huntington's disease and Kennedy's disease. All these syndromes show trinucleotide repeats.

The potential risks of this procedure will have to be decreased by the use of genetic screening and improved preimplantation diagnostics. These diagnostic procedures will become even more important once the Human Genome Project is completed. Within the next 10 years, the 60 000–100 000 genes in the human genome will have been fully decoded. This will have an enormous impact on genetic testing and preimplantation diagnostics. It will, however, bring new and difficult ethical questions to light, such as the questions of whether pregnancy becomes a matter of choosing among embryos with different traits, and whether the prospective parents have the right to know or influence the genetic make-up of their future children. These are perplexing questions and we have hardly begun to consider them and their implications for society, but the advances of genetic research are already upon us.

Early follicular development and apoptosis

The regulation of the number of follicles that reach gonadotropin dependency should also be a high priority research area. Although today we are able to control, monitor and regulate gonadotropin-dependent follicular growth and development, we do not have the theoretical know-how nor the technical ability to increase the number of follicles prior to their gonadotropin dependency. We cannot control the processes leading to degeneration, atresia or apoptosis of follicles or oocytes.

We are starting to understand the dependency of follicles on vascular components, neovasculogenesis and diverse growth factors. Designing a fine-tuned instrument to enable control of the whole span of follicular development from primordial to Graafian follicle would obviously have a significant impact on the reproductive potential of the female.

Drug development

Recombinant gonadotropins

New developments in the area of drug research will also create a significant impact on the future of reproductive medicine. With recombinant DNA technology and highly defined cell culture techniques, genetically engineered gonadotropins are now being prepared on an industrial scale, and are already on the market in most developed countries[7,8].

Besides increased safety and simpler use, comparison of the efficacy of recombinant follicle stimulating hormone (rFSH) with that of urinary follicle stimulating hormone (uFSH) in more than 2000 cycles demonstrated that the rFSH yielded more oocytes, and more embryos produced a higher pregnancy rate with lesser amounts and with less treatment days[9]. For couples who have cryopreserved embryos available, the potential for subsequent pregnancy is only slightly less than that obtained after the transfer of fresh embryos. This is a significant benefit for the couple, providing them with an additional boost in their pregnancy potential per stimulated cycle.

In patients with hypogonadotropic hypogonadism, rFSH alone was sufficient to stimulate follicular growth but was inadequate to induce competent follicular function. However, rFSH combined with recombinant luteinizing hormone (rLH) was able to produce follicular development and, following application of human chorionic gonadotropin (hCG), ovulation and pregnancy. The first birth following infertility treatment of a hypopituitary hypogonadotropic woman[10] with rFSH and rLH to stimulate follicular growth and recombinant hCG to induce ovulation was reported by Agrawal and colleagues[11].

Recombinant follicle stimulating hormone is a highly potent, safe and pure pharmaceutical-grade product, with full batch-to-batch consistency and with the additional convenience of subcutaneous self-administration, and it will hopefully replace all urinary preparations shortly.

We are starting to understand the role of subpopulations of the microheterogenetic family of gonadotropic isoforms, and the carbohydrate complexity of FSH. The change of cell culture conditions and purification techniques permits the selection of a desired proportion of gonadotropic isoforms to produce tailor-made gonadotropins for specific phases of the cycle or for specific conditions. However, one should not exaggerate the importance of isoform profiles in gonadotropic preparations until we know more about the fate and composition of these isoforms following injection. Recombinant DNA technology permits the design of potential therapeutically active gonadotropin agonists and antagonists by altering core proteins and carbohydrate moieties in the α and β subunits of FSH and LH. Using site-directed mutagenesis and gene transfer techniques, it is possible to fuse the carboxyterminal extension of hCG-β (CTP) to the 3' end of the FSH coding sequence. The FSH–CTP fusion protein retains the same biological activity as FSH but has a prolonged circulating half-life and, consequently, a higher *in vivo* potency than native FSH. This is an obvious precursor for a future long-acting FSH agonist. Alternatively, deglycosylated mutants of this chimera can be engineered, and, together with the deglycosylated α sub-unit, could serve as a model for production of various gonadotropin antagonists which would competitively bind to and desensitize gonadotropin receptors on ovarian cell membranes. A mutant FSH lacking the N-linked aspargine residue as Asn-52 on the α sub-unit exhibits ten-fold less bioactivity than the fully glycosylated wild-type. Furthermore, an FSH devoid of all four linked carbohydrates on the α and β sub-units is a potent antagonist of FSH action *in vitro*[12]. However, a word of caution may be appropriate when we produce such compounds. Elaborate changes in the protein backbone or carbohydrate panel in any of the gonadotropin sub-units might cause such preparations to provoke antibody formation.

Functional proteino-mimetic molecules

Better understanding of gonadotropin–receptor interaction combined with crystallography and sophisticated computer techniques will permit the design of proteino-mimetic orally active gonadotropin agonists and antagonists. The current challenge in biotechnology is to reduce the size of these proteins by developing small functional mimetic synthetic molecules that could be administered through the oral or transdermal route.

To achieve this objective for gonadotropins, one must first develop a working model to explain how a gonadotropin activates its receptor, then develop a high-throughput assay specific for each gonadotropin, and finally create a large number of molecules with possible agonistic or antagonistic activity to be tested.

Advances in the field of molecular reproductive endocrinology and the development of a number of molecular tools have permitted the identification of small-molecular weight FSH agonistic molecules that could interact with a catalytic region of the FSH receptor that controls G protein coupling and adenylate cyclase activation. With better understanding of FSH receptor activation, it has been possible to create small molecules predicted to induce gonadotropic signal transduction without even the necessity to bind to the extracellular domains of the membrane protein. A number of such molecules are already being actively tested. Such molecules will ultimately be converted into high-potency, orally active, therapeutic preparations to replace the dimeric glycoprotein hormones or to act as antagonists.

Gonadotropin releasing hormone analogs

Third-generation gonadotropin releasing hormone (GnRH) antagonists are in third-phase studies and will shortly appear on the market. Due to their high affinity to the GnRH receptors, these compounds lead to a suppression of gonadotropin secretion within hours. Acting through competitive binding, the duration of their effect is dose-dependent. Their immediate inhibition of gonadotropins, without the flare-up effect, may have a profound influence on their use in ovulation induction and assisted reproduction techniques. They can be administered either daily over several days in the late follicular phase, usually from day 6 of stimulation onwards (the 'multiple-dose protocol'[13]) or just at the moment when the LH surge is expected (single-dose protocol[14]).

Systematic structure–activity relationship studies of linear analogs are being performed. The development of mono- and di-cyclic analogs is being actively pursued. A number of such compounds are already available and are under active investigation.

Functional peptido-mimetic molecules

In an attempt to assess the functional relationship between GnRH and its receptor, reporter gene systems for signal transduction by the human GnRH receptor have been developed. This has permitted a better understanding of the GnRH receptor. Applying a high throughput screening has allowed the examination of thousands of potential candidates as peptido-mimetic GnRH analogs. This throughput assay is performed by using mouse fibroblasts transfected with a luciferase reporter gene plasmid and a selected cell clone super-transfected with the respective wild or mutant GnRH receptor expression plasmid. It has also enabled the identification and characterization of diverse agonists and antagonists on wild-type and site-specific receptor mutants and permitted the development of a three-dimensional model of receptor–ligand interaction. This has permitted the identification and selection of potent peptido-mimetic GnRH agonists and antagonists which could be orally active.

New directions in applied clinical research

In applied clinical research, our aim should be to improve embryo viability and implantation, and to reduce the hyperstimulation syndrome and multiple pregnancy rate. The success rates for *in vitro* fertilization (IVF) and embryo transfer (ET) depend on two major factors: embryonic viability and uterine receptivity. The nature and sequence of signals passing between the male and female pronuclei inside the freshly fertilized egg, which result in the formation of a centromere and rearrangement of male and female chromatin material, must be studied in depth in order to define the fertilization process, and to understand, and possibly to manipulate, this decisive stage of embryo development.

Implantation

The most important hurdle in obtaining a clinical pregnancy is implantation. The management of the implantation signal depends largely on our ability to understand and control neovascularization, adhesion and invasion processes, permitting the viable embryo to adhere to and invade the endometrium and to create the proper vascularization necessary for its nourishment, growth and development. We must also learn more about the immune modulation system which prevents expulsion of the fetus by the mother. Since the fetus can be considered to be an allograft, maternal immune regulatory mechanisms are set in motion to prevent the rejection of the fetus and even aid in its growth and development. A defect in this maternal–fetal tolerance is thought to result in immunologically mediated damage to the fetus. The success of embryonic implantation relies upon a perfect dialog between good-quality embryos and a receptive endometrium. In response to endometrial factors, the human embryo secretes the complete interleukin-1 system as well as other growth factors. The human blastocyst up-regulates the endometrial receptivity. Any derangement in cross-communication between embryo and endometrium can interfere with the implantation process. The consequences of pelvic inflammatory processes such as hydrosalpinx are known to reduce pregnancy rates following assisted reproduction techniques. Recently, Sharara and associates[15] have demonstrated that, in cases with hydrosalpinx, the window of implantation, which is expressed by the appearance of endometrial integrins, is impaired and might be corrected by salpingectomies.

Embryonic development

For the human embryo, a developmental block characterized by an arrest in cleavage generally occurs at the four- to eight-cell stage, as first reported by Braude and colleagues[16]. The four-cell block occurs at the point when the embryo is switching from the use of maternal ovum-derived messenger RNA (mRNA) for protein synthesis to embryonic mRNA resulting from *de novo* synthesis. If such a block occurs it may lead to degeneration or a failure of implantation. Following 'fertilization' with good and bad sperm, the resulting embryos showed equal development until the four-cell stage, but at the 16-cell stage or at the blastocyst stage the difference in development with good sperm compared to that with bad sperm became highly significant, demonstrating that, after the maternally derived mRNA is switched off, paternal factors may influence further development. Besides the important scientific contribution of these findings, they can also be applied to differentiate between maternal and paternal causes in the arrest of embryonic development.

Culture of embryos to the blastocyst stage may represent a significant advantage since it will enable selection of only those embryos with an implantation potential. It has become clear that the nutrient requirements and metabolism of the zygote and blastocyst are completely different, and that the oviduct and uterus provide different nutritional support to the human embryo as it develops[17].

The changing requirements of the embryo in this short but important period of growth and development are of utmost importance. In this period, the embryo is switching from the use of maternal, ovum-derived messenger RNA for synthesis of proteins, to embryonic mRNA resulting from *de novo* synthesis. This is crucial for the normal development and differentiation of the inner cell mass and trophectoderm.

Sequential serum-free culture media have been formulated for the development of the pronuclear and eight-cell embryo[17–21]. The benefits of providing embryologists with sufficient oocytes to enable selection among those embryos which develop to blastocysts with well-differentiated trophectoderm and inner cell mass lineage, for chromosomal normality or even metabolic capacity, could be substantial[15].

It has been clearly demonstrated for blocked four- to eight-cell human embryos that there is a lack of synthesis of a specific set of embryonic coded proteins, which are present in non-blocked embryos[16].

It is most probable that a redefinition of fertilization leading to embryo development will require the inclusion of the ability of the embryo to produce its own messenger RNA permitting production of embryo-specific proteins. It is likely that inherent viability of the embryo is a natural selection process which may be compromised by suboptimal culture conditions at the time of embryonic gene activation. Re-implantation of accurately selected blastocysts would obviously increase the pregnancy rates and enable better control of multiple gestations by allowing replacement of only one or two blastocysts. Gardner and colleagues[18–20] recently demonstrated that it is possible to obtain around 50% blastocyst development and a pregnancy rate of about 70% with the transfer

of just two blastocysts. Therefore, in order to obtain a pregnancy rate of 50%, one needs to transfer only a single blastocyst. Importantly, such blastocysts can be readily frozen and give rise to pregnancies after thawing. Gardner and Lane[20] reported a 60% survival rate of frozen embryos, with a 50% ongoing pregnancy rate following the transfer of such thawed embryos. The application of novel viability markers will help to identify those blastocysts with the highest developmental potential before transfer, therefore increasing the overall success of blastocyst transfer. This will avoid unnecessary multiple birth with increased risks and morbidity to mother and child, and requests for fetal reduction. In addition, when indicated, the longer stay of fertilized eggs in the laboratory would permit genetic studies, thus avoiding transfer of genetically inadequate embryos and also allowing the further development of the endometrium in preparation for nidation.

Recently Cohen and co-workers[22] claimed that removing cytoplasm with mitochondrial DNA from a donor ovum from a younger woman and injecting it into an ovum from an older woman contributes to the nuclear DNA and increases the chance of implantation. If substantiated, this would be a scientifically significant advance, but might raise ethical and legal implications for a child inheriting genes from two mothers.

Successful pregnancy also requires normal postimplantation embryo growth and development. The understanding of these complex events and interactions will lead to better care of the early embryo and fetus. Application of this knowledge would offer opportunities to treat the previously untreatable conditions of unexplained recurrent pregnancy loss.

Cryopreservation

To improve cryopreservation techniques, some basic biophysical research is needed. This would be useful in better freezing of embryos, freezing of oocytes, and freezing of ovarian tissue, testicular tissue and individual spermatozoa or spermatids.

Preliminary data show that similar results in terms of fertilization and clinical pregnancies can be obtained from fresh or cryopreserved testicular tissue. Such techniques could have a significant impact on the logistics, safety and expense of assisted reproductive technologies.

The *in vitro* growth, development and maturation of oocytes from cryopreserved ovarian tissue have become a reality[23]. If these techniques are improved and become routine procedures, they will permit preservation of healthy oocytes prior to irradiation or chemotherapy or even for delaying conception for personal reasons.

The freezing of eggs, although reported with occasional success, should become a reality within the next few years. This technique offers an ethically 'soft' alternative to embryo freezing. The social implications of freezing ova can also be enormous. In the 1990s, a woman who is financially independent and sexually liberated is not free of her biological clock if she wants to become a mother. The single woman in her thirties has become one of the burning social phenomena of our times as she is caught between her body clock and her career, her desire for independence and her desire to have a child. Feminism has been unable to fulfil the twin desires of a modern women – career and children – because of the ticking biological clock in each woman. However, science has come to the rescue in a way that feminism never could, and promises to take the clock out of the equation. Now it is possible for women, like men, to concentrate on their careers and put the issue of having children on hold. Human eggs can be stored for years, and, when the woman is ready, the egg can be defrosted and fertilized *in vitro* and implanted into the woman even after menopause. However, it is questionable whether this technique will or should become routine.

Reduction of the multiple pregnancy rate

In the management of infertility, our goal has to be to increase pregnancy rates and reduce abortion rates, resulting in an increase in the birth rate of normal healthy children. Furthermore, we have to decrease the occurrence of the hyperstimulation syndrome as well as the multiple pregnancy rate, with a concomitant reduction in gestational and obstetric complications. The 1995 American Society for Reproductive Medicine/Society for Assisted Reproductive Technology annual report revealed a 37% incidence of multiple deliveries with 7% being triplet or higher-order deliveries[24].

Whereas premature delivery can be expected in 24% of singleton pregnancies, it rises to 67.5% in twin pregnancies and 93% in triplet pregnancies. Admissions to neonatal intensive care units are about 15% following singleton deliveries, and about 48% following twin deliveries and 78% following triplet deliveries. The economic consequences of multiple gestations represent 'hidden costs' of infertility treatment. Goldfarb and colleagues[25] estimated the cost of triplet or greater gestations at 340 000 US$. The cost of twins has been estimated at 21 000–39 000 US$. Even this figure does not consider the cost of long-term care for children handicapped as a result of prematurity. In 40% of quadruplet pregnancies, significant developmental delay is present in at least one of the resulting children[26]. Multiple pregnancies are therefore not only a health risk to mother and child but they represent an enormous financial burden to society.

How do we proceed to reach the goals mentioned above? They could be achieved by developing stimulation and suppression techniques enabling fine-tuned follicular development, precisely timed ovulation of healthy gametes, and appropriate control of the implantation processes. Obviously, real progress in genuine improvement of the results of reproductive medicine will also be achieved with practical application of preimplantation diagnosis of genetic diseases. This would provide a substitute for early or late abortions as a means for preventing birth of disabled individuals. However, the use of such techniques to permit choice among healthy embryos with different traits is a much more complicated question which society will have to debate.

Ethical, social and political considerations

The pace at which advances are made often seems to exceed our ability to incorporate them in our lifestyles. Nearly every new advance brings a host of new ethical, social or even political changes with it. We must remember that society cannot survive without biotechnology and at the same time cannot survive its unethical use. The hopes of accumulating and applying the information needed to advance to the next phase of technological evolution in reproductive medicine must therefore also be amalgamated with the following clear directives:

(1) Public policy to restrain the population explosion, appropriate as it may be, must not be confused with the basic human right to procreation. The agony of childless couples in overpopulated areas such as India is just as painful as that of couples in industrialized nations.

(2) Infertility is a reproductive health disorder and must therefore be considered in terms of the World Health Organization definition, and the cost of its prevention and/or management should be covered by third-party providers such as national or private health insurance. It is our task to persuade political decision-makers that infertility is a medical condition and should be included in the health-care benefit package of every individual. An audit of one of the major health-care providers in the state of Massachusetts showed that the cost of infertility treatment accounts for only 0.1% of a total family premium for insurance. In Germany 0.2% of an average family total health insurance package is used for infertility treatment. Moreover, also in Germany, in 1995 the entire cost of all assisted reproduction techniques including drugs was only 0.3% of the entire cost of outpatient care and drugs. In many developed countries, infertility accounts for a large and increasing number of childless couples. This has become a problem to society in the sense of an unfortunate demographic shift. It is our duty to provide the public and politicians with information on the consequences of delaying the conception of the first child. It is also our duty to show that reproductive medicine offers a set of safe and effective solutions.

(3) Since age is the single most important factor in infertility, it is our duty to educate the public and politicians on planning for children. We should encourage an environment that allows for combining successful careers and motherhood.

(4) The public as well as regulatory agencies should be informed that infertility *per se,* as well as its causes, can be a serious and costly health risk involving hormone-dependent cancers and cardiovascular diseases and that conceptions may reduce this risk. Furthermore, infertility can cause significant emotional stress. Psychological symptom scores have been found to be comparable to those of patients with cancer, cardiac problems and chronic hypertension, and all patients studied expressed a considerable loss of well-being[27].

(5) The public as well as regulatory agencies should be informed that, with the present and emerging sophisticated technologies for induction of ovulation and assisted medical procreation, most infertile couples can expect the joy of parenthood.

(6) Attempts to prevent infertility by reducing sexually transmitted diseases, abortions and adolescent pregnancies should be a primary concern and given a high priority in educational and public health programs.

(7) Not only must short- and long-term safety of infertility therapy be of foremost importance, but also the physical, mental and social welfare of each partner of the future parents as well as that of the planned child must be taken into consideration. These considerations are particularly important when we consider the use of donor eggs or donor sperm,

or when we plan pregnancies in older women.

(8) The patients must be informed about the cost, effectiveness and short- and long-term safety of each procedure and if possible even for each specific center.

(9) Sex selection for political, economic or extraneous reasons must not be permitted.

(10) Genetic selection for ethical purification or social or political reasons must be condemned.

(11) Hundreds of thousands of embryos are steadily accumulating in tanks of liquid nitrogen in many countries. In the UK alone, 300 000 surplus human embryos have been created. These spare embryos raise a host of ethical, social and legal questions. These questions become even more complex when the people who provided the eggs or sperm divorce or die or simply lose contact with the center where the embryos are stored.

(12) Ethical aspects must be of primary concern to society and the medical profession. A line must be drawn between the theoretically possible and the practically acceptable, and between the technically feasible and the socially reasonable. Research procedures must not be confused with good medical practice.

(13) We who are near the peak of research and development in the area of reproductive medicine have to acknowledge that we must also integrate new knowledge and new technical developments into our patient information packages and into our daily practices. This should decrease the negative influence of sensational media reports, permit us to regain confidence and respect from our patients, and transform theoretical science into practical solutions to our patients' problems.

The mobile consumer society, constantly remodelled by mass media and modern explosively developing medicine must find appropriate means of communicating and developing mutual trust. To achieve this goal, the doctors must not only be scientifically competent and medically skilful, but also sensitive and honest human beings, aware of their duty to society. With these recommendations in mind, we should be able to help mankind to fulfil the first commandment in the Bible in the spirit and intent as it was bestowed: 'So God created man in His own image, in the image of God created He him; Male and female He created them. God blessed them, and God said unto them, be fruitful and multiply and replenish the Earth and subdue it' (*Genesis*; 1:27–8).

References

1. World Health Organization. *Health, Population and Development*. WHO position paper for the International Conference on Population and Development, Cairo 1994. WHO/FHE/94. Geneva: WHO

2. Westrom L. *Impact of sexually transmitted diseases on human reproduction. Swedish studies of infertility and ectopic pregnancy in sexually-transmitted diseases. Status Report of NIAID Study Group*. Washington, DC: National Institute of Health, 1980: Publication No. 81/2213:43

3. Testart J. De la spermatide au spermatozoide: quels changements necessaires au developpement? *Contracept Fertil Sex* 1996;24: 526–33

4. Cha KY, Koo JJ, Choi DH. Pregnancy after *in vitro* fertilization of human follicular fluid oocytes collected from non-stimulated cycles, their culture *in vitro* and their transfer in a donor oocyte program. *Fertil Steril* 1991;55:109–18

5. Russel JB, Knezevish KM, Fabian KF, *et al.* Unstimulated immature oocyte retrieval: early

versus mid-follicular endometrial priming. *Fertil Steril* 1997;67:616–20

6. Trounson AO, Wood C, Kausche A. *In vitro* maturation and fertilization and developmental competence of oocytes recovered from untreated polycystic ovarian patients. *Fertil Steril* 1994;62:353–62

7. Chappel S, Kelton C, Nugent N. Expression of human gonadotropins by recombinant DNA methods. In Genazzani AR, Petraglia F, eds. *Proceedings of the 3rd World Congress on Gynecological Endocrinology* 1992: Carnforth, UK: Parthenon Publishing, 1992:179–84

8. Howles CM. Genetic engineering of human FSH (Gonal-F). *Hum Reprod Update* 1996;2:172–91

9. Lunenfeld B, Lunenfeld E, Howles C. Development and use of recombinant gonadotropins. *Asian J Endocrinol* 1999;in press

10. Insler V, Melmed H, Mashiach S, *et al.* Functional classification of patients selected for gonadotropic therapy. *Obstet Gynecol* 1968;32:620–8

11. Agrawal R, West C, Conway GS, *et al.* Pregnancy after treatment with three recombinant gonadotropins. *Lancet* 1997;349:29–30

12. Keene J, Nishimori K, Boime I. Recombinant deglycosylated human FSH is an antagonist of human FSH action in cultured rat granulosa cells. *Endocr J* 1994;2:175–80

13. Diedrich K, Felberbaum R. Multiple dose protocol for the administration of GnRH antagonists in IVF: the 'Luebeck protocol'. *J Assist Reprod Genet* 1997;14(Suppl):15(abstr)

14. Olivennes F, Bouchard P, Frydman R. The use of a new GnRH antagonist (Cetrorelix) with a single dose protocol in IVF. *J Assist Reprod Genet* 1997;14(Suppl):15(abstr)

15. Sharara FI, Meyer WR, Lessey BA, *et al.* Effects of hydrosalpinx on IVF outcome. *Hum Reprod* 1997;12:2853–4

16. Braude P, Boloton V, Moore S. Human gene expression first occurs between the four- and eight-cell stages of preimplantation development. *Nature (London)* 1988;332:459

17. Gardner DK, Lane M. Culture and selection of viable blastocysts: a feasible proposition for human IVF? *Hum Reprod Update* 1997;3:367–82

18. Gardner DK, Vella P, Lane M. Culture and transfer of human blastocysts increases implantation rates and reduces the need for multiple embryo transfer. *Fertil Steril* 1998;69:84–8

19. Lane M, Gardner DK. Selection of viable blastocysts prior to transfer using metabolic criteria. *Hum Reprod* 1996;9:1975–8

20. Gardner DK, Lane M. Culture of viable human blastocysts in defined sequential serum free media. *Hum Reprod* 1998;13(Suppl):101–12

21. Servy EJ, Kaufmann RA, Liu Z, *et al.* Human pregnancies after transfer of fresh (four- to eight-cell) versus frozen-thawed blastocysts resulting from intracytoplastmic sperm injection. *J Assist Reprod Genet* 1998;15:422–6

22. Cohen J, Scott R, Schimmel T, *et al.* Birth of infant after transfer of anucleate donor oocyte cytoplasm into recipient eggs. *Lancet* 1997;350:186–7

23. Edirisinghe WR, Junk SM, Matson PL, *et al.* Birth from cryopreserved embryos following *in-vitro* maturation of oocytes and intracytoplasmic sperm injection. *Hum Reprod* 1997;12:1056–8

24. Bustillo M, Zarutskie P. Assisted reproductive technology in the United States and Canada: 1995 results generated from the American Society for Reproductive Medicine/Society for Assisted Reproductive Technology Registry. *Fertil Steril* 1998;69:389–98

25. Goldfarb GM, Austin C, Lisbona H. Cost-effectiveness of *in vitro* fertilization. *Obstet Gynecol* 1996;87:18–21

26. Evans MI, May M, Drugan A. Selective termination: clinical experience and residual risks. *Am J Obstet Gynecol* 1990;170:902–9

27. Domar D, Zuttermeister PC, Friedman R. The psychological impact of infertility; a comparison with patients with other medical conditions. *J Psychosom Obstet Gynecol* 1993;14:45–52

Endocrine, autocrine and paracrine regulation of ovarian steroidogenesis in polycystic ovary syndrome

21

L. Devoto

Introduction

Polycystic ovary syndrome (PCOS), or hyperandrogenic anovulation, is the most frequent cause of anovulatory infertility. The precise mechanisms underlying this syndrome remain to be elucidated.

Normal human ovarian follicular development and steroidogenesis are dependent on pituitary-derived follicle stimulating hormone (FSH) and luteinizing hormone (LH) which act through a cyclic adenosine monophosphate (cAMP) signalling system. However, the mitogenic and steroidogenic actions of FSH and LH are modulated by a variety of growth factors, hormones and cytokines, including insulin and insulin growth factors (IGF) I and II. These polypeptides are known to stimulate the replication of a wide variety of cells and appear to have autocrine–paracrine actions as well as classical endocrine functions. The complete IGF system, including IGF proteins, IGF receptors, IGF-binding proteins and IGF-binding protease, has been detected in the human ovary. Human granulosa cells and theca cells express IGF-I, IGF-II and insulin specific-receptors as well as IGF-binding protein, inhibin and IGF-II ligand. Interestingly, only theca cells express the gene for IGF-I[1–3].

Ovarian androgen synthesis is LH-dependent, providing an essential substrate for follicular estradiol synthesis. Additionally, ovarian androgen production directly influences ovarian follicular development. Several peptides, including insulin, IGFs and inhibin, stimulate thecal androgen biosynthesis. These peptides also amplify the LH-stimulated signal transduction pathway[4]. The aim of this study was to analyze the endocrine, autocrine and paracrine factors involved in androgen secretion in PCOS.

Dysregulation of hypothalamic–pituitary function in the development of PCOS

Abnormal LH/FSH secretion has long been identified as a common feature of anovulation in PCOS. Studies have indicated that there is an increase in gonadotropin releasing hormone (GnRH) pulse frequency and pituitary LH release in these subjects[5,6]. This central gonadotropin dysregulation results in an increase in LH and a decrease in FSH. It is thought that the change in secretion of gonadotropins causes follicular arrest, which is associated with hyperplasia of the ovarian theca and stroma, resulting in androgen hypersecretion. A number of neuroendocrine investigations have been conducted to determine if the GnRH pulse generator is intrinsically more frequent in women with PCOS. However, to date there is no definitive evidence supporting this hypothesis. For example, administration of progestins and opioidergic agents decreases LH pulse frequency in women with PCOS as well as in normal women, suggesting that the neuromodulation of GnRH release remains relatively intact in women with PCOS[7]. Ovarian wedge resection and the administration of insulin-sensitizing agents, such as metformin and troglitazone, in part restores ovarian function[8,9]. These findings suggest that the more frequent GnRH pulse frequency associated with higher LH in serum is not the primary etiology of PCOS. However, altered hypothalamic or pituitary dynamics in PCOS are important, because they contribute to elevated LH levels which result in chronic anovulation and increased androgen biosynthesis. Additionally, androgens are converted into estrogens which then suppress pituitary FSH release.

Abnormal androgen secretion in PCOS is locally regulated: $P_{450c17\alpha}$ dysregulation

Elevated levels of testosterone, free testosterone, 17-hydroxyprogesterone and androstenedione are part of the androgen biochemical phenotype of PCOS. It is well known that $P_{450c17\alpha}$ (17α-hydroxylase and 17.20 lyase) is of paramount importance in androgen biosynthesis. Assessment of this enzyme in ovarian hyperandrogenism has been clinically performed via an ovarian stimulation test, consisting of suppression of adrenal androgen production by the administration of oral dexamethasone followed by a single dose of 100 μg of the GnRH agonist nafarelin to stimulate gonadotropin release. Twenty four hours later, androstenedione and 17-hydroxyprogesterone are determined in serum. The androstenedione and 17-hydroxyprogesterone responses were two to three times greater in women with PCOS compared to normal women tested during the early follicular phase[10]. Interestingly, $P_{450c17\alpha}$ dysregulation was also present in subjects with PCOS and normal LH levels were found in adolescents with a history of premature pubarche and normal body mass index. Only one-third of these adolescents had an increased basal LH[11].

Several peptides, including LH, IGFs, insulin and inhibin, stimulate androstenedione accumulation by human thecal cell cultures from normal women and women with PCOS. Notably, in basal culture (non-stimulated conditions) as well as in stimulated conditions, the androstenedione accumulation is significantly higher in theca cell cultures from women with PCOS[5]. These *in vivo* and *in vitro* observations on androgen hyperresponsiveness may suggest an intrinsic defect of $P_{450c17\alpha}$ activity in PCOS.

Taken together, these findings suggest that LH hypersecretion is not the primary cause of $P_{450c17\alpha}$ dysregulation in most cases of PCOS. On the other hand, the autocrine–paracrine control of $P_{450c17\alpha}$ by IGFs and insulin is particularly important in obese women with PCOS and hyperinsulinemia. Insulin decreases sex hormone binding globulin (SHBG) and insulin-like growth factor binding protein (IGFBP-1) concentrations in women with PCOS. This condition may lead to an increase in the bioavailability of testosterone and IGFs, respectively. However, there is a potential for unbound testosterone to be converted to estrone and IGFs to stimulate androgen biosynthesis.

Hyperinsulinemia

The association of hyperinsulinemia with the enhancement of androgen biosynthesis in obese women with PCOS is supported by a number of *in vivo* and *in vitro* studies. However, there is no clear evidence for a role for insulin in the regulation of androgen secretion in normal women[12].

Diazoxide, an inhibitor of pancreatic insulin release, causes a decrease in insulin and androgen levels with an increase in SHBG levels in women with PCOS. Diazoxide treatment did not modify these parameters in normal women. Similarly, troglitazone, which is a novel insulin-sensitizing agent that improves oral glucose tolerance and insulin resistance in individuals with impaired glucose tolerance, reduces plasma androgen levels in women with PCOS in association with the reduction in insulin levels[13].

Collectively, these *in vivo* findings suggest that hyperinsulinemia increases $P_{450c17\alpha}$ activity in obese women with PCOS. This effect can be exerted directly by insulin on ovarian steroidogenesis or indirectly by stimulation of pituitary LH release.

In vitro studies demonstrate that insulin supports steroidogenesis in ovarian cells by acting via its own receptor[14]. However, the lack of change in androgen levels associated with changes in insulin levels in normal women can be interpreted in the following two ways:

(1) Serum insulin in normal women may be not sufficiently high to support androgen biosynthesis under physiological conditions;

(2) There exists a PCOS gene or combinations of genes, which makes the ovaries of a woman with PCOS susceptible to the steroidogenic actions of insulin.

Mechanism of insulin-dependent enhancement of ovarian androgens in PCOS

Studies of insulin action in isolated adipocytes from women with PCOS have revealed marked decreases in insulin sensitivity associated with a decrease in insulin-stimulated glucose transport. This defect can occur in the absence of obesity, glucose intolerance or changes in the waist : hip ratio. This suggests that the defect of insulin action in women with PCOS may be intrinsic[14]. On the other hand, insulin inhibits IGFBP-1 gene expression and stimulates ovarian androgen biosynthesis. These observations may reflect differences in insulin sensitivity at both hepatic and ovarian levels. Thus, there is an apparent paradox in the insulin resistance associated with PCOS. Several theoretical mechanisms may explain this apparent contradictory situation:

(1) Fibroblasts from women with PCOS showed no change in insulin binding or receptor affinity compared to normal women. However, in approximately 50% of fibroblasts from women with PCOS a diminished insulin autophosphorylation was observed. Phosphoamino-acid analysis revealed decreased insulin-dependent tyrosine phosphorylation and increased insulin-independent receptor serine phosphorylation. This defect in PCOS serine phosphorylation could be a responsible mechanism leading to hyperinsulinemia in 50% of the PCOS women[15]. This mechanism is unique in PCOS and is different to the insulin resistance found in type A and type B diabetes

(2) Recent findings postulate that the signal transduction system governing steroid biosynthesis associated with insulin could be distinct and separate from the tyrosine kinase system used for glucose transport. The inositolphosphoglycan system has been shown to serve as the signal transduction pathway for insulin's effect on steroidogenesis[16].

(3) The hypothesis that insulin can stimulate steroidogenesis via the IGF-1 receptor is unlikely, because the elevation in insulin levels in women with PCOS is rather modest. In addition, it has recently been demonstrated that the insulin-mediated effect on steroidogenesis is mediated by the insulin receptor.

The ovarian granulosa cell compartment in PCOS

The thecal cell compartment of the ovarian follicle has been targeted as the principal ovarian locus for study steroid dysregulation in women with PCOS. Abnormal androgen synthesis in women with PCOS has been suggested to be the cause of follicular arrest and anovulation. To date, there is limited information on the role of granulosa cells in the mechanisms of anovulation in PCOS. This lack of knowledge is probably associated with the fact that ovulation can be induced successfully in women with PCOS by the administration of clomiphene citrate or exogenous gonadotropins. This has led to the suggestion that anovulation is due to a failure of FSH-mediated follicular maturation in women with PCOS. Recently, specific biochemical phenotypes of granulosa cells from women with PCOS have been described, including *in vitro* hyperresponsiveness to FSH, resulting in increased progesterone and estradiol secretion, respectively. Insulin stimulates estradiol and progesterone production despite peripheral insulin resistance. In addition, insulin preincubation sensitizes human granulosa cells to LH. This suggests an *in vitro* enhancement of granulosa cell diferentiation by insulin[14].

On the other hand, granulosa cells from small follicles (> 4 mm) of anovulatory women with PCOS have a premature response to LH[17].

We recently examined the effect of insulin on steroidogenic acute regulatory protein (StAR) expression in human granulosa cells. This protein plays a pivotal role in cholesterol mobilization and particularly in the translocation of cholesterol from the cholesterol-rich outer mitochondrial membrane to the cholesterol-poor inner mitochondrial membrane. This is a rate-limiting step in the control of steroidogenesis[18]. Insulin (20 nM) increases StAR mRNA and protein levels in cultured granulosa lutein cells. Moreover, StAR protein levels in human granulosa cells are higher in women with PCOS than normal women 24 h after oocyte retrieval and after 6 days in culture[19,20].

Taken together, these data indicate that the granulosa cells from anovulatory PCOS women have specific biochemical phenotypes that may be important in the underlying mechanism of anovulation of this syndrome. This suggests that the steroidogenic abnormalities in PCOS are not only restricted to the theca cell compartment.

Acknowledgements

I gratefully acknowledge Dr K. Barnhart and Professor J. F. Strauss III for their critical revision of the manuscript.

References

1. El-Roeiy A, Chen X, Roberts VJ, *et al.* Expression of the the insulin-like growths factor (IGF-I) and the IGF-I, IGF-II and insulin receptors gene product in the human ovary. *J Clin Endocrinol Metab* 1993;77:1411–18

2. Manson H, Cwyfan-Hughes, Heinrich, *et al.* Insulin-like factor (IGF) I and II, IGF-binding proteins, and IGF-binding protein proteases are produced by theca and stroma of normal and polycystic human ovaries. *J Clin Endocrinol Metab* 1996;81:276–83

3. Yamoto M, Minamis S, Nakano R, *et al.* Immunohistochemical localization of inhibin/activin subunits in human ovarian follicle during the menstrual cycle. *J Clin Endocrinol Metab* 1992;74:989–93

4. Nahum R, Thong J, Hillier S. Metabolic regulation of androgen by thecal cell *in vitro*. *Hum Reprod* 1995;10:75–81

5. Berga SL, Guzick DS, Winters SJ, *et al.* Increased LH and α-sub-unit secretion in women with hyperandrogenic anovulation. *J Clin Endocrinol Metab* 1993;77:895–901

6. Sir T, Devoto L. Effect of clomiphene citrate on pulsatile luteinizing hormone profile in normal women and polycystic ovarian syndrome. *Horm Metab Res* 1989;21:3703–6

7. Berga L, Daniels T. Can polycystic ovary syndrome exist without concomitant hypothalamic dysfunction? *Semin Reprod Endocrinol* 1997;15:169–76

8. Nestler JE, Jakubowicz DJ. Decrease in ovarian cytochrome P450c17α activity and serum free testosterone after reduction in insulin secretion in women with polycystic ovarian syndrome. *N Engl J Med* 1996;335:617–23

9. Ehrmann D, Schneider D, Sobel B, *et al.* Troglitazone improves defects in insulin action, insulin secretion, ovarian steroidogenesis, and fibrolysis in women with polycystic ovary. *J Clin Endocrinol Metab* 1997;82:2108–16

10. Rosenfield RL, Barnes RB, Burstein, *et al.* Studies of the nature of 17-hydroxyprogesterone hyperresponsiveness to gonadotropin releasing hormone agonist challenge in functional ovarian hyperandrogenism. *J Clin Endocrinol Metab* 1994;79:1686–92

11. Barnes RB. Pathophysiology of ovarian steroid secretion in polycystic ovary syndrome. *Semin Reprod Endocrinol* 1997;15:159–67

12. Dunaif A. Insulin resistance and the polycystic ovary syndrome: mechanism and implications of pathogenesis. *Endocr Rev* 1997;18:774–800

13. Nestler JE, Barlascini CO, Matt DW, *et al.* Suppression of serum insulin by diazoxide reduces serum testosterone levels in obese women with polycystic ovary syndrome. *J Clin Endocrinol Metab* 1989;68:1027–32

14. Legro R, Spielman R, Urbanek M, *et al.* Phenotype and genotype in polycystic ovary syndrome. *Recent Prog Horm Res* 1998;53:217–56

15. Nestler JE. Role of hyperinsulinemia in the pathogenesis of the polycystic ovary syndrome, and its clinical implications. *Semin Reprod* 1977; 15:111–22

16. Willis D, Franks S. Insulin action in human granulosa cells from normal and polycystic ovaries is mediated by the insulin receptor and not the type-I insulin-like growth factor receptor. *J Clin Endocrinol Metab* 1995;80:3788–90

17. Willis D, Watson H, Manson H, *et al.* Premature response to luteinizing hormone cells from anovulatory women with polycystic ovary syndrome: relevance to mechanism of anovulation. *J Clin Endocrinol Metab* 1998;83:3984–91

18. Kallen BC, Arakane F, Christenson LK, Watari H, Devoto L, Strauss FJ III. Unveiling the mechanisms of action and regulation of the steroidogenic acute regulatory protein. *Mol Cell Endocrinol* 1998;145:39–45

19. Devoto L, Christenson LK, McAllister JM, Strauss FJ III. Insulin and insulin growth factor-I and II upregulate steroidogenesis acute regulatory protein (StAR) expression in human granulosa cells. Abstract submitted to the *1999 Scientific Meeting of the Endocrine Society*

20. Devoto L, Christenson LK, Strauss JF III. Unpublished observation

The estrogen receptor: changing concepts. Clinical lessons from molecular biology

22

L. Speroff

Introduction

The history of estrogen is a modern story. The estrogen receptor was discovered in about 1960[1]. However, even before the estrogen receptor was discovered, chemists had developed an antiestrogen[2]. This compound, called MER-25, was evaluated for the treatment of breast cancer, but caused neurological toxicity. Tamoxifen is a member of this class of compounds (as is clomiphene) called triphenylethylenes. Estrogens produce cellular responses by regulating gene activity. This action is mediated by an intracellular receptor that primarily affects gene transcription, but also regulates post-transcriptional events and non-genomic events. The estrogen receptor belongs to a superfamily of receptors. This family now includes about 50 proteins, many of which are called orphan receptors because a specific ligand for these proteins has not been identified[3].

The estrogen receptor

The estrogen receptor is translated from a 6.8-kilobase mRNA that contains eight exons. It has a molecular weight of approximately 66 000, with 595 amino acids. The receptor half-life is approximately 4–7 h, thus the estrogen receptor is a protein with a rapid turn-over. It is divided into six regions, labeled A to F.

The A/B region, or the regulatory domain, is the most variable, ranging in size from 20 amino acids in the vitamin D receptor, to 600 amino acids in the mineralocorticoid receptor. It contains the transcription activation function called TAF-1.

The C region is the DNA binding domain, containing two zinc fingers that interact with DNA leading to binding at the estrogen response element sequence GGATCNNNGATCC. This domain is responsible for target gene specificity and high-affinity DNA binding. In addition, this domain is responsible for nuclear localization of the receptor.

The D region, the hinge, contains sequences necessary for nuclear localization. This nuclear localization signal must be present for the receptor to remain within the nucleus in the absence of hormone.

The E region is the hormone binding domain, and has 251 amino acids (residues 302–553) at the C-terminal half of the receptor. In addition to hormone binding, this domain is responsible for dimerization and contains the transcriptional activation function called TAF-2. This is also the site for binding by heat shock proteins (specifically hsp 90); binding to the heat shock protein prevents dimerization and DNA binding.

The F region is a 42-amino acid C-terminal region. This region modulates gene transcription by estrogen and antiestrogen, having a role that influences antiestrogen efficacy in suppressing estrogen-stimulated transcription[4]. The conformation of the receptor–ligand complex is different with estrogen vs. antiestrogen, and this conformation is different with and without the F region. The F region is not required for transcriptional response to estrogen; however, it affects the magnitude of ligand-bound estrogen receptor activity. It is speculated that this region affects conformation in such a way that protein interactions are influenced. Thus it is appropriate that the effects of the F domain vary according to cell type and protein context. The F region affects the activities of both TAF-2 and TAF-1, which is what you would expect if the effect is on conformation[5].

The steroid family receptors are predominantly in the nucleus, even when not bound to a ligand, except for the androgen and glucocorticoid receptors where nuclear uptake depends upon hormone binding. However, the estrogen receptor does undergo what is called nucleocytoplasmic shuttling. Estrogen receptor constantly diffuses out of the nucleus but is rapidly transported back in.

Prior to binding, the estrogen receptor is an inactive complex that includes a variety of proteins, including the heat shock proteins. Heat shock protein 90 appears to be the critical protein and many of the others are associated with it. This heat shock protein is not only important for maintaining an inactive state, but also causing the proper folding and for transport across membranes. 'Activation' or 'transformation' is the dissociation of heat shock protein 90[6].

Imagine the unoccupied steroid receptor as a loosely-packed, mobile protein complexed with heat shock proteins. The steroid family of receptors exists in this complex with heat shock proteins and cannot bind to DNA until union with the ligand liberates the heat shock proteins and allows dimerization. The conformation change induced by hormone binding involves a dissociating process to form a tighter packing of the receptor. Members of the thyroid and retinoic acid receptor subfamily do not exist in inactive complexes with heat shock proteins. They can form dimers and bind to response elements in DNA, but without ligand they act as repressors of transcription.

Estrogen receptor mutants can be created that are unable to bind estradiol. These mutants could form dimers with wild type estrogen receptor, and then bind to estrogen response element, but could not activate transcription[7]. This indicates that transcription is dependent upon the result after estradiol binding to estrogen receptor, an estradiol-dependent structural

change. Dimerization by itself is not sufficient to lead to transcription. Neither is binding of the dimer to DNA sufficient.

The TAF, the transcriptional activation function, is the part of the receptor that affects other transcription factors after binding to DNA. Ligand binding produces a conformation that allows TAFs to accomplish their tasks. TAF-1 can stimulate transcription in the absence of hormone when it is fused to DNA; however, it promotes DNA binding in the intact receptor. TAF-2 is affected by the bound ligand, and depends upon estrogen binding for full activity. TAF-2 consists of a number of dispersed elements that are brought together after estrogen binding. TAF-1 in the regulatory domain is estrogen-independent. TAF-2 in the hormone-binding domain is active only in the presence of estrogen. The activities of TAF-1 and TAF-2 vary according to the promoters in target cells. These areas can act independently or with one another.

Cyclic adenosine monophosphate (cAMP) and protein kinase A pathways increase transcriptional activity of the estrogen receptor. In some cases phosphorylation modulates the activity of the receptor; in other cases, the phosphorylation regulates the activity of a specific transcription factor that in turn modulates the receptor. The steroid receptor superfamily members are phosphoproteins. Phosphorylation follows steroid binding and occurs in both the cytoplasm and nucleus. This phosphorylation is believed to enhance activity of the steroid receptor complex.

Phosphorylation of the receptor increases the potency of the molecule to regulate transcription. Growth factors can stimulate protein kinase phosphorylation that can produce synergistic activation of genes or even ligand-independent activity. The concentration of coactivators can affect the cellular response. A small amount of receptor but a large amount of coactivator can make the cell very responsive to a weak signal.

Epidermal growth factor (EGF), insulin-like growth factor-1 (IGF-1) and transforming growth factor-α (TGF-α) can activate the estrogen receptor in the absence of estrogen. This response to growth factors can be blocked by pure antiestrogens (suggesting that a strong antagonist locks the receptor in a conformation that resists ligand-independent pathways). The exact mechanism of growth factor activation is not known, but it is known that a steroid receptor can be activated by means of a chemical signal (a phosphorylation cascade) originating at the plasma membrane.

Summary of the steroid hormone–receptor mechanism

(1) Binding of the hormone to the hormone-binding domain that has been kept in an inactive state by various heat shock proteins.

(2) Activation of the hormone–receptor complex, by conformational change, follows the dissociation of the heat shock proteins.

(3) Dimerization of the complex.

(4) Binding of the dimer to the hormone-responsive element on DNA by the zinc finger area of the DNA-binding domain.

(5) Stimulation of transcription, mediated by transcription activation functions, and influenced by the protein (other transcription factors and coactivators/corepressors) context of the cell, and by phosphorylation.

Summary of factors that determine biologic activity

(1) Affinity of the hormone for the hormone-binding domain of the receptor.

(2) Target tissue differential expression of the receptor subtypes (e.g. estrogen receptor-α and estrogen receptor-β).

(3) Conformational shape of the ligand–receptor complex, with effects on two important activities: dimerization and modulation of adaptor proteins.

(4) Differential expression of target tissue adaptor proteins and phosphorylation.

Different roles for estrogen receptors-α and -β

Male and female mice have been developed that are homozygous for disruption of the estrogen receptor-α gene, and are called 'estrogen receptor-α knockout mice'[8]. Both sexes with this knockout are infertile. Spermatogenesis in the male is reduced and the testes undergo progressive atrophy, evidence of a testicular role for estrogen, because gonadotropin levels and testicular steroidogenesis remain normal. Sexual mounting behavior is not altered, but intromission, ejaculation and aggressive behaviors are reduced. Female mice with the estrogen receptor-α gene disrupted do not ovulate, and the ovaries do not respond to gonadotropin stimulation. These female animals have high levels of estradiol, testosterone and leuteinizing hormone. Follicle-stimulating hormone (FSH) β-subunit synthesis is increased, but FSH secretion is at normal levels, indicating different sites of action for estrogen and inhibin. Uterine development is normal (due to a lack of testosterone in early life), but growth is impaired. Mammary gland ductal and alveolar development is absent. Female mice with absent estrogen receptor-α activity do not display sexually receptive behaviors. This genetically engineered line of mice demonstrates essential activities for estrogen receptor-α. Relatively normal fetal and early development suggests that estrogen receptor-β plays a primary role in these functions. For example, the fetal adrenal gland expresses high levels of estrogen receptor-β and low levels of estrogen receptor-α[9]. However, nongenomic actions of estrogen are also possible and can explain some of the estrogenic responses in a knockout model.

Differential expression of the α- and β-receptors is likely in various tissues (e.g. estrogen receptor-β is the prevalent estrogen receptor in certain areas of the brain and the cardiovascular system) resulting in different and selective responses to specific estrogens. Human granulosa cells from the ovarian follicle contain only estrogen receptor-β mRNA; the human breast expresses both α- and β-receptors[10]. Some parts of the rat brain contain only estrogen receptor-β, others only estrogen receptor-α, and some areas contain both receptors[11].

The estrogen situation is further complicated by the fact that the same estrogen binding to the α- and β-receptors can produce opposite effects. For example, estradiol can stimulate gene transcription with estrogen receptor-α and a given site of the estrogen response element, whereas estradiol inhibits gene transcription with estrogen receptor-β in this same system[12]. Different and unique messages, therefore, can be determined by the specific combination of (1) a particular estrogen, (2) the α- or β-receptor, and (3) the targeted response element. To some degree, differences with estrogen receptor-α and estrogen receptor-β are influenced by activation of TAF-1 and TAF-2. Agents that are capable of mixed estrogen agonism and antagonism produce agonistic messages via TAF-1 with estrogen receptor-α, but because estrogen receptor-β lacks a similar TAF-1, such agents can be pure antagonists in cells that respond only to estrogen receptor-β. Estrogen receptor-α and -β affect the peptide context of a cell, especially coactivators and corepressors, differently.

Antiestrogens

Tamoxifen has a variety of side-effects that indicate both estrogenic activity and antiestrogenic activity. How can tamoxifen be both an estrogen agonist and an estrogen antagonist?

Mechanism of tamoxifen action

TAF-1 and TAF-2 areas can both activate transcription, but TAF-2 activates transcription only when it is bound by estrogen. The individual transactivating abilities of TAF-1 and TAF-2 depend upon the promoter and cell context. The agonistic ability of tamoxifen is due to activation of TAF-1; its antagonistic activity is due to competitive inhibition of the estrogen-dependent activation of TAF-2.

An estrogen-associated protein binds to the right-hand side of TAF-2. Estrogen binding induces binding of this protein which then activates transcription. This protein recognizes only an activated conformation of the estrogen receptor, the result of estrogen binding. Tamoxifen binding to the TAF-2 area does not activate this domain because, in at least one explanation, the conformation change does not allow binding of the estrogen-associated protein, the activating factor[13,14].

The activity of TAF-2 is negligible in the presence of tamoxifen. In cells where TAF-1 and TAF-2 function independently of each other, tamoxifen would be chiefly an antagonist in cells where TAF-2 predominates, and an agonist where TAF-1 predominates; in some cells a mixed activity is possible[15].

The contact sites of estrogens and antiestrogens with the estrogen receptor are not identical[16]. When an antiestrogen binds to the estrogen receptor, the conformational changes that are induced alter the ability of the estrogen receptor–antiestrogen complex to modulate transcriptional activity. The relative agonist/antagonist activity is determined by the specific conformation achieved by the specific antiestrogen.

Even though tamoxifen can block estrogen-stimulated transcription of many genes, its degree of antagonistic activity varies among different animals, different cell types, and with different promoters within single cells. These differences are due to differences in the relative activities of the TAFs. The extent to which an antiestrogen inhibits an estrogen-mediated response therefore depends on the degree to which that response is mediated by TAF-2 activity as opposed to TAF-1 activity or mixed activity[17].

In some cell lines TAF-1 is dominant, and in others both are necessary. No cells have yet been identified in which TAF-2 is dominant. Using mutants, the function of TAF-1 and TAF-2 has been found to depend upon promoter context. With some promoters, both TAF-1 and TAF-2 are required for transcription; with others, TAF-1 and TAF-2 can function independently.

In most cell types TAF-1 is too weak to activate transcription by itself, but of course there are now well-known exceptions: endometrium, bone and liver. In these tissues, the promoter context is right. Tamoxifen is a potent activator of estrogen receptor-mediated induction of promoters that are regulated by the TAF-1 site. Antiestrogens have no effects on TAF-1-dependent transcription in breast cells[18].

This explanation may not be the same for other mixed agonists and antagonists. Raloxifene can activate an estrogen-responsive gene through a response element separate from the estrogen response element, an action that requires specific activating peptides[19]. Estrogen metabolites also can interact with response elements other than the classical estrogen response elements. The bottom line is that there are multiple pathways to gene activation. The estrogen response elements, depending upon the ligand, can regulate more than one response element. Thus estrogen and antiestrogen actions in various tissues can reflect the presence of different response elements.

Tamoxifen treatment of breast cancer

Tamoxifen treatment achieves its greatest effect (50% reduction in recurrent disease) in estrogen receptor-positive tumors, but it is also effective in estrogen receptor-negative tumors. Most importantly, it is now recognized that acquired resistance eventually develops. Why is tamoxifen treatment effective with estrogen receptor-negative tumors? At least a part of the antiestrogenic action of tamoxifen is derived from competitive inhibition of estrogen binding to the estrogen receptor. Although the affinity of tamoxifen for the estrogen receptor is only 2–6% of estradiol affinity, the affinity for its major metabolite, 4-hydroxytamoxifen, is 200% compared to estradiol. However, besides binding to estrogen receptor and providing competitive inhibition, tamoxifen has the following actions:

(1) Tamoxifen and clomiphene inhibit protein kinase C activity.

(2) Tamoxifen inhibits calmodulin-dependent cAMP phosphodiesterase, by binding to calmodulin.

(3) Tamoxifen increases TGF-β1 and TGF-β2, as do progestins, in stromal cells surround-

ing tumor cells. TGF-β has the following actions in breast cancer cells:

(a) TGF-β inhibits growth of breast cancer cells;

(b) Tamoxifen stimulates secretion of TGF-β in breast cancer cells;

(c) Estrogen and insulin decrease the secretion of TGF-β in cancer cells; and

(d) The antigrowth effect of TGF-β can be reversed by estrogen.

(4) Tamoxifen decreases IGF-1 and IGF-2 in stromal fibroblasts.

Estrogen thus decreases TGF-β, and increases IGF-1, EGF and TGF-α[20,21].

Mechanisms for tamoxifen resistance

Generally it is believed that estrogen receptor expression is not a permanent phenotype of breast cancer cells; tumors therefore change from estrogen receptor-positive to -negative. However, more than 50% of resistant tumors retain estrogen receptors[22]. Thus far, the therapeutic response of breast cancer to endocrine therapy is not permanent; eventually all tumors progress. The conventional wisdom has therefore been that progression is associated with loss of cellular control and loss of estrogen receptor expression. However, the correlation between metastatic disease and estrogen receptor-negative state is not strong. Indeed, metastatic disease with estrogen receptor-positive cells and an estrogen receptor-negative primary tumor has been reported. The rate of estrogen receptor expression is about the same in *in situ* disease and invasive disease.

Because of the synergism between estrogen receptor and protein kinase pathways, stimulation of the protein kinase pathway can change an antagonist message to agonism. Activators of protein kinase synergize with estrogen in estrogen receptor-mediated transcriptional activation. This mechanism appears to be operating through the phosphorylation of estrogen receptor or proteins involved in estrogen receptor-mediated transcription. Stimulation of this protein kinase phosphorylation activates the agonist activity of tamoxifen-like antiestrogens. Further, the lack of response of pure antiestrogens to this phosphorylation may be part of the reason for greater efficacy.

Resistance can be due to a change in the interpretation of the tamoxifen–estrogen receptor complex and its agonist/antagonist balance. This can be a result in cross-talk with other signaling pathways[16]. Stimulation of the protein kinase A signaling pathway activates the agonist activity of tamoxifen. However, some antiestrogens fail to activate the estrogen receptor in the presence of cAMP. Activation of the protein kinase pathway may contribute to resistance development[23].

The pure antiestrogens

Binding with the pure antiestrogens inhibits DNA binding. Because the site responsible for dimerization overlaps with the hormone binding site, it is believed that pure antiestrogens sterically interfere with dimerization, and thus inhibit DNA binding. In addition, these compounds increase the cellular turnover of estrogen receptor, and this action contributes to the antiestrogen effectiveness. Estrogen and progesterone receptors exit the nucleus but are rapidly transported back. When this shuttling is impaired, receptors are more rapidly degraded in the cytoplasm. Agents that inhibit dimerization inhibit nuclear translocation and thus increase cytoplasmic degradation. The half-life of the estrogen receptor when occupied with estradiol is about 5 h; when occupied with a pure antiestrogen it is less than 1 h. This mechanism may be due to interference with nuclear localization exerted by the hinge region. Newly synthesized receptors therefore cannot be efficiently transported into the nucleus and those in the nucleus will leak back into the cytoplasm.

Because these agents function in a different manner from tamoxifen, it is not surprising that tamoxifen-resistant tumors respond to these agents[24].

New drugs

The new drugs belong to one of two classes: either they are analogs of tamoxifen or they belong to the pure antiestrogen class. Analogs of tamoxifen, such as raloxifene and droloxifene, have antiestrogenic activity in the uterus as well as in the breast[25–27].

Premarin (see Table 1) is more potent than estrone sulfate, and more potent than can be accounted for by its two major components, estrone sulfate and equilin sulfate. Estrogen-stimulated growth is the result of autocrine and paracrine activity of growth factors plus classic endocrine direct effects on cells. In addition, estrogen can modulate growth by regulating the activity of other transcription factors, e.g. TAF-1 in genes involved with growth. Also, not all estrogens affect these mechanisms in an identical fashion.

Because of the complex interactivity involved in cellular gene response, the final biologic (clinical) response of a specific estrogen is now best viewed as unpredictable until tested in appropriate clinical trials.

Table 1 Composition of Premarin

Estrone	49.3%
Equilin	22.4%
17α-Dihydroequilin	13.8%
17α-Estradiol	4.5%
Δ8,9-Dehydroestrone	3.5%
Equilenin	2.2%
17β-Dihydroequilin	1.7%
17α-Dihydroequilenin	1.2%
17β-Estradiol	0.9%
17β-Dihydroequilenin	0.5%

References

1. Jensen EV, Jacobson HI. Basic guides to the mechanism of estrogen action. *Recent Prog Hormone Res* 1962;18:387–414
2. Lerner L, Holtaus Jr FJ, Thompson CRA. A non-steroidal estrogen antagonist 1-(*p*-2-diethylaminoethoxyphenyl)-1-phenyl-2-*p*-methoxyphenyl ethanol. *Endocrinology* 1958;63:295–318
3. Parker MG. Structure and function of the oestrogen receptor. *J Neuroendocrinol* 1993;5:223–8
4. Teutsch G, Nique F, Lemoine G, *et al.* General structure–activity correlations of antihormones. *Ann NY Acad Sci* 1995;761:5–28
5. Montano MM, Müller V, Trobaugh A, *et al.* The carboxy-terminal F domain of the human estrogen receptor: role in the transcriptional activity of the receptor and the effectiveness of antiestrogens as estrogen antagonists. *Mol Endocrinol* 1995;9:814–25
6. Parker MG. Structure and function of estrogen receptors. *Vitamins Hormones* 1995;51:267–87
7. Zhuang Y, Katzenellenbogen BS, Shapiro DJ. Estrogen receptor mutants which do not bind 17β-estradiol dimerize and bind to the estrogen response element *in vivo*. *Mol Endocrinol* 1995;9:457–66
8. Lindzey J, Korach KS. Developmental and physiological effects of estrogen receptor gene disruption in mice. *Trends Endocrinol Metab* 1997;8:137–45
9. Brandenberger AW, Tee MK, Lee JY, *et al.* Tissue distribution of estrogen receptors alpha (ER-α) and beta (ER-β) mRNA in the midgestational human fetus. *J Clin Endocrinol Metab* 1997;82:3509–12
10. Enmark E, Pelto-Huikko M, Grandien K, *et al.* Human estrogen receptor-β – gene structure, chromosomal localization, and expression pattern. *J Clin Endocrinol Metab* 1997;82:4258–65
11. Shughrue PJ, Lane MV, Merchenthaler I. Comparative distribution of estrogen receptor-alpha and -beta mRNA in the rat central nervous system. *J Comp Neurol* 1997;388:507–625
12. Paech K, Webb P, Kuiper GG, *et al.* Differential ligand activation of estrogen receptors alpha and beta at AP1 sites. *Science* 1997;277:1508–10
13. Halachmi S, Marden E, Martin G, *et al.* Estrogen receptor-associated proteins: possible mediators of hormone-induced transcription. *Science* 1994;264:1455–8
14. Landel CC, Kushner PJ, Greene GL. The interaction of human estrogen receptor with DNA is modulated by receptor-associated proteins. *Mol Endocrinol* 1994;8:1407–19
15. Berry M, Metzger D, Chambon P. Role of the two activating domains of the oestrogen receptor in the cell type and promoter context-dependent agonistic activity of the antioestrogen 4-hydroxytamoxifen. *EMBO* 1990;9:2811–18
16. Katzenellenbogen BS, Montano MM, Le Goff P, *et al.* Antiestrogens: mechanisms and actions in target cells. *J Steroid Biochem Mol Biol* 1995;53:387–93
17. Tzukerman MT, Esty A, Santisomere D, *et al.* Human estrogen receptor transactivational capacity is determined by both cellular and promoter context and mediated by two functionally distinct intramolecular regions. *Mol Endocrinol* 1994;8:21–30
18. Webb P, Lopex GN, Uht RM, *et al.* Tamoxifen activation of the estrogen receptor/AP-1 pathway: potential origin for the cell-specific estrogen-like effects of antiestrogens. *Mol Endocrinol* 1995;9:443–56
19. Yang NN, Venugopalan M, Hardikar S, *et al.* Identification of an estrogen response element activated by metabolites of 17β-estradiol and raloxifene. *Science* 1996;273:1222–4
20. Colletta AA, Benson JR, Baum M. Alternative mechanisms of action of antioestrogens. *Breast Cancer Res Treat* 1994;31:5–9
21. Murphy LC. Antiestrogen action and growth factor regulation. *Breast Cancer Res Treat* 1994;31:61–71
22. Encarnación CA, Ciocca DR, McGuire WL, *et al.* Measurement of steroid hormone receptors in breast cancer patients on tamoxifen. *Breast Cancer Res Treat* 1993;26:237–46
23. Fujimoto N, Katzenellenbogen BS. Alteration in the agonist/antagonist balance of antiestrogens by activation of protein kinase A signaling pathways in breast cancer cells: antiestrogen selectivity and promoter dependence. *Mol Endocrinol* 1994;8:296–304
24. Howell A, DeFriend D, Robertson J, *et al.* Response to a specific antioestrogen (ICI 182780) in tamoxifen-resistant breast cancer. *Lancet* 1995;345:29–30
25. Jordan VC. Alternate antiestrogens and approaches to the prevention of breast cancer. *J Cell Biochem* 1995;Suppl. 22:51–7
26. Hasman M, Rattel B, Löser R. Preclinical data for droloxifene. *Cancer Lett* 1994;84:101–16
27. Geisler J, Haarstad H, Gundersen S, *et al.* Influence of treatment with the antioestrogen 3-hydroxytamoxifen (droloxifene) on plasma sex hormone levels in postmenopausal patients with breast cancer. *J Endocrinol* 1995;146:359–63

Activins and inhibins in female reproductive function

23

F. M. Reis, M. Santuz and F. Petraglia

Introduction

As early as the 1930s, pioneer experiments of McCullagh[1] demonstrated the existence of a non-steroid substance produced by the testis, which prevented the appearance of 'castration cells' in the pituitary gland. During the following decades this still mysterious gonadal product was shown to exert a selective inhibition of the release of follicle stimulating hormone (FSH) by the anterior pituitary[2]. Only the identification of similar biological activity in ovarian follicular fluid, many years later, permitted the purification and characterization of the gonadal FSH-inhibiting protein, already called inhibin[3]. The process of inhibin isolation generated the discovery of an inhibin-related protein, which owing to its ability to stimulate FSH secretion was named activin[4].

Activins and inhibins participate in the control of pituitary gonadotropin secretion, ovarian follicular development, placental function and spermatogenesis and are possibly involved in physiological mechanisms preventing the development of tumors. Inhibin and activin levels are altered in gynecological and gestational diseases, and the continuous improvement of methods for specific quantification of these proteins will make them promising diagnostic markers in reproductive medicine[5].

Structure, receptors and sources

Activins and inhibins are dimeric glycoproteins resulting from distinct combinations of α (18 kDa) and/or β (14 kDa) subunits. One variety of α subunit and two types of β subunit, named βA and βB, give rise to inhibin A ($\alpha + \beta A$), inhibin B ($\alpha + \beta B$), activin A ($\beta A + \beta A$), activin B ($\beta B + \beta B$) or activin AB ($\beta A + \beta B$). Apart from these five bioactive dimeric proteins, free α subunits and the partially processed precursor pro-α C are also present in circulation (Figure 1). Both forms of inhibin have an inhibitory effect on pituitary FSH release, whereas the three forms of activin have similar biological activity[6,7]. The availability of bioactive inhibin and activin is regulated by a binding protein also discovered in the follicular fluid and therefore named follistatin. This single-chain glycoprotein of 35 kDa is able to inhibit FSH release probably by neutralizing the effect of activin[8,9].

The biological effects of activins are mediated by the oligomerization of two types of receptor (type I and type II activin receptor) both containing an extracellular domain, a single transmembrane region, and a large serine/threonine kinase intracellular domain, the activation of which triggers a cascade of intracellular signalling events[10,11]. However, the observation that most inhibin effects are associated with antagonism to activin while some activin functions are not antagonized by inhibin suggests the existence of a specific inhibin receptor, expressed in most but not all target tissues, and required for effective inhibin action[12].

In the human ovary, activin/inhibin subunit gene expression has been demonstrated in granulosa, theca and lutein cells with a changing pattern during the menstrual cycle[13]. Activins and inhibins are also produced and secreted by extragonadal tissues, such as the pituitary gland, the adrenals and the placenta. The human placenta and fetal membranes produce considerable amounts of activin A and inhibins from early gestation[14–16] and the

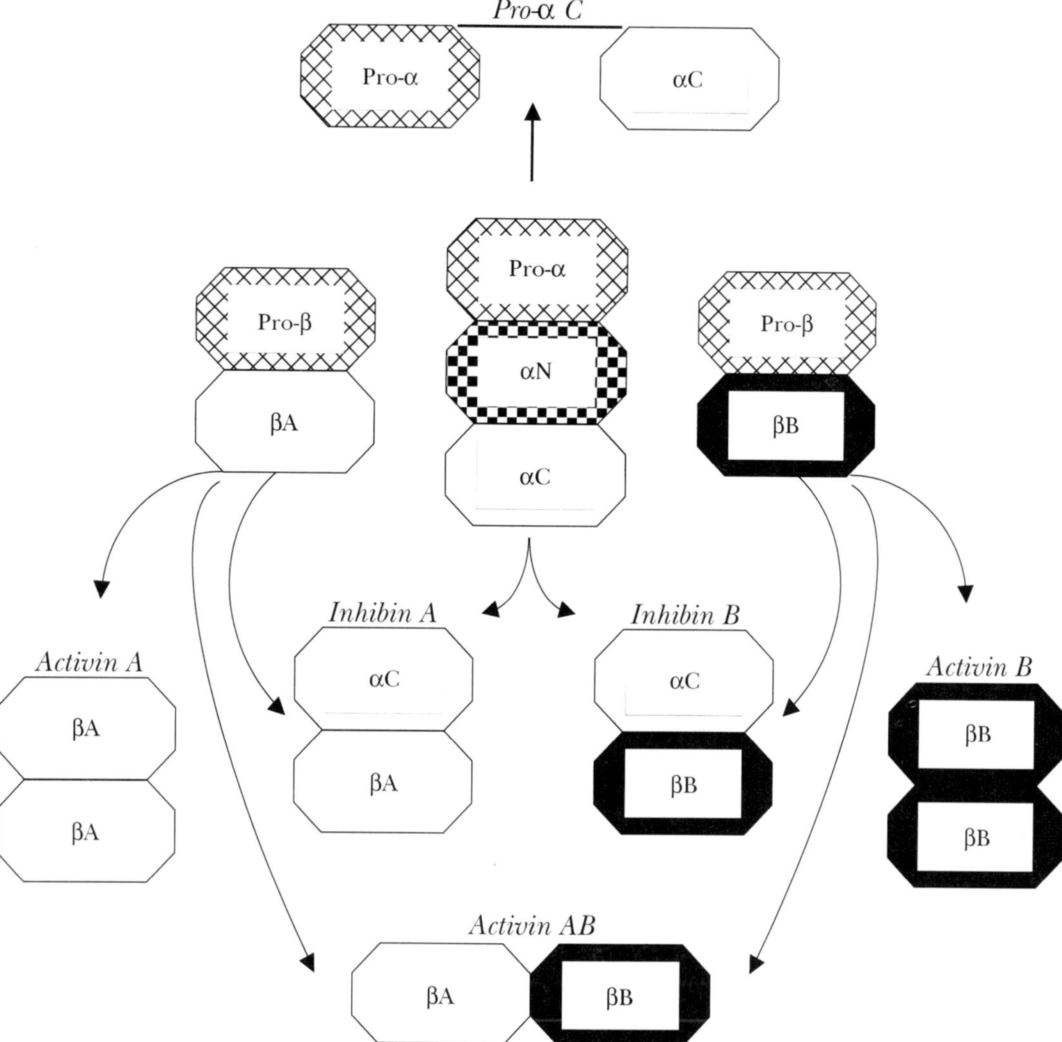

Figure 1 Schematic representation of the dimeric structure of activins, inhibins and their precursors

placenta is probably the main source of these proteins during all phases of pregnancy, apart from a minor contribution of the ovaries[17].

Endocrine function in the normal menstrual cycle

Changes in circulating levels

During the menstrual cycle, serum activin A levels change in a narrow-range, biphasic manner, with highest levels occurring around midcycle and luteal–follicular transition, and lowest levels during midfollicular and midluteal phases. From mid to late luteal phase, activin A levels increase progressively while estradiol and progesterone levels decline[18] (Figure 2).

The circulating levels of inhibin A are low in the early stage of the follicular phase and rise from the late follicular phase to peak at the midluteal phase, after a short dip coinciding with the luteinizing hormone (LH) peak. Plasma inhibin B levels rise sharply from the early follicular phase of the menstrual cycle, with a peak following the FSH rise and a progressive fall during the remainder of the follicular

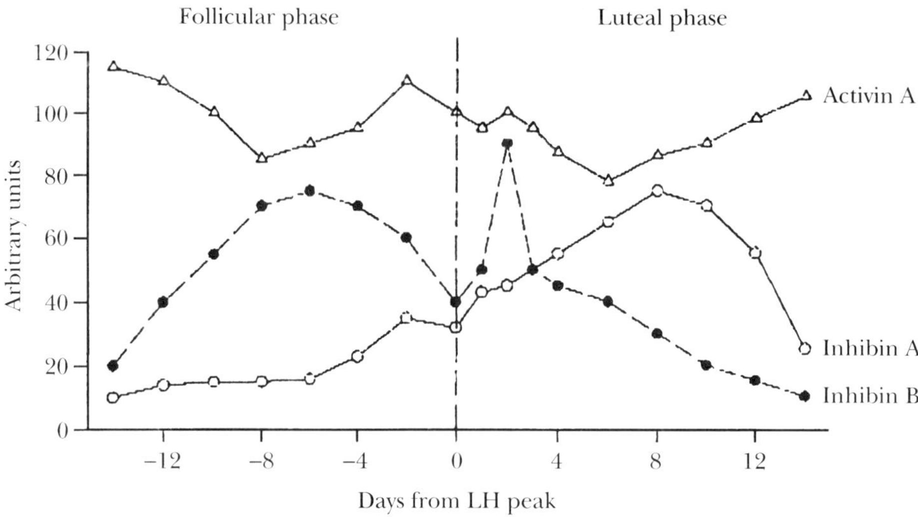

Figure 2 Relative changes of serum activin A, inhibin A and inhibin B levels throughout the menstrual cycle. Data are expressed in arbitrary units, and the three curves are plotted in different scales, so the absolute levels of one hormone are not comparable to the others. The curves were anchored by the mid-cycle luteinizing hormone (LH) peak and were drawn from original data of Muttukrishna and colleagues[18] and Groome and co-workers[19]

phase (Figure 2). Another inhibin B peak is observed 2 days after the midcycle LH peak, followed by rapid decrease and constant low levels during luteal involution[19]. These different cyclic patterns suggest that the two inhibin forms may have different physiological roles. Whereas inhibin B seems to be the major marker of follicular growth in response to FSH stimulation, inhibin A is secreted mostly by the corpus luteum and may be involved in the gradual release of ovarian negative feedback on FSH secretion during the luteal–follicular transition[20].

Evolution from puberty to menopause

Very limited data are available on inhibin secretion during pubertal transition, and no studies have correlated activin levels with the onset of puberty. Regarding female physiology, it was observed that:

(1) Both inhibin A and inhibin B are present in detectable concentrations in serum of pre-pubertal girls;

(2) Both inhibins increase through pubertal stages assessed by breast development;

(3) Both inhibins show a positive correlation with estradiol and FSH levels during puberty[21].

However, these data are not completely physiological because they were obtained from 'normal' short-stature children receiving growth hormone (GH) therapy, and direct or indirect effects of GH on inhibin secretion cannot be excluded[21].

Aging cycling women have increasing FSH levels during the follicular phase in spite of normal estrogen and LH levels and regular menstrual cycles. This FSH rise occurs many years before the menopause and accompanies the decline of ovarian follicular reserve and fertility rate. The selective FSH rise of late reproductive years might be a consequence of declining inhibin secretion by a reduced pool of ovarian follicles[22]. It was further observed that:

(1) Aging women with elevated FSH and normal estradiol levels have markedly lower inhibin B levels during the follicular phase[23,24];

(2) Luteal phase inhibin A levels are also low in aging cycling women[25];

(3) Follicular phase inhibin B levels decrease earlier than inhibin A during the process of ovarian aging[26];

(4) Both inhibin A and inhibin B levels are nearly undetectable in normal postmenopausal women[26,27].

Activin A levels in peripheral serum are nearly constant in women aged 20–90 years[28], and no significant change is observed after menopause[27]. Furthermore, no correlation exists between serum activin A and FSH levels when both hormones are quantified in a multi-age female population[28]. These findings suggest that the ovary is not the major source of circulating activin A. Serum activin AB is undetectable in normal cycling, postmenopausal and even in pregnant women, using a very sensitive and specific method[29]. With regard to circulating activin B, no data are currently available on its possible changes through reproductive life.

Secretion during normal pregnancy

The human placenta is a source and target for inhibin-related proteins[30]. Inhibin/activin subunits are present in placental cells as demonstrated by *in situ* hybridization[31] and immuno-histochemistry[32,33]. The inhibin immunoreactive sites are located in part in the cytotrophoblast and abundantly in the syncytiotrophoblast cells[32,33]. Dimeric activins and inhibins are found in placental homogenates[34,35], and dimeric activin A is localized in both cyto- and syncytiotrophoblast cells from early to term pregnancy[36]. Cultured placental cells produce activin A[37] and immunoreactive inhibin[32,38], but a precise characterization of inhibin forms produced by the placenta remains to be performed using new assay methods. Activin A and inhibins are also produced by fetal membranes[15] and decidua[39], and assayable activin A and inhibin B levels are found in amniotic and celomic fluid from early gestation[14,40]. Activin B is largely undetectable in maternal serum throughout gestation[41,42] and activin AB is undetectable in maternal serum and amniotic fluid[43].

From early pregnancy, activin A levels are higher than those measured during the menstrual cycle. Minimal changes are seen during the first and second trimesters, but an exponential increase comes with the beginning of the third trimester and is followed by an additional increase as term approaches (Figure 3)[18,41,42]. Activin A is hardly detectable in amniotic fluid from the second trimester and does not appear to change significantly in the remaining gestation period[42].

The changes in inhibin levels throughout gestation have recently been evaluated using the new generation of assays which distinguish between the two dimeric forms (Figure 3). Inhibin A is the major inhibin form in the serum of pregnant women during the second trimester[40]. Serum levels of inhibin A are constantly stable from the 10th to the 20th gestational weeks, but rise markedly during the third trimester[18]. Inhibin B is detected in maternal serum from 8 to 12 weeks of gestation and shows a dramatic increase during the third trimester, maintaining high constant levels up to term and dropping shortly after delivery[44].

The increased inhibin release from the feto-placental tissues may be the main cause of the

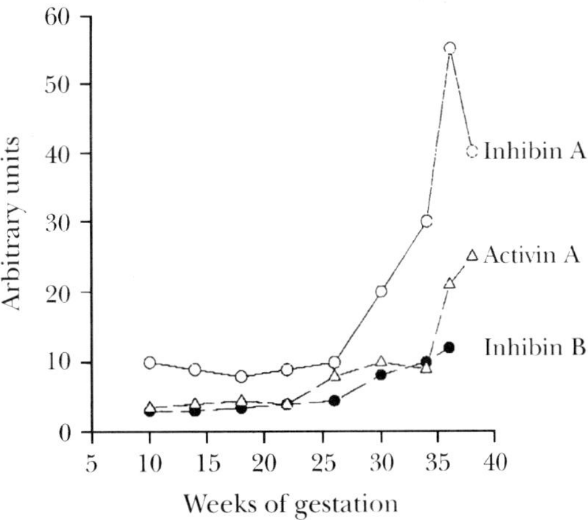

Figure 3 Relative changes of serum activin A, inhibin A and inhibin B levels during pregnancy. Data are expressed in arbitrary units, and the three curves are plotted in different scales, so the absolute levels of one hormone are not comparable to the others. According to Muttukrishna and colleagues[18] and Petraglia and co-workers[44]

suppression of FSH secretion in the pituitary during pregnancy[16]. The study of agonadal women who conceived by oocyte donation revealed the same pattern of inhibin and FSH secretion that characterizes normal pregnancy[43]. Additional effects of inhibins and activins at distant target tissues during pregnancy remain to be investigated.

Diagnostic value in reproductive diseases

Disorders of the menstrual cycle and female infertility

Amenorrheic women with deficiency of gonadotropin releasing hormone (GnRH) secretion due to hypothalamic lesions are an interesting model for studying the role of the hypothalmus–pituitary axis on inhibin secretion. When treated with exogenous GnRH at regular, physiological pulses, these patients display a normal increase of inhibin B levels during the luteal–follicular transition of induced menstrual cycles. In contrast, abnormally low frequency pulses of GnRH administered during luteal–follicular transition result in subphysiological levels of FSH and inhibin B[20]. These findings indicate that the release of inhibin B is dependent on adequate FSH stimulation and may serve to confirm the effectiveness of GnRH replacement therapy on ovarian follicular development.

Activin A levels are substantially augmented in women with hypothalamic amenorrhea of functional origin, i.e. hypogonadotropic state without evidence of hypothalamic lesion, psychiatric disease or other pituitary hypofunction[27]. The significance of this finding is still unknown, but the lack of correlation between activin A and FSH levels in these patients suggests that activin A is elevated in response to a systemic rather than a pituitary imbalance[27].

Inhibins A and B are dramatically reduced in women with premature ovarian failure[27]. Serum levels of both inhibins are as low as in normal postmenopausal women matched for time elapsed since last menstrual period, and do not correlate with patient age, length of amenorrhea or serum gonadotropin levels[27]. Conversely, follicular phase inhibin A and inhibin B levels are not altered in patients with functional hypothalamic amenorrhea[27]. These findings indicate that basal inhibin secretion does not require a normal hypothalamus–pituitary function, but may be suddenly suppressed by primary ovarian failure, regardless of senescence.

Polycystic ovarian syndrome (PCOS) is characterized by the presence of multiple follicles arrested at the early antral stage and deficient FSH pulsatile pattern. Inhibin levels are increased in PCOS patients due to the persistence of a cohort of small follicles that contribute to the pool of circulating inhibins, but the pulsatile rhythm of inhibin B secretion is blunted[45]. Treatment of PCOS patients with low doses of FSH may be sufficient to induce the development of a single dominant follicle which grows in parallel with estradiol and inhibin A levels[46]. Overall, these findings indicate that elevated circulating levels of inhibin B lead to the relative deficit of FSH in PCOS, while the disruption of inhibin B pulsatility may be an additional marker of multiple, incomplete follicular growth. Additionally, the paracrine action of inhibins on stimulating androstenedione production by theca cells may reinforce the hyperandrogenism of PCOS[47].

Inhibin B seems to predict ovarian reserve in older infertile women undergoing the clomiphene citrate challenge test. Patients with an abnormal clomiphene test have lower inhibin B and higher FSH levels, even though estradiol levels and cycle length are not altered[48]. Another test for ovarian reserve, the measurement of FSH on cycle day 3, showed that granulosa cells from patients with high day 3 serum FSH levels (over 10 IU/l) had a diminished capacity for secreting dimeric inhibins[49]. These data suggest that inhibin B is an early indicator of ovarian aging and may become a useful tool for identifying the potential ovarian responsiveness to assisted reproduction therapy.

Ovarian cancer

Experimental data strongly suggest that inhibins have a tumor-suppressing effect in physiological conditions, since knockout mice lacking the inhibin α-subunit gene develop gonadal stromal tumors[50]. However, some gynecological tumors produce and release activins and inhibins into the circulation[51–53], and this may have clinical relevance because postmenopausal women, who normally have almost undetectable serum inhibin levels, are those at greater risk of developing malignant diseases.

Immunoreactive inhibin is significantly increased in most patients with granulosa cell tumor[54,55], but only in some of the women with serous[54–56] and mucinous[57] carcinomas, which are the most frequent types of ovarian cancer. This immunoreactivity is largely due to free α and pro-α C subunits instead of biologically active inhibins. Dimeric inhibin A has poor sensitivity for the diagnosis of ovarian cancer[55,58], but it may serve as a marker for surgical completeness, remission and relapse of the disease[53,59]. Inhibin B levels are markedly increased in women with a granulosa cell tumor and they decrease after clinical remission, indicating that this inhibin form is a major secretory product of granulosa cell tumors[58]. Currently, the measurement of serum activin levels has no established role in the diagnosis of ovarian cancer, although a significant percentage of patients with epithelial (especially serous) ovarian cancer[51,58] or with granulosa cell tumor[58] have elevated serum activin A levels.

Inhibins and activins may be involved in the etiopathogenesis of ovarian tumors. Since activin is a potent mitogen for granulosa cells[60], it has been suggested that epithelial ovarian tumors have an imbalanced expression of inhibin and activin subunits, which may contribute to abnormal cell proliferation[61].

Other neoplasms of the female reproductive system

Activin/inhibin subunit mRNAs are found in endometrial and cervical malignant tumors[52]. Inhibin A and B levels are unchanged, whereas activin A is markedly increased in the serum and uterine secretion of women with endometrial adenocarcinoma[52]. However, in patients with cervical carcinoma, activin A, inhibin A and inhibin B levels either in the circulation or uterine washing do not differ from those in healthy subjects[52].

Immunoreactive inhibin is markedly elevated in molar pregnancy and has a clearance rate higher than human chorionic gonadotropin (hCG), but is a poor marker for prognosis and for detecting recurrence[5]. New studies are expected to validate the usefulness of dimeric inhibins as alternative markers for hydatiform mole and choriocarcinoma. Serum activin A levels in women with trophoblastic disease are higher than in healthy non-pregnant women even after evacuation, but chemotherapy does not seem to affect circulating levels. No correlation was found between changes in activin A and total hCG serum concentrations[62].

Gestational diseases

Activin A is increased in hypertensive complications of pregnancy[63,64], preterm labor[65] and gestational diabetes[65,66], and is particularly elevated in pre-eclampsia[63,67]. A role for activin A in the etiopathogenesis of pre-eclampsia may also be hypothesized, as we have observed an increase of activin A secretion preceding the clinical manifestations of superimposed pre-eclampsia in hypertensive patients[64].

It remains uncertain whether activin A represents a simple component of the stress response to fetal–placental disorders, or also plays a role in the establishment of some of them. Intriguingly, the finding of increased amniotic fluid activin A levels (over 95th percentile) in mid-trimester amniocentesis multiplies the risk of subsequent fetal death; this occurs in spite of unaltered amniotic fluid corticotrophin releasing hormone levels, which are supposed to increase as part of the stress response[68].

Several experimental approaches have suggested a direct involvement of activin A in the onset of preterm labor:

(1) Maternal activin A levels vary in a pulsatile pattern in patients with preterm labor, showing a pulse frequency and amplitude significantly higher than in healthy women[66];

(2) Activin A is higher in women who experience preterm delivery compared to those with preterm labor that responds to tocolytic treatment[65];

(3) Spontaneous labor and preterm labor are characterized by increased synthesis and release of activin A from amniotic and chorionic cells and by an augmented expression of the activin type IIB receptor[69].

Alterations in maternal serum inhibin levels may be indicative of several gestational diseases. Abnormally low levels of inhibin B are present in patients with chronic hypertension in later stages of gestation. Patients with pregnancy complicated by intrauterine growth retardation, pre-eclampsia, or pregnancy-induced hypertension also have lower serum inhibin B levels than gestational age matched controls[44]. Interestingly, no difference in serum inhibin B levels has been observed between healthy controls and patients at risk of, but who did not develop, hypertension[44]. On the other hand, inhibin A levels and subunit pro-α C are increased in pre-eclampsia and show a positive correlation with hCG; thus, inhibin A might be a paracrine modulator or, at least, an additional marker of the placental overgrowth which characterizes this disease[70].

Inhibin α-subunit seems to be overexpressed in the second trimester placental tissue in pregnancies affected by fetal Down's syndrome[71]. The levels of dimeric inhibin A are elevated in maternal serum of women with a Down's syndrome pregnancy[72], whereas inhibin B and pro-α C are not altered, at least between 16 and 19 weeks of gestation[73]. In contrast, inhibin A levels in amniotic fluid are abnormally reduced in this syndrome[74]. Maternal serum activin A is not significantly altered in Down's syndrome compared to an unaffected pregnancy[74].

Conclusions

Activins and inhibins are multifunctional proteins with autocrine, paracrine and endocrine functions modulating almost all aspects of the female reproductive function. Ovarian activins and inhibins are important endocrine messengers for FSH feedback, and are involved in the process of follicular growth and maturation. Pituitary activin takes part in a complex local mechanism regulating FSH release. Placental activins and inhibins are important paracrine modulators of hormonogenesis during all phases of pregnancy, and are possibly involved in the critical immune system adaptation to embryo implantation and placental invasion. Activins may also play a role in the placental signalling for the initiation of labor. Clinically, measurement of activin A, inhibin A and inhibin B levels may be indicated in the following situations:

(1) Diagnosis of granulosa cell tumor;

(2) Evaluation of amenorrhea;

(3) Test of ovarian reserve before ovulation induction.

Future perspectives for clinical use of activin and inhibin measurements include the prognosis of preterm birth in women with preterm labor, prenatal diagnosis of congenital diseases, diagnosis of hypertensive complications of pregnancy, monitoring ovarian function in aging cycling women and screening of gynecological cancer.

Acknowledgement

F.M.R. is supported by a scholarship from CAPES, Brazil.

References

1. McCullagh DR. Dual endocrine activity of the testis. *Science* 1932;76:19–20
2. Keogh EJ, Lee VLWK, Rennie GC, *et al.* Selective suppression of FSH by testicular extracts. *Endocrinology* 1976;98:997–1004
3. Robertson DM, Foulds LM, Leversha L, *et al.* Isolation of inhibin from bovine follicular fluid. *Biochem Biophys Res Commun* 1985;126:220–6
4. Vale W, Rivier C, Vughan J, *et al.* Purification and characterization of an FSH releasing protein from porcine ovarian follicular fluid. *Nature (London)* 1986;321:776–9
5. Wallace EM, Healy DL. Inhibins and activins: roles in clinical practice. *Br J Obstet Gynaecol* 1996; 103:945–56
6. Vale W, Rivier C, Hsueh AJW, *et al.* Chemical and biological characterization of the inhibin family of protein hormones. *Rec Prog Horm Res* 1988;44: 1–34
7. Robertson DM, Sullivan J, Cahir N. Inhibin forms in human plasma. *J Endocrinol* 1995;144:261–9
8. Ueno N, Ling N, Ying SY, *et al.* Isolation and partial characterization of follistatin: a single-chain Mr 35 000 monomeric protein that inhibits the release of follicle-stimulating hormone. *Proc Natl Acad Sci USA* 1987;84:8282–6
9. Mather JP, Roberts PE, Krummen LA. Follistatin modulates activin activity in a cell and tissue-specific manner. *Endocrinology* 1993;132:2732–4
10. Tsuchida K, Vaughan J, Wiater E, *et al.* Inactivation of activin-dependent transcription by kinase-deficient activin receptors. *Endocrinology* 1995;136:5493–503
11. Lebrun JJ, Chen Y, Vale WW. Receptor serine kinases and signaling by activins. In: Aono T, Sugino H, Vale WW, eds. *Inhibin, Activin and Follistatin: Regulatory Functions in System and Cell Biology.* New York: Springer-Verlag, 1997:1–20
12. Lebrun JJ, Vale WW. Activin and inhibin have antagonistic effects on ligand-dependent hetero-merization of the type I and type II activin receptors and human erythroid differentiation. *Mol Cell Biol* 1997;17:1682–91
13. Roberts VJ, Barth S, El-Roeiy A, *et al.* Expression of inhibin/activin subunits and follistatin messenger ribonucleic acids and proteins in ovarian follicles and the corpus luteum during the human menstrual cycle. *J Clin Endocrinol Metab* 1993;77:1402–10
14. Luisi S, Battaglia C, Florio P, *et al.* Activin A and inhibin B in extra-embryonic coelomic and amniotic fluids, and maternal serum in early pregnancy. *Placenta* 1998;19:435–8
15. Petraglia F, Anceschi MM, Calzà L, *et al.* Inhibin and activin in human fetal membranes: evidence for a local effect on prostaglandin release. *J Clin Endocrinol Metab* 1993;77:542–8
16. Qu J, Thomas K. Inhibin and activin production in human placenta. *Endocr Rev* 1995;16:485–507
17. Yohkaichiya T, Polson D, O'Connor AE, *et al.* Concentrations of immunoactive inhibin in serum during human pregnancy: evidence for an ovarian contribution. *Reprod Fertil Dev* 1991;3: 671–8
18. Muttukrishna S, Fowler PA, George L, *et al.* Changes in peripheral serum levels of total activin A during the human menstrual cycle and pregnancy. *J Clin Endocrinol Metab* 1996;81: 3328–34
19. Groome NP, Illingworth PJ, O'Brien M, *et al.* Measurement of dimeric inhibin B throughout the human menstrual cycle. *J Clin Endocrinol Metab* 1996;81:1401–5
20. Welt C, Martin KA, Taylor AE, *et al.* Frequency modulation of follicle-stimulating hormone (FSH) during the luteal–follicular transition: evidence for FSH control of inhibin B in normal women. *J Clin Endocrinol Metab* 1997;82:2645–52
21. Crofton PM, Illingworth PJ, Groome NP, *et al.* Changes in dimeric inhibin A and B during normal early puberty in boys and girls. *Clin Endocrinol (Oxf)* 1997;46:109–14
22. Lenton EA, de Kretser DM, Woodward AJ, *et al.* Inhibin concentrations throughout the menstrual cycles of normal, infertile, and older women compared with those during spontaneous conception cycles. *J Clin Endocrinol Metab* 1991;73:1180–90
23. Klein NA, Illingworth PJ, Groome NP, *et al.* Decreased inhibin B secretion is associated with the monotropic FSH rise in older, ovulatory women: a study of serum and follicular fluid levels of dimeric inhibin A and B in spontaneous menstrual cycles. *J Clin Endocrinol Metab* 1996;81: 2742–5
24. Reame NE, Wyman TL, Phillips DJ, *et al.* Net increase in stimulatory input resulting from a decrease in inhibin B and an increase in activin A may contribute in part to the rise in follicular phase follicle-stimulating hormone of aging cycling women. *J Clin Endocrinol Metab* 1998;83: 3302–7
25. Danforth DR, Arbogast LK, Mroueh J, *et al.* Dimeric inhibin: a direct marker of ovarian aging. *Fertil Steril* 1998;70:119–23
26. Burger HG, Cachir N, Robertson DM, *et al.* Serum inhibins A and B fall differentially as FSH rises in perimenopausal women. *Clin Endocrinol (Oxf)* 1998;48:809–13

27. Petraglia F, Hartmann B, Luisi S, *et al.* Low levels of serum inhibin A and inhibin B in women with hypergonadotropic amenorrhea and evidence of high levels of activin A in women with hypothalamic amenorrhea. *Fertil Steril* 1998;70:907–12

28. Loria P, Petraglia F, Concari M, *et al.* Influence of age and sex on serum concentrations of total dimeric activin A. *Eur J Endocrinol* 1998;139:487–92

29. Evans LW, Muttukrishna S, Knight PG, *et al.* Development, validation and application of a two-site enzyme-linked immunosorbent assay for activin-AB. *J Endocrinol* 1997;153:221–30

30. Petraglia F, Florio P, Nappi C, *et al.* Peptide signaling in human placenta and membranes: autocrine, paracrine, and endocrine mechanisms. *Endocr Rev* 1996;17:156–86

31. Petraglia F, Woodruff TK, Botticelli G, *et al.* Gonadotropin-releasing hormone, inhibin, and activin in human placenta: evidence for a common cellular localization. *J Clin Endocrinol Metab* 1992;74:1184–8

32. Petraglia F, Sawchenko P, Lim ATW, *et al.* Localization, secretion, and action of inhibin in human placenta. *Science* 1987;237:189

33. Minami S, Yamoto M, Nakano R. Immunohistochemical localization of inhibin/activin subunits in human placenta. *Obstet Gynecol* 1992;80:410–14

34. Yokoyama Y, Nakamura T, Nakamura R, *et al.* Identification of activins and follistatin proteins in human follicular fluid and placenta. *J Clin Endocrinol Metab* 1995;80:915–21

35. de Kretser DM, Foulds LM, Hancock M, *et al.* Partial characterization of inhibin, activin, and follistatin in the term human placenta. *J Clin Endocrinol Metab* 1994;79:502–7

36. Rabinovici J, Goldsmith PC, Librach CL, *et al.* Localization and regulation of the activin-A dimer in human placental cells. *J Clin Endocrinol Metab* 1992;75:571–6

37. Keelan JA, Groome NP, Mitchell MD. Regulation of activin-A production by human amnion, decidua and placenta *in vitro* by pro-inflammatory cytokines. *Placenta* 1998;19:429–34

38. Qu J, Ying SY, Thomas K. Inhibin production and secretion in human placental cells cultured *in vitro*. *Obstet Gynecol* 1992;79:705–12

39. Petraglia F, Calza L, Garuti GC, *et al.* Presence and synthesis of inhibin subunits in human decidua. *J Clin Endocrinol Metab* 1990;71:487–92

40. Wallace EM, Riley SC, Crossley JA, *et al.* Dimeric inhibins in amniotic fluid, maternal serum, and fetal serum in human pregnancy. *J Clin Endocrinol Metab* 1997;82:218–22

41. Woodruff TK, Sluss P, Wang E, *et al.* Activin A and follistatin are dynamically regulated during human pregnancy. *J Endocrinol* 1997;152:167–74

42. Petraglia F, Garg S, Florio P, *et al.* Activin A and activin B measured in maternal serum, cord blood serum and amniotic fluid during human pregnancy. *Endocr J* 1993;1:323–7

43. Santoro N, Schneyer AL, Ibrahim J, *et al.* Gonadotropin and inhibin concentrations in early pregnancy in women with and without corpora lutea. *Obstet Gynecol* 1992;79:579–85

44. Petraglia F, Luisi S, Benedetto C, *et al.* Changes of dimeric inhibin B levels in maternal serum throughout healthy gestation and in women with gestational diseases. *J Clin Endocrinol Metab* 1997;82:2991–5

45. Lockwood GM, Muttukrishna S, Groome NP, *et al.* Mid-follicular phase pulses of inhibin B are absent in polycystic ovarian syndrome and are initiated by successful laparoscopic ovarian diathermy: a possible mechanism regulating emergence of the dominant follicle. *J Clin Endocrinol Metab* 1998;83:1730–5

46. Anderson RA, Groome NP, Baird DT. Inhibin A and inhibin B in women with polycystic ovarian syndrome during treatment with FSH to induce mono-ovulation. *Clin Endocrinol (Oxf)* 1998;48:577–84

47. Pigny P, Desailloud R, Cortet Rudelli C, *et al.* Serum alpha-inhibin levels in polycystic ovary syndrome: relationship to the serum androstenedione level. *J Clin Endocrinol Metab* 1997;82:1939–43

48. Hofmann GE, Danforth DR, Seifer DB. Inhibin-B: the physiologic basis of the clomiphene citrate challenge test for ovarian reserve screening. *Fertil Steril* 1998;69:474–7

49. Seifer DB, Gardiner AC, Lambert Messerlian G, *et al.* Differential secretion of dimeric inhibin in cultured luteinized granulosa cells as a function of ovarian reserve. *J Clin Endocrinol Metab* 1996;81:736–9

50. Matzuk MM, Finegold MJ, Su JJ, *et al.* α-Inhibin is a tumour-suppressor gene with gonadal specificity in mice. *Nature (London)* 1992;360:313

51. Welt C, Lambert Messerlian G, Zheng W, *et al.* Presence of activin, inhibin, and follistatin in epithelial ovarian carcinoma. *J Clin Endocrinol Metab* 1997;82:3720–7

52. Petraglia F, Florio P, Luisi S, *et al.* Expression and secretion of inhibin and activin in normal and neoplastic uterine tissues. High levels of serum activin A in women with endometrial and cervical carcinoma. *J Clin Endocrinol Metab* 1998;83:1194–200

53. Yamashita K, Yamoto M, Shikone T, *et al.* Production of inhibin A and inhibin B in human ovarian sex cord stromal tumors. *Am J Obstet Gynecol* 1997;177:1450–7

54. Burger HG, Baile A, Drummond AE, *et al.* Inhibin and ovarian cancer. *J Reprod Immunol* 1998;39:77–87

55. Burger HG, Robertson DM, Cahir N, *et al.* Characterization of inhibin immunoreactivity in postmenopausal women with ovarian tumours. *Clin Endocrinol (Oxf)* 1996;44:413–18

56. Lambert Messerlian GM, Steinhoff M, Zheng W, *et al.* Multiple immunoreactive inhibin proteins in serum from postmenopausal women with epithelial ovarian cancer. *Gynecol Oncol* 1997;65: 512–16

57. Healy DL, Burger HG. Inhibin: a serum marker for mucinous ovarian cancer. *N Engl J Med* 1992; 326:466–71

58. Petraglia F, Luisi S, Pautier P, *et al.* Inhibin B is the major form of inhibin/activin family secreted by granulosa cell tumors. *J Clin Endocrinol Metab* 1998;83:1029–32

59. Cooke I, O'Brien M, Charnock FM, *et al.* Inhibin as a marker for ovarian cancer. *Br J Cancer* 1995; 71:1046–50

60. Mather JP, Li RH, Phillips DJ, *et al.* Inhibin and activin as paracrine regulators of gonadal function: *in vitro* model systems. In Aono T, Sugino H, Vale WW, eds. *Inhibin, Activin and Follistatin: Regulatory Functions in System and Cell Biology*. New York: Springer-Verlag, 1997:51–62

61. Zheng W, Luo MP, Welt C, *et al.* Imbalanced expression of inhibin and activin subunits in primary epithelial ovarian cancer. *Gynecol Oncol* 1998;69:23–31

62. Florio P, Luisi S, Casarosa E, *et al.* Serum levels of dimeric activin A are not a marker of placental tumors in the course of chemotherapy. *J Endocrinol Invest* 1998;21:166–9

63. Muttukrishna S, Knight PG, Groome NP, *et al.* Activin A and inhibin A as possible endocrine markers for pre-eclampsia. *Lancet* 1997;349: 1285–8

64. Petraglia F, Aguzzoli L, Gallinelli A, *et al.* Hypertension in pregnancy: changes in activin A maternal serum concentration. *Placenta* 1995;16: 447–54

65. Petraglia F, De Vita D, Gallinelli A, *et al.* Abnormal concentration of maternal serum activin-A in gestational diseases. *J Clin Endocrinol Metab* 1995;80:558–61

66. Gallinelli A, Gallo R, Genazzani AD, *et al.* Episodic secretion of activin A in pregnant women. *Eur J Endocrinol* 1996;135:340–4

67. Petraglia F, Giuntini A, Florio P, *et al.* Changes of activin A secretion in gestational diseases. In Aono T, Sugino H, Vale WW, eds. *Inhibin, Activin and Follistatin: Regulatory Functions in System and Cell Biology*. New York: Springer-Verlag, 1997: 96–103

68. Petraglia F, Gomez R, Luisi S, *et al.* Increased midtrimester amniotic fluid activin A: a risk factor for subsequent fetal death. *Am J Obstet Gynecol* 1999;180:194–7

69. Petraglia F, Di Blasio AM, Florio P, *et al.* High levels of fetal membrane activin beta A and activin receptor IIB mRNAs and augmented concentration of amniotic fluid activin A in women in term or preterm labor. *J Endocrinol* 1997;154: 95–101

70. Fraser RF II, McAsey ME, Coney P. Inhibin-A and pro-alpha C are elevated in pre-eclamptic pregnancy and correlate with human chorionic gonadotropin. *Am J Reprod Immunol* 1998;40: 37–42

71. Lambert Messerlian GM, Luisi S, Florio P, *et al.* Second trimester levels of maternal serum total activin A and placental inhibin/activin alpha and betaA subunit messenger ribonucleic acids in Down syndrome pregnancy. *Eur J Endocrinol* 1998;138:425–9

72. Wallace EM, Grant VE, Swanston IA, *et al.* Evaluation of maternal serum dimeric inhibin-A as a first trimester marker of Down's syndrome. *Prenat Diagn* 1995;15:359–62

73. Wallace EM, Crossley JA, Riley SC, *et al.* Inhibin-B and pro-alphaC-containing inhibins in amniotic fluid from chromosomally normal and Down syndrome pregnancies. *Prenat Diagn* 1998;18: 213–17

74. Wallace EM, Crossley JA, Ritoe SC, *et al.* Inhibin-A in amniotic fluid in chromosomally normal and Down's syndrome pregnancies. *J Endocrinol* 1997;152:109–12

Involvement of interleukin-1 and interleukin-1 receptor antagonist in *in vitro* embryo development among women undergoing *in vitro* fertilization–embryo transfer

24

S. D. Spandorfer, A. Neuer, H.-C. Liu, L. Bivis, R. Clarke, L. Veeck, Z. Rosenwaks and S. S. Witkin

Introduction

Despite major advances in *in vitro* fertilization–embryo transfer (IVF–ET), most patients are not successful in an initial cycle of IVF–ET. Enhancing the development of human embryos *in vitro* has remained a major concern for IVF–ET. Many strategies have been utilized, which have included assisted hatching[1], improved culture media[2] and co-culture techniques[3,6]. Co-culture techniques appear to improve the pre-embryonic development *in vitro*[3].

A number of studies have evaluated the effect of various somatic cell lines on human pre-embryo development. A significant decrease in embryo fragmentation was found in embryos grown on co-culture when compared to conventional medium[4]. Higher rates of blastocyst formation when embryos were co-cultured on Fallopian tube epithelium, compared to conventionally cultured embryos, indicates improved pre-embryo development[5]. In a randomized trial, Weimer and colleagues found that, utilizing bovine oviductal cells for co-culture, the embryos in co-culture had significantly more blastomeres and fewer cytoplasmic fragments than conventionally grown embryos[6].

We have also recently demonstrated that human autologous endometrial co-culture improves pre-embryo development in human IVF–ET[7]. The fragmentation rate was significantly less for the pre-embryos in the co-culture

system, compared to non-co-cultured pre-embryos. Also, at the time of pre-embryo replacement, the mean number of blastomeres per pre-embryo was greater for the co-cultured pre-embryos, compared to the non-co-cultured pre-embryos.

Mechanisms to explain the actions of co-culture to improve embryonic development include cell–cell interactions, cytokine and growth factor elaboration and detoxification of the culture medium[8,9]. In this study, we evaluated the role of interleukin-1 (IL-1) and interleukin-1 receptor antagonist (IL-1ra) production by human endometrial cells on *in vitro* embryo development and IVF outcome.

The IL-1 system is composed of a family of peptides. There are two agonists, IL-1α and IL-1β, and one antagonist, IL-1ra. Endometrial cells secrete IL-1[10]. IL-1 receptors are located on the early human embryo[10]. Thus, there exists the potential for interactions between the IL-1 secreted by the endometrium and the early embryo. In this study, we evaluated the potential role of IL-1 and IL-1ra in early human embryo development.

Specifically, we examined the communication in the human endometrial co-culture system between the IL-1 cytokines and the human pre-embryo. Furthermore, because embryos are often cultured in media supplemented with maternal serum, we also investigated the effect of IL-1α, IL-1β and IL-1ra in maternal sera in patients undergoing conventional IVF without utilizing co-culture techniques.

Materials and methods

This study was divided into two parts. First, we evaluated 160 patients undergoing conventional IVF. The second part of the study involved patients with a history of multiple implantation failures undergoing IVF and utilizing autologous endometrial co-culture.

IL-1 cytokines in maternal serum

We retrieved stored maternal serum (from matched pregnant and non-pregnant patients after IVF) that had been used to supplement human tubal fluid (HTF) medium for *in vitro* embryo growth. We analyzed for IL-1α, IL-1β and IL-1ra and correlated the findings with embryonic development and IVF outcome. These patients were matched for age, stimulation protocol, number of previous attempts, stimulation response and the number of embryos transferred. Sera collected for medium supplementation drawn 1 day before oocyte retrieval (or 1 day post-human chorionic gonadotropin (hCG) administration) were assayed utilizing commercial enzyme linked immunosorbent assay (ELISA) kits. Embryo grade was on a scale of 1–5 (1 = best). High-quality embryos were defined as grade 1 or 2.

IL-1 cytokines in autologous endometrial co-culture

Twenty-nine patients with a history of multiple implantation failures (at least two) after IVF–ET were enrolled in our autologous endometrial co-culture (AECC) study. Patients had previously undergone at least two embryo transfer cycles without success.

Endometrial co-culture

Endometrium was obtained from each patient in a non-medicated cycle prior to her IVF attempt. The endometrium was obtained by a luteal phase endometrial biopsy using a Pipelle endometrial suction curette (Unimar, Wilton, CT, USA). The biopsy was performed 3–10 days after the luteinizing hormone (LH) surge was detected by a urinary ovulation predictor kit. The digestion and separation of the endometrium has been previously described[11].

In brief, the tissue was then minced into small pieces (1–2 mm^3) and washed with Hank's balanced salt solution (HBSS) (Gibco BRL, Grand Island, NY, USA) supplemented with 5000 μg/100 ml penicillin–streptomycin (Gibco BRL, Grand Island, NY, USA) to remove excess red blood cells and mucus.

Incubation of the tissue pieces for 5 min at 37 °C in a shaking water bath in 10 ml of HBSS containing 0.2% collagenase type 2 (SIGMA, St Louis, MO, USA) was then performed. Cell clumps were dispersed by brisk aspiration through a sterile transfer pipette. The digested tissue pieces were then allowed to settle by differential sedimentation at unit gravity for 5 min. After sedimentation, the supernatant, containing a mixture of single stromal cells and small intact glands, were transferred into a separate 15-ml polyethylene test-tube and centrifuged at 400g for 5 min. The pellet was resuspended in RPMI Medium 1640 (Gibco BRL, Grand Island, NY, USA) supplemented with 10% patient's serum (RPMI/10% serum) and 5000 μg/100 ml penicillin–streptomycin. The above steps were repeated four times, resulting in a combined 4 ml of single stromal cells mixed with small glands. This stroma and small gland sample underwent another differential sedimentation at unit gravity for 45 min to separate the majority of small glands from the single stromal cells remaining in solution. The supernatant, containing the stroma-enriched fraction, was centrifuged at 400g for 5 min and the cell pellet was resuspended in RPM/10% patient serum. A small aliquot of the sample was diluted 1:1 with Trypan blue stain 0.4% (Gibco BRL, Grand Island, NY, USA), and cell yield and viability were determined quantitatively on a hemocytometer. Tissue culture flasks (25 cm^2) were seeded with approximately 5×10^5 cells.

The tissue pieces, which remained after the four digests, contained predominately intact glands mixed with undigested connective tissue and stromal clumps. Concurrently, the glands were further purified by resuspension in 10 ml of HBSS. After approximately 30 s, the largest fragments (stromal clumps, undigested tissue) settled to the bottom of the 15-ml test tube and the top 8 ml, which had a 'snowflake' appearance (glands and single stromal cells), was transferred to another 15-ml test tube and allowed to settle for 30 min at unit gravity. This sedimentation allowed the majority of glands to form a pellet at the bottom of the test-tube while leaving the remaining single stromal cells in the supernatant that was removed and discarded. This glandular-enriched pellet was then resuspended in RPMI/10% serum and plated into one 25-cm^2 tissue culture flask. After several hours of incubation for the glandular-enriched pellet, the supernatant was removed and replated in a new tissue flask. This was done to improve the purity of the glandular component, based on the fact that stromal cells plate quickly and glands are much slower to attach to the tissue flask.

The seeded tissue flasks were maintained at 37 °C in a 5% CO_2 air atmosphere and the culture medium was changed every 2–3 days. After approximately 1 week, the cells reached confluence and were released with Trypsin–ethylenediaminetetra-acetic acid (EDTA) (Gibco BRL, Grand Island, NY, USA). The cells were cryopreserved in a 15% glycerol solution and frozen at –70 °C overnight then transferred to liquid nitrogen storage.

Approximately equal mixtures of the glandular and stromal cells were thawed 3 days prior to placement of the human embryos on the co-culture cells. Cell count and viability were determined, and about 4×10^5 cells were seeded into a four-well tissue culture plate containing 800 µl of Ham's F-10 with 15% human serum. Usually, three wells were plated. In general, about 90% confluence was achieved when the human embryos were placed into the co-culture system. Conditioned medium was changed every 1–2 days prior to exposure to human embryos.

Embryos were placed on AECC the day after oocyte retrieval when fertilization was determined. Fresh medium consisting of Ham's F-10 with 15% human serum was utilized prior to placement of the embryos on the co-culture. Embryos were grouped and placed in one or two of the wells. The embryos remained on AECC until just prior to the embryo transfer. During this 2-day period, the medium was not changed. Immediately after removing the embryos from the AECC wells preparation for embryo transfer, the conditioned medium was collected, centrifuged and stored at –20 °C. For each of the 29 patients in this study, conditioned medium was collected from AECC wells that were and were not exposed to human embryos.

IVF methods

Patients were treated with standard ovulation induction protocols and underwent IVF–ET as previously described[12]. In brief, most women were treated with luteal phase leuprolide acetate (Lupron; Tap Pharmaceuticals, Deerfield, IL, USA), 1 mg subcutaneously daily until ovarian suppression was achieved. Women not treated with luteal leuprolide acetate began stimulation on day 2 of their treatment cycle. Ovarian stimulation was then effected with a combination of gonadotropins (human menopausal gonadotropin (hMG) and/or pure follicle stimulating hormone (FSH): (Pergonal or Metrodin; Serono, Waltham, MA, USA), employing a step-down protocol[5]. Human chorionic gonadotropin (hCG) was administered (3300–10 000 IU) when at least two follicles reached or exceeded 16–17 mm mean diameter as measured by transvaginal ultrasound. Oocytes were harvested by transvaginal ultrasound-guided follicular puncture, 35–36 h after hCG administration.

Conventional oocyte insemination or micromanipulation was performed as indicated. Morphologically normal embryos were transferred into the uterine cavity approximately 72 h after retrieval. The number of embryos transferred was dependent on maternal age, according to our standard protocol. In general, three embryos were transferred to patients under 35 years of age, patients 35–40 years of age received four embryos, and patients over 40 underwent transfer of up to five embryos when available. Methylprednisolone (16 mg/day) and tetracycline (250 mg every 6 h) were administered for 4 days to all patients commencing on the day of oocyte retrieval. Progesterone supplementation was initiated on the third day after hCG administration (25–50 mg/day intramuscularly), and was continued until the sonographic assessment of the pregnancy.

IL-1 ELISA

IL-1 (IL-1α, IL-1β, IL-1ra) ELISA was performed on all 29 samples utilizing commercially available kits. For IL-1α, the interassay and intra-assay variation was 5.2% and 3.5%, respectively. The minimum level of detection was 0.5 pg/ml. For IL-1raβ, the interassay and intra-assay variation was 5.5% and 5.5%, respectively. The minimum level of detection was 14 pg/ml. For IL-1β, the interassay and intra-assay variation was 5.4% and 3.9%, respectively. The minimum level of detection was 0.5 pg/ml. Curves were generated from standards provided in the kit, and the values were determined from these curves. IL-1 (IL-1α, IL-1β, IL-1ra) was measured in each of the supernatants as well as medium alone (Ham's F-10 supplemented with 15% patient's serum). Prior to performing the assay, the supernatants were brought to room temperature. Cross-reactivity with other cytokines was insignificant.

Statistical analysis

Data are presented as mean (± standard deviation). The data were not normally distributed, and, therefore, continuous data were compared utilizing non-parametric tests. Categorical data were compared utilizing χ^2 analysis. A p value of < 0.05 was considered significant.

Results

IL-1 cytokines in maternal serum

All of the patients underwent a luteal leuprolide stimulation cycle and had normal random day-3 levels before beginning their stimulation. There were no differences in the pregnant and non-pregnant patients with respect to age, number of previous stimulations, peak estradiol levels, number of oocytes retrieved and number of embryos transferred (Table 1). Of the 80 patients with a positive pregnancy test, 69 progressed to a viable ongoing pregnancy (beyond 20 weeks), five underwent a clinical miscarriage (pregnancy loss after fetal cardiac activity was confirmed) and six had a biochemical pregnancy (no fetal cardiac activity confirmed).

IL-1α was detected in only one patient's serum. No differences were found in the mean values of the cytokines based on the etiology of infertility. Table 2 indicates the relationships of IL-1β and IL-1ra with embryo quality and pregnancy outcome. Relative antagonism of the IL-1 cytokines was positively associated with *in vitro*

Table 1 Characteristics of patients analyzed for maternal serum presence of interleukin 1 (IL-1) cytokines. Values are expressed as mean ± SD

	Pregnant ($n = 80$)	Not pregnant ($n = 80$)
Age (years)	33.2 ± 2.1	33.0 ± 2.2
Previous stimulations (n)	1.3 ± 0.5	1.3 ± 0.3
Oocytes (n)	12.6 ± 4.3	13.0 ± 4.6
E_2 level (pg/ml)	1222 ± 121	1262 ± 117
Embryo transfers (n)	3.2 ± 1.1	3.3 ± 1.2

E_2, estradiol

Table 2 Relationships of interleukin-1β (IL-1β) and interleukin-1 receptor antagonist (IL-1ra) with embryo quality and pregnancy outcome

	IL-1β			IL-1ra		
	> 10 pg/ml	< 10 pg/ml	p Value	> 900 pg/ml	< 900 pg/ml	p Value
High-quality embryos*	2/22 (9%)	69/125 (55.2%)	0.001	36/51 (70.6%)	48/109 (44%)	0.003
Clinical pregnancy[†]	2/22 (9%)	61/125 (48.8%)	0.001	33/51 (64.7%)	41/109 (37.6%)	0.003

*High-quality embryos, grade 1 or 2 from scale grades 1–5 (1 = best, 5 = worst); [†]clinical pregnancy, presence of fetal cardiac activity

embryonic development and IVF outcome. Detectable levels of IL-1β were negatively associated with *in vitro* embryonic development and IVF outcome. Conversely, lower levels of IL-1ra were negatively associated with *in vitro* embryonic development and IVF outcome.

IL-1 cytokines in autologous endometrial co-culture

The average age of the patients was 38.3 ($\pm$ 3.8) years and each had an average of 3.3 ($\pm$ 1.9) prior attempts at IVF–ET. The etiologies of infertility were as follows: male (11), idiopathic (8), tubal (9) and endometriosis (1). Twelve of the 29 patients (41.4%) established a clinical pregnancy after IVF–ET when utilizing AECC.

Effect of co-culture on embryo development

Embryos grown on AECC demonstrated a significant improvement in number of blastomeres and less fragmentation when compared to embryos grown in conventional medium without ECC (6.4 ± 1.3 vs. 5.5 ± 1.2 blastomeres and $14.6 \pm 9.3\%$ vs. $18.4 \pm 9.8\%$ fragmentation; $p < 0.008$ and 0.003, respectively).

Interleukin-1 levels in co-culture

Table 3 gives IL-1 (IL-1α, IL-1β, IL-1ra) levels in the supernatant of the wells utilized for AECC. IL-1 levels were not different with regard to exposure or non-exposure to an embryo. However, the IL-1 levels in both groups of supernatants (exposed or non-exposed to embryos) were greater than that found in the medium alone (15% Ham's F-10).

Interleukin-1 levels and outcome

When IL-1α and IL-1β were undetectable in the conditioned medium, the embryos grown in ECC were of improved quality, compared to the embryos grown only in conventional medium (IL-1α: 6.5 vs. 5.5 blastomeres, $p = 0.03$, Wilcoxon signed rank test; IL-1β: 6.6 vs. 5.3 blastomeres, $p = 0.002$, Wilcoxon signed rank test). Conversely, IL-1ra levels in the conditioned medium were positively associated with embryo quality (IL-1ra: 6.7 vs. 5.7 blastomeres, $p = 0.04$, Wilcoxon signed rank test). Mean IL-1β levels were inversely correlated with pregnancy outcome (3.3 pg/ml vs. 27.1 pg/ml; $p = 0.008$, Mann–Whitney test). IL-1α and IL-1ra levels were not associated with pregnancy outcome.

Discussion

This study suggests a role for the IL-1 cytokines in early pregnancy. The presence of the IL-1 cytokines in maternal serum, when utilized to supplement the medium for *in vitro* early embryo growth, was strongly associated with outcome. Relative antagonism of the IL-1 system was associated with higher-quality embryos and higher clinical pregnancy rates. This would suggest that the IL-1 cytokines may play an important role at the very early stage of development of the embryo (1–8 cells).

We have also demonstrated the importance of IL-1 production by endometrial cells. There was an overall clinical pregnancy rate of 41.4% when embryos from patients with a history of multiple IVF failures were grown on AECC. Similarly, there was an improvement in embryo quality when comparing AECC to conventional medium. Although many authors[4–7] have shown

Table 3 Interleukin-1 (IL-1) cytokines in autologous endometrial co-culture (AECC). Values are expressed as mean $\pm$ SE

	IL-1α (pg/ml)	IL-1β (pg/ml)	IL-1ra (pg/ml)
AECC + embryo	10.4 ± 6.9	17.4 ± 9.7	419.9 ± 135.9
AECC − embryo	10.8 ± 5.3	16.4 ± 8.9	420.8 ± 133.3
15% Ham's F-10*	2.4 ± 6.7	5.4 ± 1.2	128.0 ± 34.6

AECC + embryo, AECC exposed to an embryo; AECC − embryo, AECC not exposed to an embryo; *15% Ham's F-10 was medium utilized for AECC and embryos beneficial results when utilizing AECC techniques, the mechanism of this action remains largely unknown. Given the potential for interactions between the IL-1 cytokines secreted by the endometrium and the early embryo, which contains receptors for IL-1, we evaluated the potential role of IL-1 communication in the human endometrial co-culture system.

We have demonstrated that the IL-1 cytokines are elaborated in our autologous endometrial co-culture system. Furthermore, the antagonism of IL-1 activity by IL-1ra in early embryo development appears to be beneficial. De Los Santos and colleagues demonstrated, in a single embryo that developed into a blastocyst, that antagonism of the IL-1 system occurred with development of the embryo (i.e. the IL-1α + IL-1β/IL-1ra decreased as the embryo progressed from the four-cell to the blastocyst stage)[10]. They also demonstrated that the elaboration of IL-1 cytokines required the presence of co-culture with either endometrial epithelium or conditioned medium from endometrial epithelium. This suggested an obligatory role of the endometrium in regulating the embryonic IL-1 system.

In the present study, we were unable to determine whether the IL-1 cytokines were elaborated from the AECC cells or from the embryos or a combination of the two. However, given the vast differences in numbers of cells contained in each, it seems reasonable to attribute the IL-1 levels to the AECC.

While we have found overall associations between embryonic development and IL-1 cytokines in our autologous endometrial co-culture system, this does not establish that the improvement is a direct effect of these cytokines. IL-1ra is predominantly produced in the endometrial epithelium[13]. Therefore, IL-1ra may simply be a marker for the importance of endometrial epithelium in our co-culture system. Our previous work evaluating granulocyte–macrophage colony-stimulating factor (GM-CSF) has suggested the importance of the endometrial epithelium in the co-culture system[14]. IL-1β is, on the other hand, produced in the stromal tissue in the endometrium[13]. Therefore, co-culture cells with higher levels of IL-1ra and lower levels

of IL-1β may simply reflect the best combination of epithelium and stroma that we utilize in our co-culture system.

In addition, other work has suggested that IL-1β production by the stroma significantly increases by cycle day 23, with decidualization of the stroma[15]. The relatively poor performance of co-culture with elevated IL-1β levels may suggest that biopsies performed after this date are not as effective. However, this is not in agreement with our previous work that demonstrated autologous endometrial co-culture was effective in both the mid- and late luteal periods[16]. When embryos were randomly assigned to AECC or conventional medium, embryonic development was improved only when utilizing mid- and late luteal endometrial biopsies, while early (day 1 to day 4 after the LH surge) luteal biopsies were not associated with improved embryonic development. Furthermore, the pregnancy rate was significantly higher in patients undergoing endometrial co-culture with tissue utilized from a mid- or late luteal biopsy. Thus, the associations with IL-1β do not appear to be as a result of decidual changes to the endometrium.

In contradistinction to our findings of a positive correlation with IL-1ra, in mice, high levels of exogenous IL-1ra have been shown to block implantation[17]. This may reflect a varying concentration of the antagonist : agonist or may reflect a differing function of the IL-1 system at a later point in embryonic development.

Finally, IL-1β levels are elevated in local infections as this cytokine recruits and activates macrophages. Therefore, the elevated IL-1β levels may reflect an underlying, clinically asymptomatic, endometritis. We are currently investigating this possibility.

Conclusion

The IL-1 cytokines are intimately involved with early embryo development. Relative IL-1 antagonism in maternal serum utilized to grow embryos was associated with the quality of the embryos and pregnancy outcome. Autologous endometrial co-culture is beneficial for the patient with a history of multiple IVF failures. The IL-1 cytokines are produced by our autologous endometrial co-culture system. In confirming our work on maternal serum utilized to supplement embryo media, we have demonstrated a positive association between antagonism of the IL-1 cytokines and improved embryonic development when utilizing autologous endometrial co-culture. This study further demonstrates the importance of the IL-1 cytokines in early embryo development.

References

1. Liu H-C, Cohen J, Alikani M, Noyes N, Rosenwaks Z. Assisted hatching facilitates earlier implantation. *Fertil Steril* 1993;60:871–5
2. Gardner DK, Lane M. Culture and selection of viable blastocysts: a feasible proposition for human IVF? *Hum Reprod Update* 1997;3:367–82
3. Thibodeaux J, Godke R. *In vitro* enhancement of early stage embryos with coculture. *Arch Pathol Lab Med* 1992;116:364–72
4. Nietro FS, Watkins WB, Lopata A, Baker HWG, Edgar DH. The effects of coculture with autologous cryopreserved endometrial cells on human *in vitro* fertilization and early embryo morphology: a randomized study. *J Assist Reprod Genet* 1996;13:386–9
5. Vald M, Walker D, Kennedy RC. Nuclei number in human embryos cocultured with human ampullary cells. *Hum Reprod* 1996;11:1678–86
6. Wiener KE, Hoffman DI, Maxson WS, *et al.* Embryonic morphology and rate of implantation of human embryos following coculture on bovine oviductal epithelial cells. *Hum Reprod* 1993;8:97–101
7. Barmat LI, Liu H-C, Spandorfer SD, *et al.* Human preembryo development on autologous endometrial coculture versus conventional medium: a randomized trial. *Fertil Steril* 1998;70:1109–13
8. Bongso A, Ng SC, Fong C-Y, Ratnam S. Co-cultures: a new lead in embryo quality improvement for assisted reproduction. *Fertil Steril* 1991;56:179–91
9. Dirnfeld M, Goldman S, Gonene Y, Koifman M, Calderon I, Abramovici H. A simplified coculture system with luteinized granulosa cells improves embryo quality and implantation rates: a controlled study. *Fertil Steril* 1997;67:120–2
10. De Los Santos MJ, Mercarder A, Frances A, *et al.* Role of endometrial factors in regulating secretion of components of the immunoreactive human embryonic interleukin-1 system during embryonic development. *Biol Reprod* 1996;54:563–74
11. Liu H-C, Tseng L. Estradiol metabolism in isolated human endometrial epithelial glands and stromal cells. *Endocrinology* 1979;104:1674–8
12. Davis OK, Rosenwaks Z. *In vitro* fertilization. In Adashi E, Rock JA, Rosenwaks Z, eds. *Reproductive Endocrinology, Surgery, and Technology*. Philadelphia: Lippincott-Raven, 1996: 2319–34
13. Simon C, Frances A, Piquette G, Hendrickson M, Milki A, Polan ML. IL-1 system in the materno-trophoblast unit in human implantation: immunohistochemical evidence for autocrine/paracrine function. *J Clin Endocrinol Metab* 1994;78:847–54
14. Spandorfer SD, Barmat LI, Liu H-C, Mele C, Veeck L, Rosenwaks Z. Granulocyte macrophage-colony stimulating factor production by autologous endometrial co-culture is associated with outcome for IVF patients with a history of multiple implantation failures. *AJRI* 1998;40:xx
15. Kauma S, Matt D, Strom S, Elerman D, Turner T. IL-1β, hLA-DRα, and TGF-β expression in endometrium, placenta and placental membranes. *Am J Obstet Gynecol* 1990;163:1430–7
16. Spandorfer SD, Barmat LI, Liu H-C, Mele C, Veeck L, Rosenwaks Z. The day of the luteal phase endometrial biopsy (EBx) is an important predictor of success when autologous endometrial coculture (AECC) is utilized in IVF-ET. Presented at the *American Society of Reproductive Medicine* San Francisco, CA, October 1998:O-333
17. Simon C, Frances A, Piquette G, *et al.* Embryonic implantation in mice is blocked by IL-1ra. *Endocrinology* 1994;134:521–8

Menstruation suppression in the treatment of catamenial diseases

25

E. M. Coutinho

Introduction

In a previous publication, concern was expressed over the role played by incessant menstruation in the causation or exacerbation of women's diseases[1]. Among the various medical conditions directly associated with menstruation are iron-deficiency anemia, endometriosis and premenstrual syndrome, which together affect over 50% of all women of reproductive age. Other conditions that may be aggravated by menstruation include epilepsy, asthma, rheumatoid arthritis, diabetes and migraine. During menstruation, women may also experience an aggravation of chronic disorders that hinder blood coagulation, such as von Willebrand's disease, sickle-cell anemia and porphyria.

Conditions affected by menstruation

Anemia

In terms of absolute numbers of women, iron-deficiency anemia is the disease most affected by menstruation. For malnourished women around the world already suffering from chronic iron deprivation, the blood loss associated with normal menstruation causes depletion of iron stores, worsening the condition[2].

It is estimated that approximately 30% of the world population of 6 billion are anemic. About half of those suffering from anemia, around one billion individuals, have iron-deficiency anemia. In less developed regions of the world, most of the population is anemic. Even in developed countries such as the United States, 20% of menstruating women are also anemic. Among the women at risk of developing anemia we should include those having uterine fibroids, because of the metrorrhagia associated with most of these tumors[3].

Endometriosis

Endometriosis is the most common cause of pelvic pain in women of reproductive age. It is also a major cause of infertility. The overall global rate of endometriosis is estimated at 10%. With the present world population of 6 billion, the United Nations estimates that there are 1.5 billion women of reproductive age. Consequently, about 150 million probably have endometriosis. As the population grows and women desire fewer children, they menstruate more frequently than their mothers did, becoming more susceptible to developing endometriosis. The disease is now a major health problem, and since curing endometriosis is difficult because recurrence is common, the situation is bound to worsen[4].

Premenstrual syndrome

Premenstrual syndrome (PMS) is a physical condition involving biological changes in the brain, hormone levels and the immune system that occur in the days preceding menstruation. It is estimated that 30–40% of women experience symptoms such as pelvic discomfort, bloating, fatigue, backache and headache during the premenstrual period. For 3–7% of women premenstrual syndrome is incapacitating. The expression 'premenstrual dysphoric disorder' (PDD) has been adopted to characterize the symptoms linked to behavioral changes such as depression, introspection, anxiety and irritability. The American Psychiatric Association labeled PMS as a mental disorder in 1987 and it was only recently that we began to understand the causes of the behavioral symptoms.

The effects of PMS on mood and behavior can create problems in all aspects of a woman's life and can be devastating, not only for the woman herself but also for those around her. Marital conflicts, mistreatment and rejection of children, aggressiveness at work (directed towards subordinates and superiors alike), excessive food intake and alcohol abuse, suicide attempts and other acts of violence including murder are alleged to be consequences of the altered mental state of PMS victims[5].

The most frequent PMS symptoms are tiredness (92%), irritability (91%), abdominal distention (90%), nervous tension (89%), breast tenderness (85%), mood changes (81%), depression (80%), increased appetite (78%) and sleep disturbances (78%).

Migraine

Menstrual migraine may be considered a separate entity from PMS or part of the syndrome. Sixty per cent of women with migraine associate the attacks with menstruation. True menstrual migraine occurs in 8–14% of women who suffer migraines exclusively at the time of menstruation and not at any other time of the menstrual cycle.

Estrogen withdrawal occurring at the end of the menstrual cycle seems to initiate the vascular changes associated with menstrual migraine. The initial vasoconstriction, followed by vasodilation, which characterizes the headache, seems to be provoked by an abnormal platelet aggregation, altered platelet content of serotonin, abnormal neurotransmitter activity and central opioid deregulation[6].

Menstrual thrombocytopenia

Thrombocytopenia is a reduction in the number of platelets. Several types of thrombocytopenia have long been recognized but catamenial or menstrual thrombocytopenia was first described only in 1989. The platelet count falls only during a woman's period, causing a longer

and heavier menstrual flow than usual. The platelet count returns to normal at midcycle, around the time of ovulation. Women with a deficiency of other important clotting factors, such as factor V, risk excessive bleeding during menstruation which may require blood transfusion.

Excessive bleeding, which may endanger a woman's life, may also develop in thrombocytopenic individuals whose uteri are overdistended by leiomyomas[7].

Dysmenorrhea

As with menstrual migraine, dysmenorrhea may be considered a separate entity or a component of PMS. Dysmenorrhea, the most common disorder associated with menstruation, is defined as painful menstruation. Cramping, which can be so intense as to require hospitalization, is usually the result of prolonged uterine contractions. Congenital malformations, tumors in the reproductive organs, such as leiomyomas, endometriosis, and adhesions resulting from pelvic inflammatory disease or from previous pelvic surgery can cause or aggravate dysmenorrhea[8].

Dysmenorrhea can be classified as either spasmodic or congestive. Spasmodic dysmenorrhea occurs mainly in young women, usually appears on the first day of bleeding, and lasts as long as menstruation. Congestive dysmenorrhea, on the other hand, is characterized by intense pain prior to the onset of bleeding.

Epilepsy

A relationship between epilepsy and menstruation has been well established. Menstruation-related seizures occur in approximately 70% of epileptic women. At least 50% of women with epilepsy experienced their first convulsive seizure with the onset of their first menstrual period. Both estrogens and progesterone influence seizure disorders. Estrogens lower the excitability threshold of both nerve and muscle cells, and therefore increase the susceptibility to the development of seizures. Progesterone has the opposite effect. The occurrence or worsening of seizures should be associated either with increasing estrogen levels or progesterone withdrawal.

Women with catamenial epilepsy are first treated with conventional anti-epilepsy drugs for controlling menstruation-related seizures. However, ovulation and menstruation suppression with Depo-Provera® improves catamenial seizure control, reducing the requirement for conventional anti-epilepsy drugs[9].

Treatment of catamenial diseases

All these conditions, as well as a few others which are associated with menstruation, are usually treated with medication aimed at controlling or alleviating symptoms or correcting deficiencies. Iron-deficiency anemia, for example, is treated with iron supplementation. Pain of dysmenorrhea, endometriosis and menstrual migraine is currently treated with inhibitors of pain-producing substances. Aspirin, which inhibits prostaglandin synthesis, is widely used. Diuretics and anti-inflammatory drugs, which eliminate salt and excessive fluid from congested areas, are also used. Mental anguish, irritability, insomnia and depression occurring during the premenstrual phase are treated with anti-depressive drugs, tranquilizers and hypnotics[10].

Traditional medicine has kept a hands-off attitude towards menstruation over the last 2000 years, demonstrating an unshakeable loyalty in the medical profession to the teachings of Hippocrates and Galen who hailed menstruation as a remedy for all ailments and used it as an example of therapeutic blood-letting. It was only in the last 20 years that a few doctors, recognizing the harmful effects of menstruation in some of their patients, decided to experiment with menstruation suppression[1,11].

Natural menstruation suppression

Menstruation suppression may be achieved either by natural means or by medical intervention[7]. Natural suppression of menstruation occurs during pregnancy, lactation and vigorous exercise. Patients with endometriosis who intend to have children should be encouraged to become pregnant early and to breast-feed for

as long as possible in order to avoid future infertility caused by the progression of the disease. They can also take advantage of the long menstruation-free (and pain-free) periods afforded by pregnancy and lactational amenorrhea, which may bring about the additional benefit of endometriomata regression.

The inhibition of ovulation caused by breast-feeding is very efficient in the first 6 months following delivery. In the following months, 50% of women restart ovulation even when they are still breast-feeding on demand because other food is usually given to the infant during this period[12].

Natural menstruation suppression for women who do not plan to have children may be achieved by regular exercise. Runners, ballet dancers, gymnasts, weight-lifters, skaters and swimmers frequently experience athletic amenorrhea resulting from ovulation and menstruation suppression. Many body changes occur with exercise, including loss of body fat and the production of endorphins, which inhibit luteinizing hormone release from the pituitary, preventing ovulation. It is possible that the high levels of cortisol resulting from the psychic stress provoked by competition may also interfere with ovulation in athletes[13].

Inhibition of ovulation and menstruation by regular physical exercise requires perseverance, discipline and good health. Those who are willing to undertake the practice of exercise, either sport or dance, before the first menstrual period can delay the onset of menarche for several years. For each year of exercise the onset of menstruation is delayed for an average of 5 months. For the suppression of menstruation in adult women who menstruate regularly, and who wish to do this by running, it is necessary to run 5 km daily. In order to avoid loss of calcium and development of osteopenia, amenorrheic runners are advised to take a low dose of estrogen (or estrogen–progestin) or calcium supplementation.

Medical suppression of menstruation

The medical suppression of menstruation may be achieved either by surgical or non-surgical intervention. Hysterectomy, ovariectomy and endometrial resection are widely used to treat bleeding problems in older women who do not wish or are unable to have children. Endometrial resection is the least radical of the three methods[14,15].

The most convenient and efficient medication currently used to suppress ovulation and menstruation is medroxyprogesterone acetate injection, marketed worldwide as Depo-Provera. A dose of 50 mg inhibits ovulation for 1 month; 150 mg inhibits ovulation for 3 months and a dose of 400 mg inhibits ovulation for 6 months[16]. The effect is reversible. Following discontinuation of therapy, women have ovulation and menstruation restored within a short period of time, usually 2 months. Menstruation is suppressed in over 70% of Depo-Provera users.

Contraceptive implants are another convenient method of menstruation suppression through ovulation inhibition. An implant of elcometrine (ST-1435) inhibits ovulation for 6 months. The method has recently been registered in Brazil. The first single implant of elcometrine containing 50 mg of the compound induces ovulation inhibition for 6 months in 100% of subjects. With the first implant, amenorrhea occurs in 55% of subjects. With the second implant, amenorrhea occurs in 70% of users, and with a third implant amenorrhea occurs in over 80% of patients[17].

Oral contraceptives used continuously can be a good alternative for those women who are concerned about a very long menstruation-free interval or who want to get acquainted with the concept of menstruation suppression. Long-term ovulation and menstruation inhibition can be maintained for months or years by the continuous use of oral contraceptives. The same results can be obtained by vaginal administration of contraceptive pills. Symptom-free amenorrhea can be maintained for years using contraceptive pills vaginally on a continuous daily schedule[18].

Gestrinone and danazol may in appropriate doses inhibit ovulation and menstruation. Although they act similarly, gestrinone has the advantage of being more potent. The amount of gestrinone required to maintain a patient in amenorrhea for 1 year (400 mg) corresponds to 1 day of danazol therapy. Gestrinone should be administered at the dose of 2.5 mg every other day. Both gestrinone and danazol are widely used in the clinical management of endometriosis but their use can be extended to other menstruation-related conditions[19].

Gonadotropin-releasing hormone analogs, both agonists and antagonists, can be used to suppress menstruation by inhibiting luteinizing hormone-releasing hormone (LHRH) and the creation of a reversible menopause. Limitations of their use include the need for simultaneous estrogen replacement therapy to prevent menopausal symptoms and consequences. In developing countries, cost may be another limitation[20,21].

Menstruation suppression through ovulation inhibition should be considered not only for the treatment of catamenial diseases but also as prevention for those diseases in women at risk[4].

References

1. Coutinho EM. *Menstruação: Sangria Inútil.* São Paulo: Editora Gente, 1996
2. Kent SP, Stuart-Macadam AS, Kent S. *Anemia Through the Ages: Changing Perspectives and Their Implications in Diet, Demography and Disease.* New York: Aldine de Gruyter, 1992
3. Barer AP, Fowler WM. The blood loss during normal menstruation. *Am J Obstet Gynecol* 1936;31: 979–86
4. Coutinho EM. Induced amenorrhea in the prevention of endometriosis: A proposal for the third millenium. In Coutinho EM, Spinola P,

Moura L, eds. *Progress in the Management of Endometriosis.* London and New York: Parthenon Publishing, 1995:437–40

5. Keye WR Jr. *The Premenstrual Syndrome.* Philadelphia: WB Saunders, 1998
6. Linet MS, Stewart WF. Migraine headache: epidemiological perspectives. *Epidemiol Rev* 1984;6: 107–39
7. Tomer A, Schreiber AD, McMillan R. Menstrual cycle thrombocytopenia. *Br J Haematol* 1989;71: 519–23
8. Lark S. *Menstrual Cramps.* Los Altos, CA: Westchester Publishing Co., 1993
9. Newmark ME, Penry JK. Catamenial epilepsy. *Epilepsy* 1980;21:281–90
10. Smith S, Schiff I. *Modern Management of Premenstrual Syndrome.* New York: Norton Medical Books, 1993
11. Case AM, Reid RI. Effects of the menstrual cycle on medical disorders. *Arch Intern Med* 1998;158: 1405–12
12. McNeilly AS, Tay CC, Glasier A. Physiological mechanisms underlying lactational amenorrhea. *Ann NY Acad Sci* 1994;709:145–55
13. Diddle AW. Athletic activity and menstruation. *South Med J* 1983;76:619–24
14. Pokras R, Hufnagel VG. Hysterectomy in the United States 1965–1984. *Am J Public Health* 1988; 78:852–61
15. Magos AL, Baumann R, Turnbull ACB. Transcervical resection of endometrium in women with menorrhagia. *Med J* 1989;298:1209–12
16. Coutinho EM, de Souza JC, Csapo AI. Reversible sterility by medroxyprogesterone injections. *Fertil Steril* 1966;17:261–6
17. Coutinho EM, Carreira C, Bastos GJO. ST-1435, a new alternative for medical therapy of endometriosis. In Coutinho EM, Spinola P, Hanson de Moura L, eds. *Progress in the Management of Endometriosis.* New York and London: Parthenon Publishing Company, 1995:333–6
18. Coutinho EM, O'Dwyer E, Barbosa IC, *et al.* A comparative study of intermittent versus continuous use of a contraceptive pill administered by the vaginal route. *Contraception* 1995;51:355–9
19. Coutinho EM. Conservative treatment of uterine leiomyomas with the anti-estrogen, antiprogesterone, R-2323. *Int J Gynecol Obstet* 1981; 19:357–9
20. Bergquist C, Nillius SJ, Wide L. Inhibition of ovulation in women by intranasal treatment with luteinizing hormone-releasing hormone agonist. *Contraception* 1979:19:497–506
21. Schmidt-Goldwitzer M, Hardt W, Schmidt-Goldwitzer K. Influence of the LH-RH analogue buserelin on cyclic ovarian function and the endometrium. A new approach to fertility control? *Contraception* 1981;23:187–96

Section IV
Endoscopy

Retroperitoneal endometriosis

26

C. P. Roberts and J. A. Rock

Introduction

Retroperitoneal endometriosis has a classic presentation of pelvic pain and dyspareunia that is unresponsive to conservative medical management and laparoscopic therapy. Recent literature has recognized retroperitoneal endometriosis as a separate form of endometriosis. This paper addresses the clinical presentation and surgical treatment of this evasive subtype of endometriosis.

Background

Endometriosis is a common condition in women of reproductive age in which abnormal growths of endometrial tissue are present in locations other than the uterine cavity, and should be suspected in any patient of reproductive age complaining of pain and infertility. Endometriosis is present in at least 1% of all women of reproductive age and is found in 20% of women operated upon for pelvic pain.

Retroperitoneal endometriosis usually causes severe pain, dysmenorrhea and dyspareunia in patients. A characteristic examination will reveal tender nodules in the cul-de-sac, uterosacral ligaments, rectosigmoid junction and rectovaginal septum. Often the uterus is retroverted and fixed posteriorly. The origin of endometriosis of this deep-infiltrating endometriosis is not from retrotubal flow of endometrial cells but from metaplasia of Müllerian rests[1–3].

Extensive retroperitoneal disease often is not easily accessible by the laparoscope. Removal of disease requires retroperitoneal dissection, which may be facilitated by placing a bougie in the rectum, sponge forceps in the vagina and a Foley catheter in the bladder. The pararectal and paravaginal spaces may be exposed by applying traction in the appropriate direction.

Clinical presentation

The diagnosis of endometriosis is suggested by a patient's history. Most describe constant pelvic pain or a low sacral backache that subsides after menses begins. Dyspareunia is the most striking symptom, particularly with deep penetration. Lesions within the urinary tract or bowel may result in bloody urine or stool in the perimenstrual period. Implantations on or near the external surfaces of the cervix, vagina, rectum or urethra may cause pain and bleeding with defecation, urination or intercourse at any time of the menstrual cycle. A sensation of pelvic pressure may result if large masses are present.

Classically, pelvic examination reveals tender nodules in the posterior vaginal fornix and pain upon uterine motion. The uterus may be fixed and retroverted due to cul-de-sac adhesions, and tender adnexal masses may be felt if endometriomas are present. Careful inspection may reveal implants in healed wounds, especially in episiotomy and Cesarean section incisions, in the vaginal fornix or on the cervix. Biopsy may be required to prove the lesions are due to endometriosis. The staging system most commonly used for documentation of the progression of endometriosis is the revised American Fertility Society (AFS) classification[4,5]. The point system for the revised AFS classification is heavily weighted toward ovarian and peritoneal involvement and adhesions as indicators of more severe disease.

Different morphologic types of endometriotic lesions have been shown to have different biosynthetic capabilities and may have varying potential for pelvic pain[6]. The 'early' papular, atypical lesions exposed to peritoneal fluid might cause functional pain, whereas 'older' pigmented, nodular lesions embedded in infiltrating scars might cause organic pain[7]. In addition, although it is now known that peritoneal, ovarian and retroperitoneal disease are three distinct endometriotic lesions, the current classification system does not incorporate retroperitoneal disease or varying morphological types into the staging process[8].

Cornillie and associates reported that the cul-de-sac and uterosacral ligaments were frequent sites for deeply infiltrating lesions often associated with pelvic pain. Endometriosis infiltrates through loose connective tissue but stops at the junction of adipose tissue. Because the depth of subperitoneal connective tissue is more substantial in the posterior cul-de-sac and uterosacral ligaments, these areas tend to harbor deeper lesions. There is retroperitoneal fat in the ovarian fossae and deep infiltrating lesions are rarely found. Deeply infiltrating lesions (2–5 mm) were frequently associated with painful symptoms. Very deep (> 10 mm) lesions were exclusively found in patients with pelvic pain. These deep lesions were also more likely to be histologically active and in phase with the endometrium[9]. Koninckx and colleagues[10] found that the degree of pelvic pain was not related to total surface area of endometriosis. Ripps and Martin[11] studied the ability to correlate focal tenderness on pelvic examination with the presence of endometriotic lesions. In this study, the presence of focal tenderness was associated with endometriosis at that site in approximately 66% of patients. Of those patients with focal tenderness and endometriotic involvement, 96% of these lesions were fibrotic in nature. The average depth of infiltration was 5.4 mm for these types of lesions[11].

Koninckx and Martin further described deep endometriotic lesions and subdivided them into three groups. Type I lesions were conical shaped with the largest area lining the peritoneal cavity. These lesions were suspected to be formed by local infiltration. Type II lesions represented deeper lesions, which had been covered by dense adhesions. These lesions were felt probably to be formed by retraction. Type III lesions were the most severe and the largest lesions and were represented by spherical nodules in the rectovaginal septum. These lesions had their largest area of involvement underneath the peritoneal surface. At laparoscopy, these latter lesions may only appear superficially as small, typical pigmented lesions. In some patients, these lesions can only be identified by digital palpation. Type III lesions were speculated to arise from either closed Allen–Masters defects or from Müllerian rests. A poor correlation between the types of deep endometriotic lesions and the revised AFS classification was noted in this report. The most severe type III lesions were actually most frequently associated with patients who had been classified as Stage I (39.1%)[12].

To address the limitations of the revised AFS classification with respect to pelvic pain, a panel of international experts recently recommended a clinical instrument to be in the documentation of the extent of endometriosis and pelvic pain[13].

Surgical treatment

Conservative resection of endometriosis

Laparotomy is required for any patient with persistent pain after a trial of expectant management, medical management or laparoscopic treatment and when severe disease has invaded the bowels, ureters or other surrounding structures. It is also necessary when the extent of disease exceeds the operative skill of the surgeon or the availability of laparoscopic instrumentation.

Conservative surgery is best accomplished with the use of microsurgical techniques. The pelvis is copiously irrigated throughout the operation to maintain moist tissues. Ringer's lactate with 5000 IU of heparin and 1 g hydrocortisone added to each liter is recommended. Adhesions are removed without damage to underlying tissues and sent for pathological documentation of endometriosis. If hemostasis cannot be maintained by bipolar cautery, a bioabsorbable suture should be used.

Palpation is often necessary for deeper lesions and these should be excised rather than ablated to avoid surrounding healthy tissue damage and to enable complete resection. Deep nodules of endometriosis are not uncommon; in one study, 25% of patients with clinical disease had lesions that penetrated deeper than 5 mm. The pouch of Douglas and the uterosacral ligaments are two areas that need careful inspection and palpation for deeper implants of endometriosis[9,11]. Retroperitoneal fibrosis is often encountered involving the uterosacral ligaments, ureters and the rectum. In difficult cases, a careful dissection of pararectal and rectovaginal spaces accompanied by ureterolysis is necessary to isolate the uterosacral ligaments. Once free of surrounding structures, the uterosacral ligaments are held under tension and resected either sharply or with electrocautery. Postoperative adhesion formation is reduced by reperitonealization of the posterior cul-de-sac.

Presacral neurectomy

The sensory pathways from pelvic viscera involve the lumbar and lower thoracic sympathetic ganglia, as well as the superior, middle and hypogastric plexus. Pain impulses from the cervix, uterine corpus and proximal portions of the Fallopian tubes are transmitted through afferent fibers that accompany the sympathetic nerves into the spinal cord at T10, T12 and L1. These afferent sensory fibers course through the uterosacral ligaments and the posteriolateral portions of the pelvis to mesh together in the midline as the presacral nerve prior to turning cephalad to enter the spinal cord at the lower thoracic and upper lumbar nerve roots. It is the ovarian plexus, however, which receives afferent sensory fibers from the ovary, broad ligament, and distal Fallopian tube. This plexus follows the blood supply, trailing up the ovarian artery to blend with the meshwork of nerves arising from the aortic and renal plexus.

Presacral neurectomy is an adjunctive procedure at laparotomy for treatment of central dysmenorrhea due to endometriosis. Patient selection is important for effectiveness of the procedure. One study showed that patients with midline pain had excellent results after presacral neurectomy but patients with adnexal pain symptoms had a quite variable relief of pain[14]. Interestingly, Chen and Soong have reported laparoscopic presacral neurectomy as an effective alternative for patients wishing to avoid laparotomy[15].

The immediate but rare complications of presacral neurectomy include damage to ureter and blood vessels but the risk is greatly diminished with proper surgical technique. Side-effects include constipation, vaginal dryness and bladder dysfunction. As a rule, these symptoms will resolve over several months.

Conclusion

Endometriosis remains a challenging disease after years of study towards medical and surgical management. Its elusive nature supports subtypes of disease that are yet unclassified and encompass infertility and pain. Although we have been able to slow the disease process with hormonal suppression in those patients with dyspareunia and recurrent painful symptoms from endometriosis, it is only a temporizing method. While absolute curative treatment is not yet available, conservative surgery at laparotomy, combined with adjunctive measures such as presacral neurectomy, has proven effective when medical and laparoscopic management has failed.

References

1. Donnez J, Nisolle M, Casanas-Roux F, Brion P, Da Costa N. Stereometric evaluation of peritoneal endometriosis and endometriotic nodules of the rectovaginal septum. *Hum Reprod* 1995;11:224–8

2. Donnez J, Nisolle M, Smoes P, Gillet N, Beguin S, Casanas-Roux F. Peritoneal endometrioisis and

'endometriotic' nodules of the rectovaginal septum are two different entities. *Fertil Steril* 1996;66: 362–8

3. Nisolle M, Connez J. Peritoneal endometriosis, ovarian endometriosis and adenomyotic nodules of the rectovaginal septum are three different entities. *Fertil Steril* 1997;68:585–96

4. The American Fertility Society. Classification of endometriosis. *Fertil Steril* 1979;32:633

5. The American Fertility Society. Revised American Fertility Society classification of endometriosis. *Fertil Steril* 1985;43:351

6. Vernon MW, Beard JS, Graves K, Wilson EA: Classification of endometriotic implants by morphologic appearance and capacity to synthesize prostaglandin F. *Fertil Steril* 1986;46:801

7. Verceliini P, Bocciolone L, Vendola N, Colombo A, Rognoni M, Fedele L. Peritoneal endometriosis: morphologic appearance in women with chronic pelvic pain. *J Reprod Med* 1991;36:533

8. Chapron C, Dubuisson JB, Tardif D, Fritel X, Lacroix S, *et al.* Retroperitoneal endometriosis and pelvic pain: results of laparoscopic uterosacral ligament resection according to rAFS classification and histopathologic results. *J Gynecol Surg* 1998;14:51

9. Cornille FJ, Oosterlynck D, Lauweryns JM. Deeply infiltrating pelvic endometriosis: histology and clinical significance. *Fertil Steril* 1990;53:978

10. Koninckx PR, Meuleman C, Beneyere S, *et al.* Suggestive evidence that pelvic endometriosis is a progressive disease, whereas deeply infiltrating endometriosis is associated with pelvic pain. *Fertil Steril* 1991;55:750

11. Ripps BA, Martin DC. Focal pelvic tenderness, pelvic pain and dysmenorrhea in endometriosis. *J Reprod Med* 1991;36:470

12. Koninckx PR, Martin DC. Deep endometriosis: a consequence of infiltration or retraction or possibly adenomyosis externa? *Fertil Steril* 1992; 58:924

13. The American Fertility Society. Management of endometriosis in the presence of pelvic pain. *Fertil Steril* 1993;60:952

14. Tjaden B, Schlaff WD, Kimball A, Rock JA. The efficacy of a presacral neurectomy for the relief of midline dysmenorrhea. *Obstet Gynecol* 1990;76: 89

15. Chen FP, Soong YK. The efficacy and complications of laparoscopic presacral neurectomy in pelvic pain. *Obstet Gynecol* 1997;90:974

27

Recurrence rate after laparoscopic excision of ovarian endometriomas

M. Busacca, R. Marana, B. Agnoli, P. Caruana, M. Candiani, G. F. Catalano, C. Calia, S. Bianchi and M. Vignali

Introduction

Laparoscopy is the best treatment for ovarian endometriomas. Comparative studies have shown that the results in terms of pregnancy rates or recurrence are comparable to or better than those obtained with laparotomy[1-3]. One of the aspects that is not yet clear is the percentage of recurrence of endometriomas over time. The data in the literature are not sufficiently indicative: the results reported depend on the technique used, the medical therapy given and above all, on the duration of follow-up[4-10].

The real incidence of endometriosis recurrence is uncertain because the criteria used to define it are different: some authors consider the recurrence of symptoms as disease recurrence, whereas in a few studies ultrasonographic and/or surgical findings have been used. The recurrence and adhesion rates after laparoscopy are comparable to those of laparotomy[1,11,12].

The incidence of recurrence of endometriosis, and especially of endometriomas, is linked to the etiology of the disease and the persistence, due to estrogen stimulation, of those factors which are linked to a change in local and general immunological mechanisms[13,14]. It is, however, possible that there is not only one origin of ovarian endometriosis; both superficial and deeper origins may exist[15], due to superficial implants or metaplasia. The problem of recurrence is therefore difficult to resolve because the origin may vary. It is logical that the recurrence of endometriomas occurs over a significantly long and variable period of time for each condition. In the data reported in the literature the duration of follow-up varies from 2 months to several years[1,4,5]. When follow-up is longer, the recurrence of the disease is essentially based on the reappearance of symptoms rather than laparoscopic findings of cysts.

One of the more controversial points is the efficacy of the various surgical techniques for laparoscopic treatment of endometriomas. Excluding needle aspiration, which appears to be totally ineffective[16], there are no large randomized studies which allow for the comparison between excision of the cyst by capsular stripping and laser vaporization or excision diathermy. In 1991 Fayez and Vogel[17] presented a non-randomized prospective study which assessed the different methods of laparoscopic treatment of endometriomas: there were no significant differences between stripping the capsule and laser ablation, in terms of recurrence of endometriosis and adhesions. The study was, however, performed on a limited number of cases and the follow-up was too short (6 months).

Brosens and colleagues have recently presented a two-step endosurgical procedure for the treatment of endometriomas, with excision at the stigma of inversion of the cyst, eversion through the site of inversion, low-power bipolar coagulation and ovarian suppressive therapy with gonadotropin-releasing hormone (GnRH) agonist[18]. This technique, like the more traditional laser ablation or diathermic excision of the capsule, has been developed on the basis of morphological and histological studies which seem to indicate that an endometrioma is not an intraovarian cyst but rather an extraovarian pseudocyst and that functionally active endometriotic implants and neovascularization are located on the surface of the 'inverted cortex'. The same authors found no recurrence in a follow-up that varied from 26 to 42 months. This case study is, however, rather limited (18 cases).

A study by Donnez and colleagues of 814 patients, using the combined technique of GnRH agonists with laser CO_2, found recurrence in 8% of the women with a follow-up varying from 2 to 11 years[4]. There is no report of a cumulative curve of recurrence, however. In common with other authors[7,9,11], we believe that the removal of the capsule through stripping is the most correct and complete surgical method which does not necessarily require pre- or post-surgical additional medical therapy and gives to the pathologist an adequate specimen to exclude the rare risk of a carcinoma. Nevertheless, in a recent multicenter randomized clinical study, Beretta and associates[19] assessed the efficacy of two laparoscopic methods for the management of endometriomas: cystectomy, and drainage and bipolar coagulation of the inner lining. The 24-month cumulative recurrence rates of dysmenorrhea, deep dyspareunia and non- menstrual pelvic pain were lower after cystectomy: the median interval between the operation and the recurrence of moderate to severe pelvic pain was longer when the capsule of the cyst was removed. Large randomized studies are needed to assess objectively the effectiveness and reliability of the two techniques. There are at least three advantages in using pre-surgical medical therapy: (a) reduction of the mass, thus facilitating removal; (b) reduction of vascularization, thus decreasing blood loss; and (c) reduction of the risk of endometriotic cellular implants due to intraoperative dissemination. However, at present there are no reported findings which uphold these theories. The reduction of the endometrioma is dubious and limited to 50% of the initial mass[20,21], and there is no demonstration that this makes surgery more simple. The main surgical difficulties are related to adhesions, and it is well-known that medical therapy does not modify the adhesion score[22,23]. Preoperative medical therapy can reduce the cleavage between the cyst and the ovarian parenchyma. Muzii and colleagues[24], in a controlled clinical study, compared 20 patients treated preoperatively with GnRH agonists for 3 months and 21 patients who had not had any form of presurgical therapy: no difference was found between the two groups in total time of surgery, time of cyst excision, time necessary to control bleeding and the complexity of the various stages. Moreover, the use of preoperative medical therapy increases the costs of surgery and the time delay before the operation. For these reasons we do not administer preoperative medical therapy. The main purpose of post-operative therapy would be to eradicate any remaining disease or to prevent implants spreading at operation. At the moment, there is no published paper that demonstrates that medical therapy after excision of endometriomas prevents recurrence or improves fertility. In a previous randomized study on the use of GnRH agonists after surgery for third- or fourth-stage endometriosis, no advantage was shown in terms of pain recurrence or improved fertility[25]. Post-operative medical therapy must be personalized.

Study of laparoscopic excision

Our study included all the patients who underwent laparoscopic treatment for ovarian endometriotic cysts of more than 3 cm in diameter at the 2nd Department of Gynecology and Obstetrics at the University of Milan and the Department of Gynecology and Obstetrics at the Università del Sacro Cuore in Rome, between January 1990 and June 1997. A total of 458 patients were treated with laparoscopy (655 cysts). The surgical technique consisted of excision of the ovarian capsule of the cyst as described.

The cysts were all found to be endometriotic at histological examination. The patients who had a minimum of 6 months of post-operative follow-up, or follow-up for 6 months after the suspension of medical therapy following surgery, were included in the analysis. Patients were re-examined and vaginal ultrasound was performed with a 7.5-MHz probe at 3, 6 and 12 months after surgery and subsequently at least once a year. The diagnostic criteria adopted for ovarian endometrioma were those reported by Kupfer and co-workers[26]: (1) homogeneous contents of low echogenicity; (2) echoes present in one cyst or in various cysts in different positions; and (3) confirmation of the suspected mass by repeated ultrasound in the early follicular phase.

In 14 cases (3.8%) laparotomy was necessary because of technical difficulties during the laparoscopy. These patients were excluded from the analysis. We selected 366 patients on the basis of these criteria. Patient characteristics are reported in Table 1. The mean duration of follow-up was 27.7 ± 17.9 months. Sixty-three (17.2%) patients had previously undergone surgery for endometriosis.

In all the patients the capsule was stripped away from the ovarian stroma. After the introduction of the laparoscopic fiber optic and two or three 5-mm ancillary routes, and after inspection of the pelvis and of the cyst, the latter was isolated and freed from any adhesions and the contents were aspirated. When no suspect vegetations were seen, the capsule of the cyst was stripped completely, applying an adequate traction with two forceps. In no case was the ovarian parenchyma sutured. The cysts were removed from the abdominal cavity using an endobag. No preoperative medical therapy was given. Post-operative medical therapy was given in 119 cases (33.5%) according to the specific needs of the patients.

Statistical analysis

The analysis of the incidence of pain recurrence, of the clinical findings and of repeat surgery, as well as pregnancy rates, was performed using the Kaplan Meier method. The curves we obtained were stratified according to age, stage of disease, previous surgery for endometriosis, the diameter of the larger endometriotic cysts, and adhesion score. The comparison between the curves thus obtained was carried out with the logarithmic rank test. Univariate analysis of the possible risk factors for pain recurrence, of clinical findings and of repeat laparoscopy was carried out by χ^2 analysis and the t-test. Six variables (stage, previous surgery for endometriosis, adhesion score, number of endometriotic cysts, diameter of largest cyst and pregnancy after laparoscopic surgery) were evaluated to assess their effect on two separate outcomes, the recurrence of clinical and instrumental signs and the need for reintervention. Categories were defined as follows: stage (stage III, $n = 239$, and stage IV, $n = 127$); previous surgery for endometriosis (no, $n = 303$, and yes, $n = 63$); adhesion score (up to 3, $n = 87$, between 4 and 20, $n = 229$, above 21, $n = 50$); and number of cysts and diameter of largest cyst (single cyst, $n = 230$, >1 cyst, $n = 136$; < 4 cm, $n = 209$, > 4 cm, $n = 157$). Pregnancy after laparoscopic surgery occurred in 85 women whereas 281 did not conceive. These variables were inserted into an unconditional logistic regression. The reference group for each analysis was the first of each of the above variables. A p-value of < 0.05 was considered significant.

Results

The characteristics of the disease at surgery are reported in Table 2. During follow-up we observed recurrence in 26 (7.1%) cases and surgery was repeated in 12 (3.3%) cases. The cumulative rate of ovarian endometrioma recurrence at clinical and instrumental investigation over 48 months was 11.7%, while the cumulative rate of second surgery was 8.2%. In most cases recurrence was observed on the same ovary as in previous surgery (21 cases), while in five cases the recurrence was found on the contralateral ovary. Ultrasonographic cyst recurrence was associated with pain recurrence in 73% of cases, whereas in the remaining 27% the recurrence was asymptomatic. The cumulative pregnancy

Table 1 Characteristics of patients

Number of patients	366
Mean age (years)	30.25 ± 6.11
Previous surgery for endometriosis	63 (17.2%)
Dysmenorrhea	265 (72.6%)
Pelvic pain	118 (32.2%)
Infertility	91 (24.9%)
Length of follow-up (months)	27.7 ± 17.9
Conversion to laparotomy	14 (3.8%)
Post-operative medical therapy	119 (33.5%)

rate in infertile patients at 48 months after surgery was 55.4%.

Table 3 illustrates the differences between patients with recurrence in terms of stage, total score, adhesion score, implant score, number of cysts, diameter of largest cyst, previous surgery for endometriosis, age and pregnancy after laparoscopy, compared to those in whom recurrence was not observed. Patients in whom recurrence was observed were given total, adhesion and implant scores that were significantly higher than in patients in whom there was no recurrence. Age, number of cysts, cyst volume at initial surgery or pregnancy during the postoperative period did not differ in patients with disease recurrence compared with those without. According to univariate analysis significant factors related to recurrence of endometriomas would appear to be the stage of disease ($p = 0.03$) and previous surgery for endometriosis ($p = 0.003$).

Patients who underwent second surgery had significantly higher total scores and adhesion scores and larger cyst diameter compared to those who had no further operation, while the stage of disease was only slightly higher ($p = 0.08$). The effect of prognostic variables on recurrence of clinical signs and instrumental findings appears to be limited. Neither stage, adhesion score, number and diameter of endometriotic cysts or pregnancy after surgery significantly influenced disease recurrence. However, patients who had undergone previous surgery for endometriosis showed a higher probability of recurrence with respect to patients who did not (odds ratio 1.75, 95% confidence interval 1.13–2.72, $p < 0.02$).

Only the diameter of the larger cyst was a significant predictive factor for reintervention. Patients who had endometriotic cysts larger than 4 cm had a higher probability of reintervention with respect to patients with smaller cysts (odds ratio 1.96, 95% confidence interval 1.01–3.85, $p < 0.05$).

Discussion

In our case series, 27.5% of recurrence was totally asymptomatic and discovered only through clinical follow-up and ultrasound. The data reported in this study show that the trend of the cumulative recurrence rate depends on the months of follow-up and increases over time: it is possible to say that 11.8% of recurrence at

Table 2 Disease severity at laparoscopy

Stage III disease	239 (65.3%)
Stage IV disease	127 (34.2%)
Total score	38.4 ± 21.3
Implant score	25.9 ± 8.4
Adhesion score	13.1 ± 17.5

Table 3 Recurrence of clinical signs and reoperation according to clinical characteristics of patients

	Recurrence of clinical signs (n = 26)	Non-recurrence of clinical signs (n = 340)	Reoperation required (n = 12)	Reoperation not required (n = 354)
Stage of disease				
stage III	5%	95%	2%	98%
stage IV	11%*	89%	5.4%	94.6%
Previous endometriosis				
yes	16.4%**	83.6%	4.7%	95.3%
no	5.4%	94.6%	3%	97%
Pregnancy				
yes	4.7%	95.3%	2.4%	97.6%
no	7.9%	92.1%	3.6%	96.4%
Age (years)	31 ± 5	30.2 ± 6.2	30.2 ± 6.0	30.3 ± 6.1
Cyst size (mm)	56.8 ± 18.0	52.3 ± 21.8	68 ± 18.7[†]	51.9 ± 21.6
Number of cysts	1.6 ± 0.7	1.6 ± 0.9	1.7 ± 0.8	1.6 ± 0.9
Implant score	29 ± 8.9[†]	25.5 ± 8.5	26.9 ± 9.1	25.7 ± 8.6
Adhesion score	19.9 ± 22.9[†]	12.2 ± 16.3	24.2 ± 24.8[†]	12.4 ± 16.5
Total score	48.9 ± 27.3[‡]	37.7 ± 20.7	51 ± 29[†]	38 ± 20

[†]$p < 0.05$; [‡]$p < 0.01$ by Student's t-test; *$p < 0.05$, **$p < 0.005$ by χ^2 analysis

48 months from surgery may increase over time, although in 15% of cases recurrence of endometrioma was found in the other ovary. This indicates a new pathological factor.

One of the limits of this study in the majority of cases is the lack of histological and laparoscopic confirmation of cyst recurrence, as second-look laparoscopy was not always performed. However, we scrupulously respected the ultrasound criteria proposed by Kupfler and colleagues[26], and ultrasound was repeated in the post-menstrual phase for two successive cycles.

The aim of our study was to analyze the risk factors which might influence the recurrence rate of endometriomas. Age does not seem to be significant. The diameter of the cyst removed does not seem to influence the possibility of recurrence. It has been repeatedly reported that the stripping of the cyst capsule is not always complete, especially in large endometriomas. The correct surgical technique therefore limits these risks to a considerable extent and means that the diameter of the cyst has little influence on the rate of recurrence. The rate of recurrence is not dependent on the number of cysts removed or on the advent of pregnancy after surgery. The unfavorable data for prognosis seem to be the extent of the disease and previous surgery for endometriosis. In both cases the lowest common denominator seems to be the extent and the progression rate of the disease. It has previously been reported that, without specific reference to endometriomas, the advanced stage of the disease is worsened by recurrence[13]. The less favorable prognosis for women who have already had surgery for endometriosis may be explained by the progressive nature of the disease. At the moment there are no parameters which are able to predict with any accuracy the development of the illness or to separate currently active from inactive endometriosis. It is possible that the reason for the less favorable prognosis for women who have already had surgery for endometriosis is that the disease itself is more aggressive. In patients who have repeat surgery, on the other hand, the cyst volume $(p = 0.05)$ and the adhesion score $(p = 0.03)$ assume different values. This fact seems to be related to the need for further functional recovery in patients who desire conception. The statistical analysis of the clinical factors which can influence the recurrence of endometriosis in our patients gave results which differed for univariate and multivariate analysis. While in accordance with the univariate analysis many factors were distributed in a significantly different way among the patients who had had recurrence and/or repeat surgery and those who had not, only previous surgery for endometriosis and cyst volume seem to have a predictive significance according to logistic regression. The reason for this divergence should be sought, on the one hand, in the marked correlation between certain factors (scores for disease stage, for example) and on the other, in the number of events (recurrences or repeat surgery) recorded.

The percentage of repeat surgery in our case series (8.2%) is higher than that reported by Ahmed and Barbieri (2.9%)[27]: the longer follow-up (48 months vs. 32 months) might partially explain the difference.

Conclusion

Laparoscopic treatment of endometriomas seems to be both effective and reliable. The rate of recurrence appears to be correlated to the duration of follow-up. The stage of the disease and previous surgery for endometriosis are unfavorable prognostic factors. Cyst volume and adhesion scores are important for patients who have repeat surgery. Large randomized clinical studies are needed to determine the most advantageous technique (capsular stripping as opposed to laser vaporization) and the effectiveness of pre- and post-operative medical therapy.

References

1. Bateman BG, Kolp LA, Mills S. Endoscopic versus laparotomy management of endometriomas. *Fertil Steril* 1994;62:690–5
2. Catalano GF, Marana R, Caruana P, *et al.* Laparoscopy versus microsurgery by laparotomy for excision of ovarian cysts in patients with moderate or severe endometriosis. *J Am Assoc Gynecol Laparosc* 1996;3:267–70
3. Adamson GD, Subak LL, Pasta DJ, *et al.* Comparison of CO_2 laser laparoscopy with laparotomy for treatment of endometriomata. *Fertil Steril* 1992;57:965–73
4. Donnez J, Nisolle M, Gillet N, *et al.* Large ovarian endometriomas. *Hum Reprod* 1996;11:641–6
5. Sutton CJG, Ewen SP, Jacobs SA, *et al.* Laser laparoscopic surgery in the treatment of ovarian endometriomas. *J Am Assoc Gynecol Laparosc* 1997;4:319–23
6. Reich H, McGlynn F. Treatment of ovarian endometriomas using laparoscopic surgical techniques. *J Reprod Med* 1986;31:577
7. Nezhat C, Crowgey SR, Nezhat F. Videolaparoscopy for the treatment of endometriosis associated with infertility. *Fertil Steril* 1989;51:237–40
8. Cook AS, Rock JA. The role of laparoscopy for the treatment of endometriosis. *Fertil Steril* 1991;55:673–80
9. Martin DC. Laparoscopic treatment of ovarian endometriomas. *Clin Obstet Gynecol* 1991;34:452–9
10. Daniell JF, Kurt BR, Gurley LD. Laser laparoscopic management of large endometriomas. *Fertil Steril* 1991;55:692–5
11. Canis M, Mage G, Wattiez A, *et al.* Second-look laparoscopy after laparoscopic cystectomy of large ovarian endometriomas. *Fertil Steril* 1992;58:611–19
12. Redwine DB. Conservative laparoscopic excision of endometriosis by sharp dissection: life table analysis of reoperation and persistent or recurrent disease. *Fertil Steril* 1991;56:628–34
13. Dmowsky WP, Braun D, Gebel H. The immune system in endometriosis. In Thomas EJ, Rock J, eds. *Modern Approach to Endometriosis.* London: Kluwer Academic Publishers, 1991: 97–111
14. Busacca M, Viganò P, Magri B, Vignali M. The adhesion molecules on human endometrial stromal cells: immunological implication. *Ann NY Acad Sci* 1994;734:43
15. Brosens IA, Puttemans PJ, Deprest J. The endoscopic localization of endometrial implants in the ovarian chocolate cyst. *Fertil Steril* 1994;61:1034–8
16. Donnez J, Nisolle M, Gillerot S, *et al.* Ovarian endometrial cysts: the role of gonadotropin-releasing hormone agonist and/or drainage. *Fertil Steril* 1994;62:63–6
17. Fayez JA, Vogel MF. Comparison of different treatment methods of endometriomas by laparoscopy. *Obstet Gynecol* 1991;78:660–5
18. Brosens IA, Van Ballaer P, Puttemans P, Deprest J. Reconstruction of the ovary containing large endometriomas by an extraovarian endosurgical technique. *Fertil Steril* 1996;66:517–21
19. Beretta P, Franchi M, Ghezzi F, *et al.* Randomized clinical trial of two laparoscopic treatments of endometriomas: cystectomy versus drainage and coagulation. *Fertil Steril* 1998;70:1176–80
20. Doberl A, Berqvist A, Jeppson S, *et al.* Regression of endometriosis following shorter treatment with or without lower dose danazol: comparison of pre- and post-treatment laparoscopic findings. *Acta Obstet Gynecol Scand* 1984;123:51–9
21. Rana R, Thomas S, Rotman C, Dmowsky WP. Decrease in the size of ovarian endometriomas during ovarian suppression in stage IV endometriosis. Role of preoperative treatment. *J Reprod Med* 1996;41:384–93
22. Kennedy SH, Williams IA, Brodribb J, *et al.* A comparison of nafarelin acetate and danazol in the treatment of endometriosis. *Fertil Steril* 1990;53:998–1003
23. Marana R, Muzii L, Muscatello P, *et al.* Gonadotrophin-releasing hormone agonist (buserelin) in the treatment of endometriosis: changes in the extent of the disease and in CA 125 serum levels after 6-month therapy. *Br J Obstet Gynaecol* 1990;97:1016–19
24. Muzii L, Marana R, Caruana P, Mancuso S. The impact of pre-operative gonadotropin-releasing hormone agonist treatment on laparoscopic excision of ovarian endometriotic cysts. *Fertil Steril* 1996;65:1235–7
25. Parazzini F, Fedele L, Busacca M, *et al.* Post-surgical medical treatment of advanced endometriosis: results of a randomized clinical trial. *Am J Obstet Gynecol* 1994;171:1205–7
26. Kupfer MC, Schiwimer RS, Lebovic J. Transvaginal sonographic appearance of endometriomata: spectrum of findings. *J Ultrasound Med* 1992;11:129–32
27. Ahmed MS, Barbieri RL. Reoperation rates for recurrent ovarian endometriomas after surgical excision. *Gynecol Obstet Invest* 1997;43:53–4

Computers and robotic devices in endoscopic gynecological surgery

28

L. Mettler

Introduction

Over the last two decades, minimally invasive surgery has become increasingly popular and has been demanded by both surgeons and patients. Its benefits lie predominantly in reducing pain and providing a more rapid recovery for patients compared to traditional surgery. Today, many advanced techniques are being performed in gynecology, urology, cardiac surgery, brain surgery and orthopedic surgery, as well as in general surgery. To control the surgeon's visual field, it is either necessary for the surgeon to hold the laparoscope and camera attachment or rely on assistance. At present and in the imminent future, improvements in efficiency and safety in minimally invasive surgery will include the disciplines of robotics, computer assistance, three-dimensional optics and mechanics. The benefits of sophisticated technologies will be measured by factors such as shortened operating times, improved outcomes, lesser morbidity, diminished use of personnel and elimination of other instrumentation. Utilizing robotic technology called 'Computer Motion', offered by a company in Santa Barbara, USA, a robot has been designed for endoscopic surgeons specifically for the purpose of holding and maneuvering the laparoscope under the direct control of the surgeon. AESOP (Automated Endoscopic System for Optimal Positioning) has been tested in a variety of laparoscopic procedures and has already proved to perform at least as well, as if not better, than a human assistant in terms of camera holding, with less erroneous camera motion and accidental contact of the endoscopic lens with internal organs. Robotic control of the laparoscopic camera scope and visual field has improved efficiency and shortened

operative procedures in minimally invasive surgery. About 1 year ago, voice control of the robotic arm became clinically available and has been used successfully. AESOP offers the possibility of hand control, foot control and voice control. It was the aim of the present study to compare voice with foot control in so-called solo surgery using the AESOP.

Materials and methods

The Automated Endoscopic System for Optimal Positioning (AESOP) from Computer Motion Inc. of Goleta, California, holds and moves the laparoscope during surgery[1-4]. The surgeon can direct the articulated metal arm by means of a foot pedal or hand control or by using the voice control. In addition, laparoscopic views can be saved for repeated viewing by using the memory feature which is available for three visual positions. With careful movements of the foot or hand, the surgeon can smoothly shift the laparoscope in any direction – left, right, up, down, forwards or backwards. The pressure applied by the surgeon controls the speed. At all times the vertical and horizontal orientation is maintained. This system eliminates unwanted movements of the laparoscope caused by the assistant's heartbeat, breathing or sudden sneezes. AESOP is controlled by a computer with read-only memory software. With the robotic arm as an assistant, laparoscopic procedures, including hysterectomy, adnexectomy, ovarian cyst enucleation, ectopic pregnancy treatment, omenectomy and other types of surgery, can be performed by a solo surgeon. Even telesurgery can be performed controlling an AESOP computer linked to a telephone line.

Telerobotic surgery with AESOP was pioneered in the USA by Dr Louis Kavoussi, Director of the Brady Institute of Urology at the John Hopkins University School of Medicine and it was also performed in Europe by the urologist Professor Janetschek in Innsbruck. Figure 1 gives a picture of the AESOP control arm hooked to a special storage carriage with which it can easily be adapted to the operating table. A voice-control card for the individual surgeon has to be established and inserted at the beginning of the procedure. Figure 2 shows the AESOP control arm attached to the operating table during an endoscopic gynecological procedure at the Department of Obstetrics and Gynecology, University of Kiel, Germany. It also demonstrates the use of the voice-activated headset used by the surgeon.

Voice control works according to the following principles:

(1) The surgeon carries a small voice receiver around the head;

(2) AESOP responds to short commands, such as 'AESOP move in; move out; move back; move down; move up; move right; move left; left; right; up; down; back; in; save 1; save 2; save 3; return 1; return 2; return 3 and quit'.

During the procedure the computer also gives commands, such as 'press manual mode button'. No noise in the operating theater distracts the direct voice control of the surgeon.

Patients

As the control arm of the AESOP is used as a camera holder only, no patient consent for this robotic device had to be obtained. Twenty-five patients were treated in gynecological procedures using the foot and hand control and 25 patients were treated using the voice control.

Results

No mishaps occurred in any of the surgical procedures. The number of personnel required during laparoscopic surgery using the robotic arm attached to the operating table dropped

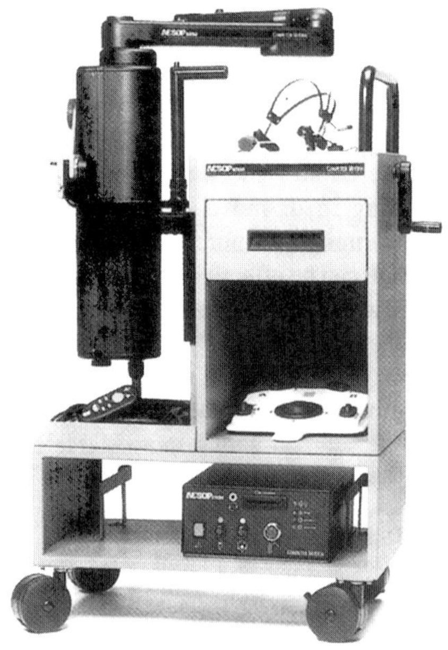

Figure 1 AESOP 2000 (Automated Endoscopic System for Optimal Positioning) as a voice-controlled robotic assistant for endoscopic surgery in its mobile carriage

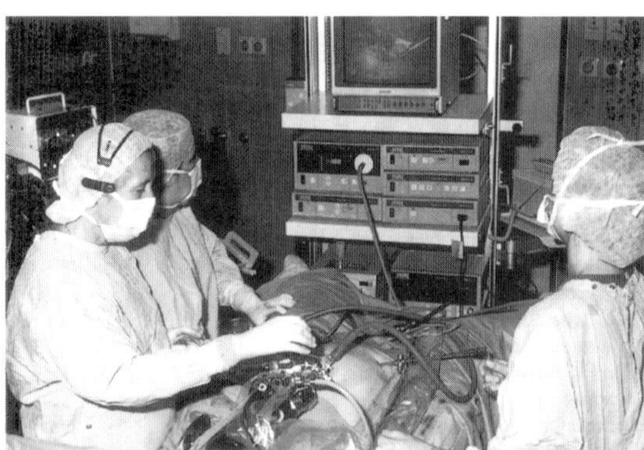

Figure 2 Position of surgeons using AESOP 2000 as camera holder during a hysterectomy at the Department of Obstetrics and Gynecology, University of Kiel, Germany

from three to two. The visual field was found to be completely steady. In our experience the foot and hand control was superior to interactions by the first assistant and the voice control of the visual field was best directed by the operating surgeon. Voice control increased the surgeon's concentration and proved to be superior to foot or hand control of the robotic arm.

Table 1 compares the length of the operating times of those procedures performed by foot/hand control, by voice control and with an assistant camera holder.

The elimination of the camera holder allows two gynecologists, or one gynecologist and a nurse, to perform complex laparoscopic gynecological surgical procedures, such as ovarian cyst enucleation, myomectomies and hysterectomies using the classic intrafascial supracervical hysterectomy technique[5,6]. In cases with three additional ports, in addition to the optical trocar, the assistant can help with a third arm thereby adding to the surgeon's two arms in action. At the Department of Obstetrics and Gynecology, University of Kiel, Germany, a nurse always assists in all surgical procedures. The use of the robotic arm to hold the laparoscope and camera, along with its ability to provide an absolutely steady visual field, increases the concentration and efficiency of the surgeon. As the application of the hand piece limits the surgeon to using the two arms for the laparoscopic procedure, foot control seems preferable; however, in our experience this procedure takes longer as we had to first control the foot piece by the eye as the eye/foot co- ordination was not always optimal. The robot with the voice control enables us to ask the robotic arm to move up, down, left, right, in, and out, to save one, two and three pictures and to return to these pictures. It allows a safer and more secure movement of the laparoscope. Data specified in Table 1 demonstrate the decrease in the operating time of the procedure. Certainly, less fogging and smudging of the scope lens was observed. As a result, it was seldom necessary to clean the laparoscope in heated water (50 °C) during the procedure.

In the solo surgery model, the surgeon performed both simple and complex tasks more rapidly and without error using voice control of the robotic arm (and visual field) when compared to foot control or hand control of the visual field. The studies demonstrated clear trends in favor of voice control of the visual field both in humans and our previous porcine subjects during laparoscopic surgery.

Discussion

Industrial robots have displaced workers in many fields. Will surgeons be sidelined as robotic devices advance in their operative capabilities? We think not. AESOP, for example, is a sophisticated tool to assist the surgeon only in moving the laparoscope. In no way does it replace the surgeon. It supports the surgeon in doing his best and enables him to give a more powerful approach than was possible in the past. Technology is developing and we as doctors need to be part of it. We need to identify the appropriate use of new technologies in our field of medicine. Patients' outcomes do, of course, take first place. Using the solo surgery model, the surgeon can perform both simple and complex procedures, as described here, more rapidly and without error using voice control of the robotic arm (and visual field) compared to using foot control and hand control. Our studies have demonstrated trends in favor of voice control of the visual field both in humans

Table 1 Use of a robotic arm in 50 gynecological endoscopic surgical procedures: a comparison between foot/hand and voice control and gynecological endoscopic surgery with an assistant camera holder. Times are rounded up to the nearest 5 min and comprise the whole preoperative preparation time after the anesthetized patient has been taken into the operating theater, including the time taken to fix and set up the robotic tool

			Length of operation with robotic arm (min)	
Surgical procedure	Number of cases	Length of operation without robotic arm (min)	Hand/foot	Voice
Ovarian cyst enucleation	29	95	70	60
Myomectomy	17	70	50	40
Hysterectomy	4	60	50	40

and in our previous porcine subjects during laparoscopic hysterectomy, ovarian cyst resection and myomectomy. It is definitely the conclusion of our working group that at the present time, the fixation of the robotic tool to the operating table takes some time and the whole procedure requires more concentration of the surgeon; however, the possibility of working more steadily in a confined field is greatly appreciated. At the present time, the limitations of the device are seen in cases of adhesions, where movements of the robotic arm over larger distances are required. In such cases, the robotic arm takes longer to respond to the voice control than it takes to perform the procedure by hand. A robotic assistant is seen to be a cost-effective device, taking the place of the traditional assistant if so wished by the surgeon. This type of surgery is best applied in smaller clinics where less personnel are available. In larger university hospitals where, for educational reasons, more personnel are available, these techniques are used to support the technological development.

The cost of AESOP 2000, described here, and the newer version AESOP 3000, which has more joints and is easier to move, amounts to US$60 000. This is well within the price range of other tools, such as lasers, which are also used in endoscopic surgical procedures. In the long run, the cost-benefit is indeed more favorable, as AESOP reduces the number of personnel required in the operating theater and can be used for solo surgery. With regard to teaching possibilities, AESOP increases the input of an assistant who can be very helpful using this modern technology. For example, by moving the camera with the hand or foot control the assistant can help during the procedure to advance or move away the camera while the surgeon is performing a suture. Teaching possibilities are increased. AESOP can effectively be used in telerobotic surgery, where surgeons working at different places can communicate by voice over the video screen.

In conclusion, in the long run a robotic assistant is seen to be a cost-effective device replacing the traditional assistant and providing the surgeon with a more stable operating field.

References

1. Harding R. Gearing up for a new era in surgery: robotic assistance. *Same-Day Surg* 1994;18:86–8
2. Kavoussi L, Moore R, Adams J, Partin A. Comparison of robotic versus human laparoscopic camera control. *J Urol* 1995;154:2134–5
3. Geis P, McAfee P, Kim C, Brennan E. Robotic arm enhancement to accommodate improved efficiency and decreased resource utilization in complex minimally invasive surgical procedures. Presented at the *IV International Symposium Medicine Meets Virtual Reality*, San Diego, USA, 17–20 January 1996
4. Garcia C. Clinical utility of a robotic assistant during laparoscopic cholecystectomy. Presented at the *8th Annual International Conference of the Society for Minimal Invasive Therapy*, Como, Italy, 16–20 September 1996
5. Mettler L, Semm K, Lütpes JE, Panandikar D. Pelviskopische intrafasciale Hysterektomie ohne Kolpotomie (CISH). *Gynäkol Prax* 1993;17:509–26

29

Computerized robotics: is this the final stage of development in surgery?

K. Semm

Introduction

General surgery has changed. A large incision no longer implies a 'big' surgeon. Endoscopic surgery has finally put an end to the unco-ordinated, free-style battle of the ten fingers within the opened recesses of the human body. The endoscopic principle has been accepted throughout the world and is based on the idea that the instruments follow the longitudinal lines allowed for by trocars of different diameters placed in positions to permit easy access to the organ being surgically treated. All instruments used to perform sutures, ligation and cutting are limited in their range of movement to forward–backward motion and axial rotation. These simple movements may also be executed by a robot. The direction of the robot's arm and the axial rotation of the instrument it is controlling can be modified.

A perfect example of this principle can be found in the automobile industry, in which highly complicated cars are assembled by the linear function and rotation of the robotic arms. Human anatomy is practically constant, and the surgical procedures are described in teaching manuals. Operations on organs such as the appendix and now the gall bladder and heart bypass vessels will be the first to be performed by robots in the 21st century.

Endoscopy has irrevocably changed surgery at the end of the 20th century, marking its fifth and perhaps final stage of development. Following an era of open surgery, operative endoscopic surgery began in the 1960s. This 'keyhole' surgery has perhaps become the 'key' to the newly developing computer robotic surgery which will undoubtedly reign in the 21st century. In order to fully appreciate the importance of computer robotic technology, it is necessary to examine the milestones in surgery up to this point.

Pre-anesthesiological era of surgery (BC–1846)

Operations were being performed as early as 6000 years ago in the Tigris–Euphrates Valley of the Babylonian Empire. There are similar reports from China. From the first millennium AD, many reports from Central American cultures (i.e. the Toltecs, Incas, Mayans, Aztecs) exist.

To perform specific surgical procedures, an exact knowledge of the regional anatomy was mandatory. During the Middle Ages, scientists such as Leonardo da Vinci and Gabriel Falloppius risked their lives to exhume fresh cadavers from cemeteries. Teams of scientists then dissected the bodies and produced excellent anatomical sketches and descriptions.

Even at this time, theft among scientists existed, and many scientists protected themselves by devising secret codes to record information. Leonardo da Vinci, for example, wrote from right to left in mirror writing. Other scientists named organs after themselves, such as Gabriel Falloppius who first described the human salpingus as the Fallopian tube. Johann Wolfgang von Goethe (1820) was also a part of this competitive scientific game, and was the last to give his name to a bony fissure in the maxilla.

Anatomists at this time developed the descriptive anatomy we still learn today. Their fight was not a simple one, as they were vehemently criticized by the rather fanatical scholastic thinkers who wished to ignore any of the basic 'hands-on' knowledge obtained by exhuming cadavers. These 'scholars' believed that all information regarding the human body could be derived from the study of etymology. This ended in the 17th century, by which time specific operations following very clear anatomical guidelines were being performed.

Many of the greatest innovations in surgery began in the field of obstetrics and gynecology. Obstetrics gave us a pure and noble reason to perform surgery in the case of the Cesarean section, which was performed at that time as a life-saving operation. This was particularly true for patients with bony abnormalities, either congenital or caused by osteomalacia, and rickets, as these conditions, which caused significant cephalopelvic disproportion, were ultimately considered a death sentence for mother or child, or both. At that time, it was quite normal for a man to become a widower following the first five pregnancies, owing to the extremely high perinatal mortality rate. Obstetricians had an exceedingly difficult task. Although the anatomy of both mother and child were well known at this time, Cesarean section resulted most often in death. The impenetrable enemy was not the high degree of pain asociated with the procedure, but a worse enemy not known as yet, bacterial infection.

In Kiel, Germany between 1826 and 1836, Mrs Adametz survived four Cesarean sections[1] without anesthesia and without wound closure. She was attended by the obstetrician Gustav Adolph Michaelis. This success was in no way reproducible. Following the first section, the patient had peritonitis, which she survived following 9 months hospitalization. At the subsequent operations, Michaelis opened the uterus each time exactly in the longitudinal scar. Underneath the visceral peritoneum of the uterus had become adherent to the parietal peritoneum, which was adherent to the scar. Cesarean section became the first operation to have clear indications, so much so that Professor Osiander of Göttingen, Germany wrote in 1826, 'If you indicate Cesarean section for a patient you must prepare her for death and allow her the time to make a last will and testament.'

All operative procedures were, at this time, clouded by the risk of wound infection. The teachings of I. P. Semmelweis were recognized. It had been shown through the work of Semmelweis of Vienna, Austria and Michaelis from Germany that puerperal fever could be arrested if first, the obstetricians were instructed to avoid attending postmortems and second, they washed their hands with chlorinated water prior to performing a Cesarean section. This thinking, however, had not yet progressed through to the realm of surgery, and many patients still died of postoperative sepsis.

Post-anesthesiological era (1846/7–1945)

True surgery as we know it today began with the development of anesthesia using ether in Boston, Massachusetts, USA in 1846 and with the development of anesthesia by the young obstetrician J. Y. Simpson in 1847 in Edinburgh, Scotland. Chloroform was used, and proved to be so effective that it could be used at the delivery of the new Queen Victoria, and the method became known as the 'narcose à la Reine'. From this time on, chloroform anesthesia dominated over the ether that had been introduced 1 year earlier by a Bostonian dentist. The first demonstration in Boston was a disaster, as the patient screamed more than ever before.

The combination of chloroform and ether allowed surgery to progress to a level whereby operations such as resection of limbs, laparotomy, thoracotomy and craniotomy could be performed. The entire spectrum of possible surgical procedures developed very quickly, and surgeons believed themselves to be the 'gods' of medicine. Despite advances such as the acceptance of the Semmelweis teaching of washing the hands with chlorinated water, the introduction of steam sterilization and the use of rubber gloves produced by the Goodyear Tyre Company, the risk of wound infection was still seen as an inconquerable hurdle.

The solution came with a discovery which has its origin dating back to Roman times.

Gladiators rubbed the moss from trees into their wounds because, unbeknown to them, it contained penicillin. This was discovered 2000 years later in 1928 by Alexander Fleming, who was awarded the Nobel Prize in 1938.

Era of auxiliary-supported surgery: antibiotics, transfusions and intensive care medicine (1945–75)

Parallel to the introduction of antibiotics came the knowledge of the necessity for and development of pre-, intra- and postoperative infusion therapy. The blood-groups were discovered in 1900 by Landsteiner, and we were now at a stage where almost any blood loss could be compensated. The stage was set for the first transplantation operations. Knowledge regarding the immune system and its importance exploded in medicine, and this culminated in 1968 with the first heart transplant by Dr Christian Barnard. This occurred a remarkable 120 years after the development of anesthesia and 20 years after the introduction of penicillin, infusion therapy, transfusions and intensive care medicine.

Era of reducing trauma (1975–85)

In the 1960s, new techniques in surgery began to reduce trauma and minimalize operations, leading to microsurgery. Once proficiency in macrosurgery had been achieved, microsurgery began[2,3]. Gynecologists were the first to make practical use of these procedures for infertility surgery on the Fallopian tubes. Industry became involved by creating operative microscopes, and microsurgical societies were established to promote the new operative techniques, particularly in the field of reproductive medicine.

These developments led to greater successes in the area of reproductive surgery, which culminated in operations to remove ova for what would become our greatest invasion into nature: *in vitro* fertilization. The first *in vitro* ovum was fertilized following the method demonstrated by veterinary surgeons.

Era of endoscopic surgery (since 1964)

Parallel to these developments was the foundation of the School of Endoscopic Surgery in Kiel, Germany[2,3]. Initially, ova were retrieved at laparotomy, and in Kiel this was replaced by laparoscopy. The surgical indications for laparoscopy at this time were sterilization or sterility surgery involving the Fallopian tubes.

In Kiel, endoscopic surgery matured to its present status. Here, 80% of the classic operations in gynecology and some classic surgical procedures were adapted into endoscopic techniques[3]. The necessary equipment and instruments were developed in Kiel, meeting the requirements to perform the procedures. Little change has occurred since with regard to operative techniques and instrumentation. With time, the steps of classic surgery became endoscopic procedures. The large incisions required at laparotomy became a symbol of the past.

Since 1983, radical as well as conservative operations have been performed, including surgery for ectopic pregnancy, myoma enucleation, ovarian cyst enucleation, salpingectomy and salpingo-oophorectomy. Initially, when these operations were reported at scientific meetings, the reaction was not only criticism but even ridicule. Classical surgeons considered the operations unethical and the work of a charlatan. Some colleagues, in addition, saw the great imminent danger: 'if this man proves to be correct, macrosurgery via laparotromy is doomed.' A new epoch in surgery had begun.

At this point, it is fitting to refer to a great scientific mind, Werner von Braun, who was, in mid-1954, convinced that it was possible to pull away from the force of gravity and fly to the moon. His plans had been laid, but the Second World War robbed him of his possibilities. His laboratories in Peenemuende, Germany were divided between the USA and the USSR following the war, thus ultimately setting the stage for the ensuing cold war. The Americans brought von Braun, following the war, to the USA, and then decided to abandon his theory. Braun believed that burning a few thousand kilograms of gas would produce enough energy to push 5 kg beyond the pull of gravity. The Americans had developed the atom bomb, and were convinced that their theory of 'plasma flow' would produce the necessary energy to overcome gravity.

The Russians took control of the reasearch workers who had worked closely with von Braun at Peenemuende, and with them, the German Research Center for Weapons and Jet Propulsion. Using the methods of their mentor, they were able to send the 5-kg Sputnik into orbit on 4 October 1957. For scientists today, all this is self-evident. However, the present author debated with scientists in Buenos Aires at the 13th World Congress for Physiology that the plasma theory was not believable, and that the Russians would be the first to send a satellite into space if they followed the ideas of von Braun. The Americans had now lost 1 year in the race to the moon. As the Russians were indeed first into space, the Americans re-established Werner von Braun, and thus began their success story at NASA. Von Braun became the first head of NASA with the Explorer 1 on 31 January 1958.

Man soon realized that the human brain had not the capacity to calculate the ecliptic in which we are moving. Computers were required to establish the exact orbits that would lead us to the moon. When on the moon, a robot would be required to drive a car, take photographs and pick up stones. At that time (1960s), no one dared to think that this technique would take over surgery.

Since its early development, endoscopic surgery has been refined. Appendectomy[4], cholecystectomy and endoscopic hysterectomy[5] have all now become routine procedures. This •became possible when the image seen by the endoscope could be transmitted in color. The first endo-video camera used in Kiel weighed 35 kg. At NASA, smaller and smaller cameras were constantly being produced, as was necessary for the space program. From year to year, the progress was followed and integrated into medicine, ultimately producing a video image so true that one could operate from the video screen: a dream became reality.

The developments of one man in Kiel between 1970 and 1995 had changed the entire spectrum of surgery in the abdomen (laparoscopy), thorax (thoracoscopy) and joints (arthroscopy).

The equipment necessary to produce a pneumoperitoneum[6] and to perform hemostasis matured into highly differentiated mechanisms and was developed by Semm in Munich and Kiel in Germany. In the space program, centers for development realized that they could also make inroads in the new area of endoscopic surgery.

What began with anesthesia and the auxiliary-supported era with antibiotics, transfusions and intensive care medicine has changed the entire realm of surgery and put the concept of 'better quality of life' forever on the surgical map. Endoscopic surgery was the final development of this concept. For many, it remains unclear whether endoscopic surgery is indeed a great improvement when compared to the open procedure. However, it can now be said that the freestyle battle of the ten fingers into the open cavity of the human body is finished. The manual dexterity required to perform the techniques established through the basic endoscopic surgery practiced today is the keystone of the future: robotic surgery.

Until now, the human brain has dictated control over the hands and fingers, so that the commands it gives can be realized on the patient. The various equipment and instruments used at endoscopic surgery, together with the two-dimensional aspect, is proving to be almost too much for the human brain. It is a logical consequence that a computer would come between the human brain and the inexact finger movements, allowing the precision necessary to perform intricate endoscopic surgery both accurately and routinely.

In the automobile industry, we have long become accustomed to the fact that manual production is a thing of the past. Computers and robots determine the quality of the product. The quality of a surgeon's work is determined by his manual dexterity, which is a result of his experience. Manual dexterity is variable, and dependent on physical and psychological components. Should not this irregular component also be improved upon by the precision only a computer can achieve? The surgeon no longer stands bent over the operating table but sits comfortably in front of the computer screen. The computer can demonstrate in seconds each minute detail of the operative site. The surgeon manipulates virtual instruments which are then processed by the computer to steer robots that actually move the classic instruments such as scalpels, scissors and clamps. This is already the standard used daily in air travel, where it has long been known that the human brain is not in a position to control and co-ordinate all movements required to operate a jet-liner effectively.

A geographical powered system (GPS) allows us to map out via satellite the exact position of planes, boats, cars and even taxis, and allows their movements down to the last decimeter to be continually monitored. Hospitals in the future will constantly know the whereabouts of each patient using this same system.

All prerequisites currently exist; only the initiative to co-ordinate the matter is missing. The seed for this idea has already been sown: it is computer motion, the precursor of computerized robotic surgery.

A small group in Santa Barbara, California have continued the work of a surgeon from Kiel, Germany. His first requirement to perform operative endoscopic surgery was the necessity to work with both hands[2,3]. Initially, the endoscope was held with one hand and the second was used to operate. Later, an assistant held the endoscope so that the surgeon could operate with both hands.

The first stage of using computer motion was AESOP (automated endoscopic system for optimal positioning), the optic holder. Its movements are controlled by voice commands ('voice-controlled'). The surgeon decides the visual field he wishes to see. Both hands are free throughout the entire procedure, and his voice commands the optic holder to 'advance', 'go back', 'go left', 'go right', 'up', etc.

The second stage in the use of computer motion was the program HERMES. The number of pieces of equipment required at endoscopic surgery has greatly increased over time, for example the CO_2-insufflator[7], the aquapurator, the endo-coagulator[7], etc. To use all this equipment at the correct time, 'circulators' are required to be present in the operating room at all times to switch items on and off and regulate their intensity when required. Using the HERMES program, these functions are taken over by the voice-controlled system.

The third stage of computer motion is use of the ZEUS program (robotic system for microsurgery). In this program, the brain itself coordinates the movements of the hands and fingers to move virtual instruments that give an impulse to the computer which, in turn, translates the finger movements into the language of one or more robots. Furthermore, complete knowledge about the actual surgery is input into the computer.

This all sounds very Utopian, but is actually routine in the airline and automobile industries. Here, robots work the assembly line. Human brains in the construction office make the software and the actual mechanical work is performed by robots in the construction hall.

The financial background for the ZEUS program will be provided by heart surgery, for example the endoscopic bypass operation. An endoscopic coronary bypass graft (E-CABG) may be performed through a 4-cm space between two ribs, replacing thoracotomy. Two robot arms simplify this operative procedure. Tests of computer motion in Santa Barbara show that ZEUS can perform the end-to-end anastamosis on the heart vessels with great ease and perfection. Another technique, to stop heart movements during the operation time, is already complete in Germany. Progress in heart vessel surgery is rapid. If money was no object and what we spend for investigation of our neighboring planets could be spent on people, using the ZEUS program for E-CABG, around 700 000 cases world-wide per annum would before long be routine.

References

1. Semm K, von Hassel MW. *Kiel University Hospital of Gynecology and Michaelis School of Midwifery.* 1985:196
2. Semm K. *Pelviscopy and Hysteroscopy. Color Atlas and Reference Book.* Stuttgart, New York: Schattauer, 1976:340
3. Semm K. *Operative Manual for Endoscopic Abdominal Surgery.* New York: Year Book Medical Publishers, 1987:485
4. Semm K. Hysterektomie per laparotomiam oder pelviscopiam ohne Colpotomie. *Geburtsh Frauenheilkd* 1992;51:737–77
5. Semm K. Advances in endoscopic surgery (endoscopic appendectomy). In *Current Problems in Obstetrics and Gynecology.* Chicago, London: Year Book Medical Publishers, 1982;
6. Semm K. Die Technik des Pneumoperitoneum. *Endoscopy* 1969;1:68–70
7. Semm K. *Interfascial Subtotal Hysterectomy, C*IS*H, TUMA, IVH. Macro-Morcellation,* 3rd edn, 1997:152

30

The role of hysteroscopy in the evaluation of the mechanism of carcinogenesis in endometrial polyps

H. Maia, A. Maltez, M. Oliveira and E. M. Coutinho

Introduction

Endometrial atypical hyperplasia is a precursor lesion for endometrial carcinoma. Usually this is the result of the longstanding unopposed action of estrogens on the endometrium. The association between hyperestrogenism, endometrial hyperplasia and carcinoma has been known for a long time. The endometrial carcinoma is usually of a low-grade, endometrioid type and has a favorable clinical course[1]. However, not all endometrial neoplasias follow this pattern and 10% of endometrial carcinomas are not associated with longstanding unopposed exposure to estrogens. These carcinomas are usually of a non-endometrioid type, are high-grade, and are associated with less favorable survival rates. They occur more frequently in elderly patients in a background of endometrial atrophy[2]. Endometrial hyperplasia is not a precursor lesion for this kind of neoplasm. It is known that the process of carcinogenesis involves the accumulation of random mutations affecting both oncogenes and tumor suppressor genes. These events occur during cell division and it is unlikely that an atrophic non-proliferating endometrium can be the precursor lesion for these neoplasms. Endometrial polyps, on the other hand, are found in the uterine cavity during both the pre- and postmenopausal periods. They are frequently associated with the origin of high-grade endometrial carcinomas in tamoxifen users[3]. Another highly aggressive neoplasm, the serous papillary endometrial carcinoma, frequently arises in endometrial polyps, particularly in elderly patients[4]. However, the role of endometrial polyps as precursor lesions for some forms of endometrial carcinoma is not totally understood. Here we discuss the diagnosis and hysteroscopic treatment of endometrial polyps and the mechanism of carcinogenesis in these lesions.

Pathology and hysteroscopy in the diagnosis of endometrial polyps in premenopausal patients with menorrhagia

Endometrial polyps are a relatively common cause of abnormal uterine bleeding during the reproductive years, although a significant number of them are either asymptomatic or not clinically suspected. Despite their frequency, the diagnosis of endometrial polyps is greatly underestimated when blind biopsies or dilatation and curettage are used, because they may be missed by any procedure that samples only portions of the endometrium[5]. The use of hysteroscopy or sonohysterography can make the diagnosis of endometrial polyps more accurate. However, there are frequent discrepancies in the diagnosis of polyps based on their microscopic or hysteroscopic appearance, reflecting the absence of a gold standard for hysteroscopic diagnosis. The term 'endometrial polyp' as used in hysteroscopy is a clinical rather than a pathological one, indicating a growth attached by means of a pedicle or stem. From the pathological point of view the diagnosis of a polyp requires the presence of a fibrous stroma, thick-walled blood vessels and an altered glandular pattern[6]. The uninvolved endometrium is often histologically normal, and it may be in any phase of the cycle. However, not all polypoid lesions within the uterine cavity, detected by hysteroscopy, fulfil all the necessary criteria for the microscopic diagnosis of a polyp. Indeed, some polypoid projections of endometrial mucosa present during the luteal phase are simply localized overgrowths of histologically normal secretory endometrium[7]. Since endometrial polyps have distinct glandular and stromal abnormalities, it is important to determine the accuracy of hysteroscopic diagnosis when compared to histopathology. This was studied in 72 premenopausal patients (31–51 years) with menorrhagia and a hysteroscopic diagnosis of endometrial polyps. These patients were submitted to polypectomy followed by endometrial resection in an unprepared endometrium. After the uterine cavity was visualized, the polypoid lesion was sliced with the resectoscope all the way down to the base. When this was completed, an 8-mm Karman curette was introduced into the uterine cavity. A vacuum curettage was then performed to remove the functional layer of the endometrium[8], followed by the reintroduction of the resectoscope to remove the basal layer of the endometrium and upper part of the myometrium. The endometrium and polyp were fixated with formalin 4% and submitted to routine hematoxylin–eosin stain. They were examined separately by the same pathologist (A.M.). The histopathological results of the excised polypoid lesions are summarized in Table 1. Eighteen per cent of the polypoid projections of the endometrium were mucosal folds histologically indistinguishable from the rest of the secretory endometrium. These polypoid projections lacked both thick-walled blood vessels and fibrous stroma which are characteristic of polyps. The glandular architecture was preserved. In 8% of the cases, the polyp represented a focal area of simple hyperplasia that was devoid of thick-walled blood vessels and fibrous stroma. This area of hyperplasia appeared at hysteroscopy as a sessile polypoid projection of the mucosa. The surrounding endometrium was normal, showing either proliferative or secretory changes according to the phase of the menstrual cycle. Two patients in this group, who were using an oral combination

Table 1 Histopathological findings in endometrial polypoid lesions diagnosed by hysteroscopy and polypectomy specimens

Diagnosis	n	%
Normal endometrial tissue	13	18
Focal hyperplasia	6	8
Endometrial polyps	53	74
Total	72	100

of estrogens and progestin to control bleeding, had secretory changes and stromal decidualization in the endometrium but not in the polypoid lesion. The presence of thick-walled blood vessels and a fibrous stroma was detected by pathology in 74% of the hysteroscopically diagnosed polyps. The glandular epithelium was non-functional in 46 out of 53 cases (87%), displaying different degrees of architectural disarray and cystic dilatation of the glands. This epithelium was out of phase with the adjacent endometrium which showed normal secretory changes. The stroma in the polyps was fibrous and did not show decidualization in any of the cases. In some of these polyps it was possible to follow the immature endometrium downwards as a broad zone to the basalis. In seven patients (13%), the polyps were made up of functional endometrium that responded to progesterone, showing normal secretory changes in the glandular epithelium that were identical to those observed in the adjacent endometrium. There was no architectural disarray of the glandular epithelium. The connective stalk and the thick-walled blood vessels in these polyps were similar to those observed in the non-functional polyps, and their presence was important to differentiate these lesions from the normal mucosal folds of the luteal-phase endometrium. Hysteroscopy could not distinguish between these two types of polyps with accuracy even though cystic dilated glands could be observed frequently when the non-functional polyp was sliced with the resectoscope. These results indicate that not all endometrial polyps diagnosed by hysteroscopy fulfil all histopathological criteria for their diagnosis. Polypoid projections of the luteal-phase mucosa can easily be mistaken for endometrial polyps[7]. Focal areas of endometrial hyperplasia unresponsive to progesterone can have a polypoid appearance at hysteroscopy. However, these lesions lack both the connective stalk and the thick-walled blood vessels. From the standpoint of responsiveness to ovarian steroid hormones, true endometrial polyps, on the other hand, can be divided into two groups, according to the morphology of endometrial glands. In the great majority of polyps, the endometrial glands are non-functioning, showing a pattern of simple and, less commonly, complex hyperplasia, which does not respond to progesterone even when a full secretory response is present in the glands of the adjacent endometrium[6]. This type of polyp is made up of endometrium capable only of proliferation but not of functional differentiation. The origin of this immature endometrium can be traced to the basalis. Because these areas of mucosa do not respond adequately to progesterone they are not shed during menstruation. In time they move upward without differentiating and present in the uterine cavity as polyps. Recent cytogenetic studies have revealed chromosome aberrations confined only to the mesenchymal component of endometrial polyps[9]. Changes affecting genes involved in cell proliferation have been described in endometrial polyps. The lack of response to progesterone, on the other hand, may be caused by a decrease in the number of receptors for this hormone in the stroma of endometrial polyps[10]. Without proper action on stromal cells the response of the glandular epithelium to progesterone is impaired, favoring an unopposed action of estrogens[10]. However, progesterone unresponsiveness is not observed in all cases and some polyps can display secretory changes in their glandular epithelium during the luteal phase of the menstrual cycle. These polyps have thick-walled blood vessels and a connective axis similar to that of the non-functional polyps. It is evident that the term 'endometrial polyp' encompasses a variety of different pathologies. It is not known, for example, whether functional or non-functional polyps harbor the same cytogenetic or genic aberrations.

The histogenesis of non-functional endometrial polyps can be traced downward to the basal layer of the endometrium, which is normally unresponsive to progesterone. Whether the observed chromosome aberrations are responsible for the alterations observed in the maturation of the glandular epithelium is only speculative at the moment. However, the secretory changes of the endometrial glands depend on their interaction with the underlying stroma. The decrease in the number of progesterone receptors in stromal cells of polyps may impair the response of the glandular epithelium to this hormone. This might explain the lack of effect of progesterone on glandular hyperplasia present in polyps[10]. Without the antiproliferative action of progesterone, estrogens act unopposed on these lesions, favoring the appearance of carcinomas in the polyp even though the adjacent endometrium is secretory. The concomitant presence of endometrial carcinoma and secretory endometrium has been reported, and when this occurred the neoplasia was confined to a polyp or to areas unresponsive to progesterone. This is in agreement with our findings that there are areas in the endometrium that do not respond adequately to progesterone, resulting in the formation of polypoid lesions that represent foci of refractory hyperplasia.

Hysteroscopic management of abnormal uterine bleeding in postmenopausal patients

Progestins are administered to postmenopausal patients under hormone replacement therapy (HRT) in order to prevent the occurrence of endometrial hyperplasia, which is one of the consequences of the unopposed action of estrogens on the endometrium. However, the use of progestins does not prevent the occurrence of uterine pathology, including endometrial carcinoma, in all patients. Measurement of endometrial echo by transvaginal sonography in these patients is a reliable method for monitoring endometrial safety during the use of HRT[11]. These studies have shown that postmenopausal women can develop an increase in endometrial thickness while using HRT despite the use of progestins. This increase in endometrial thickness occurs between 6 and 36 months after initiation of therapy and is usually associated with abnormal uterine bleeding. The hysteroscopic findings in these patients are shown in Table 2. The most common cause of abnormal uterine bleeding in HRT users was endometrial polyps, followed by atrophic endometrium and submucous myoma. The occurrence of carcinomas was observed in only 2% of cases and those had their origin in polyps. Comparison between hysteroscopy and suction curettage for evaluation of uterine cavity during menopause has revealed low rates of positive diagnosis for polyps and submucous myomas when curettes with a diameter less than 4 mm were used[7]. However, the percentage of positive diagnoses of endometrial polyps increased to 80% when the diameter of the suction curette was at least 5 mm. This indicates that suction curettage can be a reliable method for the diagnosis of endometrial polyps if curettes of large diameter are used. Suction curettage using 8-mm cannulae can be used prior to resectoscopic surgery to remove large parts of endometrial polyps, thus facilitating polypectomy and endometrial resection. In HRT patients, endometrial resection is effective in controlling bleeding and in removing intrauterine lesions. One of the advantages of this procedure is that it can be carried out on an out-patient basis using paracervical block and intravenous propofol with minimal trauma to elderly patients. Whenever indicated, conjugated estrogens are given preoperatively in the form of vaginal cream to soften the cervix and facilitate cervical dilatation to 9 mm[5]. Resectoscopic surgery can be used safely to perform polypectomies, myomectomies and endometrial resection in HRT patients. Histopathological examination of polypectomy specimens revealed the presence of different degrees of hyperplasia inside endometrial polyps while the adjacent endometrium displayed only atrophic or functional changes. In early cases endometrial polyps appeared as a localized unevenness of endometrial mucosa frequently associated with hematometrium. Pathology showed the presence of basal-cell hyperplasia in these lesions. The glandular epithelium in endometrial polyps often displayed a persistent hyperplasia with the glands showing cystic dilatation and architectural disarray. Complex hyperplasia, sometimes with atypia, was observed in 10% of the polyps from HRT users. The rest of the endometrium was usually atrophic or showed functional changes. Cases of endometrial carcinoma were observed in our series of menopausal patients using HRT despite the use of progestins. In these patients the carcinomas were usually confined to endometrial polyps and they were frequently of high grade or non-endometrioid type (Figure 1). This contrasts with the well-differentiated endometrial carcinoma observed in menopausal patients using unopposed estrogens. This suggests that endometrial polyps may be precursor lesions for some forms of carcinomas. Because of the frequent association of polyps with carcinoma, endometrial resection should always be carried out whenever polypectomy is performed during the menopause. This may reduce the

Table 2 Hysteroscopic findings in postmenopausal patients with abnormal uterine bleeding after using hormone replacement therapy

Finding	n	%
Atrophic uterine cavity	30	25
Submucous myoma	13	11
Endometrial polyp	69	57
Endometrial hyperplasia	6	5
Endometrial carcinoma	3	2*
Total	121	100

*Two carcinomas were confined to polyps

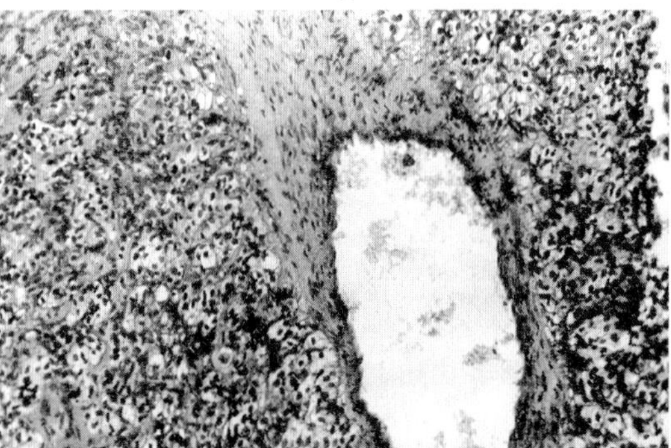

Figure 1 Clear-cell carcinoma developing in an endometrial polyp from a postmenopausal patient using conjugated estrogens with medroxyprogesterone acetate. Note the presence of cancerous cells surrounding the thick-walled blood vessels of the base of the polyp

recurrence not only of polyps but also of endometrial carcinoma, particularly in patients using HRT for a long period of time[4]. Amenorrhea rates were over 95% after resectoscopic surgery in patients who chose to continue using HRT. The use of progestins was not discontinued in these cases and recurrence of polyps occurred in less than 5% of the patients after 2 years.

Steroid receptors and p53 overexpression in endometrial polyps

Progestins are effective agents in opposing the stimulatory effect of estrogens on the endometrium, thus preventing the hyperplasia induced by the use of estrogen alone during menopause. The antiproliferative effects of progestins on endometrium are achieved through several mechanisms acting on both glandular and stromal components. They involve a reduction in the number of estrogen receptors in the glandular epithelium, activation of 17β-hydroxysteroid dehydrogenase, which converts estradiol to less potent estrogens, and synthesis of insulin-like growth factor binding proteins by the stromal cells. The presence of progesterone receptors in the endometrial stroma is necessary for the full secretory response of the glandular epithelium to progestins. Whenever they are administered sequentially or continuously to postmenopausal patients taking estrogens, the end result will be either endometrial sloughing or atrophy. In the absence of cell proliferation, endometrial thickness will be less than 4 mm. A persistent thick endometrial echo in menopausal patients using HRT, on the other hand, is suggestive of the presence of intrauterine pathology. In these cases, hysteroscopy has revealed the presence of polyps in the uterine cavity that were missed by endometrial biopsies[11]. One characteristic of endometrial polyps is that they respond only to the stimulatory effects of estrogens, showing very little response to progesterone. The glandular epithelium in polyps displays a pattern of hyperplasia that is not reversed by progestins. The lack of response to progesterone leads to an unopposed action of estrogens on these lesions. This may favor the appearance of carcinomas in endometrial polyps. It has

been reported that when there is coexistence of secretory endometrium and carcinoma, the neoplasia is always confined to a polyp or to areas of the endometrium unresponsive to progesterone[12]. A similar situation may occur in HRT patients who develop endometrial polyps after treatment. We have, in fact, recently observed the occurrence of endometrial carcinomas confined to polyps in menopausal patients using HRT. The mechanisms of carcinogenesis in endometrial polyps are not completely understood but they may involve a p53 pathway. Alterations in the p53 tumor suppression gene can antedate the appearance of carcinoma in colonic polyps[13]. A retrospective study was carried out by us to evaluate steroid receptors and p53 in postmenopausal patients who developed endometrial polyps after using HRT for at least 1 year. These patients were referred to our center for evaluation because of abnormal uterine bleeding in the presence of endometrial thickness greater than 5 mm. The diagnostic work-up included transvaginal sonography, hysteroscopy and endometrial biopsy. Twenty-two of these patients had endometrial polyps and they were submitted to an endometrial resection using the 27F resectoscope. Determinations of estrogen, progesterone receptors and p53 overexpression were carried out by histochemical methods in the endometrial polyps. Pathological examination of these polyps revealed the presence of simple hyperplasia with cystic dilated glands and a fibrous stroma in 20 out of 22 cases. The blood vessels at the base of the connective stalk were thick-walled. There was no evidence of stromal decidualization or glandular secretion in the polyp even when the adjacent endometrium showed secretory glands and decidual changes (Figure 2). In one patient, the polyp had a pronounced stromal hyperplasia. Histochemical methods revealed the presence of estrogen receptors in both stroma and glandular epithelium in all polyps. The progesterone receptor, on the other hand, was not detected in the stroma of the polyp in 15 of the 22 patients. A faint positivity for this receptor was detected in the glandular epithelium in the polyp in 12 patients (50%), while in the

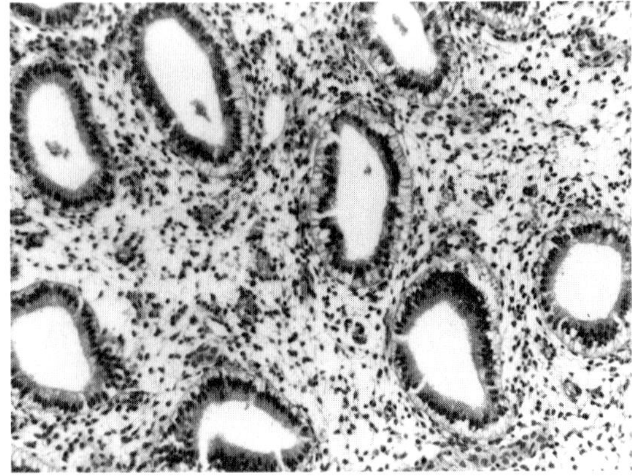

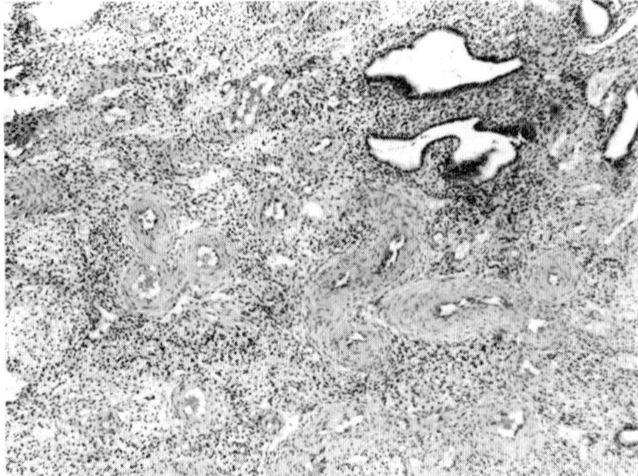

Figure 2 Lack of effect of medroxyprogesterone acetate on an endometrial polyp. Note the signs of glandular secretory exhaustion and intense stromal decidualization in the adjacent endometrium (upper panel), while in the polyp the glands are non-functional and the stroma is fibrous (lower panel)

Table 3 Distribution of progesterone receptors in endometrial polyps from postmenopausal patients using hormone replacement therapy

Distribution	n	%
Stroma positive, glandular epithelium positive	2	9
Stroma positive, glandular epithelium negative	5	23
Stroma negative, glandular epithelium negative	5	23
Stroma negative, glandular epithelium positive	10	45
Total	22	100

remaining cases the glands were completely negative (Table 3). Focal isolated over-expression for p53, sometimes involving only a cell nucleus in the gland, was observed in 13 of 22 patients. This focal over-expression of the p53 tumor suppression gene occurred before the appearance of nuclear atypia and did not show any correlation with the degree of architectural disarray in the glandular epithelium. The pathological meaning of these focal changes in p53 over- expression is not known but they may reflect areas of genomic instability in the polyp. Accumulation of p53 in the cell nucleus may also occur as a result of point mutation or loss of heterozygosity[14]. In both circumstances this may result in a defective DNA repair

mechanism that can lead to an accumulation of deleterious mutations in the cell, favoring its transformation into cancer. It is worthy of mention that carcinomas arising in endometrial polyps have aggressive biological behavior[4]. They are usually of higher grade or non-endometrioid types such as papillary, serous or clear-cell. Over- expression of p53 is detected in these tumors at an early stage of the disease and this correlates negatively with survival[14]. Alterations in the p53 tumor suppression gene in the polyp favor the abrupt transition from simple hyperplasia to carcinoma. This is in contrast with what occurs in the process of carcinogenesis in the endometrium when alterations in the p53 gene occur only in more advanced stages of the disease. In patients using tamoxifen, most of the cases of endometrial carcinoma arise in polyps and they are high-grade tumors[3]. These findings suggest that endometrial polyps may be precursor lesions of some forms of endometrial carcinomas. Polyps have areas of hyperplasia that are unresponsive to progesterone while the adjacent endometrium is either atrophic or displays normal secretory changes. The relative insensitivity of endometrial polyps to progestins present in HRT regimens may be due to a decreased expression of progesterone receptors in their stroma[10]. This may impair the response of the glandular epithelium to progesterone in terms of secretory changes and final differentiation. *In vitro* studies have shown that endometrial glandular epithelium cannot respond to progesterone unless stromal cells are added to the culture. This indicates that the interaction between these two cell types is necessary for the full effect of progesterone on the endometrium. The presence of estrogen receptors in endometrial polyps explains the growth-promoting effects that HRT can exert on these lesions when they are present in the uterine cavity[11]. The proliferative effect of estrogens on polyps cannot be opposed effectively by progesterone, which may increase the risk of carcinomas, particularly if alterations in the p53 tumor suppressor gene occur in these lesions.

References

1. Silveberg SG, Mullen D, Faraci A. Endometrial carcinoma: clinicopathologic comparison of cases in postmenopausal women receiving and not receiving exogenous estrogens. *Cancer* 1980; 45:3018–26
2. Deligdish L, Holinka C. Progesterone receptors in two kinds of endometrial carcinoma. *Cancer* 1986;57:1385–7
3. Magriples U, Naftolin F, Schwartz PE, Carcangiu ML. High grade endometrial carcinoma in tamoxifen-treated breast cancer patients. *J Clin Oncol* 1993;11:485–90
4. Silva EG, Jenkin R. Serous carcinoma in endometrial polyps. *Mod Pathol* 1990;3:120–8
5. Maia H Jr, Calmon LC, Marques D, *et al.* Polypectomy and endometrial resection in postmenopausal patients. *J Am Assoc Gynecol Laparosc* 1997;4:577–82
6. Hendrickson M, Kempson R. Surgical pathology of the uterine corpus. In Bennington J, ed. *Major Problems in Pathology*, Vol. 12. Philadelphia: WB Saunders, 1980
7. Maia H Jr, Maltez A, Calmon LC, *et al.* Comparison between suction curettage, transvaginal sonography and hysteroscopy for the diagnosis of endometrial polyp. *Gynecol Endosc* 1998;7:127–82
8. Maia H Jr, Calmon LC, Marques D, *et al.* Endometrial resection after vacuum curettage. *Gynecol Endosc* 1997;6:353–7
9. Vanni R, DalCin P, Moermam P, *et al.* Endometrial polyp: another benign tumor characterized by 12q13-q15 changes. *Cancer Genet Cytogenet* 1996;90:14–16
10. Maia H Jr, Maltez A, Calmon LC, *et al.* Histopathology and steroid receptors in endometrial polyps of postmenopausal patients under hormone replacement therapy. *Gynecol Endosc* 1998; 7:267–72
11. Maia H Jr, Barbosa IC, Marques D, *et al.* Hysteroscopy and transvaginal sonography in women receiving hormone replacement therapy. *J Am Assoc Gynecol Laparosc* 1997;4:13–18
12. Risberg B, Grontof O, Westholm B. Origin of carcinoma in secretory endometrium: a study using a whole organ sectioning technique. *Gynecol Oncol* 1983;15:32–41
13. Ohue M, Tomita N, Monden T, *et al.* A frequent alteration of p53 gene in carcinoma adenoma of colon. *Cancer Res* 1994;54:4798–804
14. Zheng W, Cao P, Zheng M, *et al.* P53 over-expression and bcl-2 persistence in endometrial carcinoma: comparison of papillar, serous and endometrioid subtypes. *Gynecol Oncol* 1996;61: 167–74

Fertiloscopy 31

A. Watrelot, J. M. Dreyfus, J. P. Andine and M. Cohen

Introduction

Following the work of Gordts and colleagues[1] on transvaginal hydropelviscopy, we have recently developed the concept of fertiloscopy[2,3] as an approach to the diagnosis of tuboperitoneal infertility. The aims of this chapter are to explain the technique, to describe the imagery obtained and to detail the indications for and the results of this procedure.

Technical data

We define fertiloscopy as the combination of transvaginal hydropelviscopy, dye testing, salpingoscopy and microsalpingoscopy as described by Marconi and Quintana[4], and hysteroscopy, performed in this order, on one occasion, under local or general anesthesia.

The different steps in the procedure are as follows (carried out on the patient in normal gynecological position, a speculum being inserted):

(1) Vaginal asepsia with polyvinyl–pyrolidone (Betadine®; Astra Medica, France);

(2) Exposition of the cervix, with use of a Pozzi tenaculum attached at the 8 o'clock position;

(3) Local anesthesia using Xylocaine: 5 ml are injected in each uterosacral ligament;

(4) Introduction of a uterine balloon catheter (Fertiloscopy FH 1–29®; Soprane SA, France) of diameter 2.9 mm: the balloon is inflated with 2–3 cm^3 of air; the trocard is removed, so the flexible catheter can be fixed on the patient's thigh;

(5) Introduction of a Veres needle 1 cm below the cervix: the axis of introduction is strictly median, parallel to the axis of the vaginal posterior wall;

(6) Instillation of 200 ml of saline solution preheated to 34–35 °C: the Veres needle is then removed;

(7) Introduction of the transvaginal catheter in the same manner (Fertiloscopy FTO 1–40®; Soprane SA, France): the balloon is inflated with 4 cm^3 of air; irrigation is continued via the third channel of the catheter;

(8) Introduction of a Fertiloscope of 2.9 mm diameter with a 30° lens (Storz SA, Germany).

(9) Examination of the peritoneal cavity, ovaries, tubes, peritoneum and posterior uterine wall;

(10) Dye testing using methylene blue is then performed via the operative channel of the uterine catheter;

(11) Salpingoscopy can be carried out at the next step: a forceps (5 French) is inserted through the operative channel enabling the fimbria to be grasped, to introduce the scope into the ampulla; at this stage, tubal irrigation is made via the sheath of the miniscope, to distend the tube moderately. Making use of the dye test, we can also perform a microsalpingoscopy, using the magnification given by the scope (up to ×150); the appearance and the number of stained nuclei of tubal cells give a good appreciation of the functionality of the tube; if a peritoneal or ovarian biopsy is needed, the biopsy forceps is also introduced via the operative channel of the catheter;

(12) The transvaginal catheter is then removed after evacuation of the saline solution: it is not necessary to try to remove all the saline solution;

(13) No vaginal stitches are required;

(14) Hysteroscopy is performed last using the same scope inserted through the uterine catheter, without its sheath; irrigation is performed via the operative channel;

(15) The patient is discharged immediately, except if she has asked for general anesthesia; in this case she can leave the hospital during the following hours; if a surgical laparoscopy appears necessary, it can be performed at the same time if the patient is under general sedation and has agreed that the surgeon do so;

(16) The patient is asked not to use a tampon or to have intercourse for 5–6 days.

Anatomical and pathological aspects

The image of the pelvis is inverted, compared to that obtained by laparoscopy. Even if it seems a great advantage to have a physiological view of the ovaries and tubes without the need to move them, it is also a difficulty at first because this is not the habitual aspect of these structures. We can compare the differences between fertiloscopic and laparoscopic views with those observed between abdominal and vaginal ultrasonography. The image is also enlarged: on the one hand it is an advantage to make the diagnosis more precise but, on the other hand, we have to be careful not to overestimate the size of the findings and the pathological aspects. If there is any doubt, it is necessary to compare the size of an abnormality found with, for instance, the known size of a structure such as an ovary, previously visualized by preoperative ultrasonography.

Another potential disadvantage is that the view obtained is not panoramic. It seems necessary to perform 5–10 procedures to obtain an accurate picture. It is also important to be systematic in observation, to achieve completeness. The guideline at the entrance of the pelvis is the posterior concavity of the uterus. It is the 'roof' of the space explored, and by moving alternately to the left and to the right, it is possible to find the utero-ovarian ligament and the ovary when the ligament is followed. It is possible to observe the entire ovarian surface. At the external part of the ovary, the fossa ovarica is explored and the peritoneal aspect can be noted.

Between the ovary and the uterus, the fimbria is found spread around the posterior pole of the ovary (Figures 1 and 2). The fimbrial appearance is well evaluated by fertiloscopy, and it is possible to follow the variations in the mucosa during the normal menstrual cycle. The congestion of the fimbrial fringe around the pre-ovulatory follicle is spectacular, and ovulation can be observed in some cases if fertiloscopy is well programmed. In these cases, follicular fluid comes by transudation from the follicle and seems to be attracted by the fimbria. At the same time, the fimbria moves slowly to encompass the ovarian surface. This phenomenon can be observed during a period of more than 40 min. It is at present difficult to know exactly at which time the oocyte is picked up by the fimbria.

After examination of the fimbria, the ampulla and the isthmus can be reached.

Then, chromopertubation is performed. It is important to check for spillage of the methylene blue from the tube, to detect any phimosis or ampullary dilatation. For this reason, methylene blue has to be sufficiently diluted not to 'blacken' the entire peritoneal cavity at this stage. In all cases, a very acute inspection of the fimbria is important, to detect subtle abnormalities. Next, salpingoscopic evaluation takes place. Salpingoscopy has to be performed as often as possible, to evaluate the ampullary mucosa, and systematically if any post-pelvic inflammatory disease (PID) lesions are found. As outlined by Brosens[5], it is also important to detect any intra-ampullary adhesions, which give a very poor prognosis on the ability of the tubes to have a normal function. So, the presence and quality of folds are noted, and intra-ampullary adhesions are sought. In addition dye-stained nuclei of tubal epithelium are checked according to classifications of

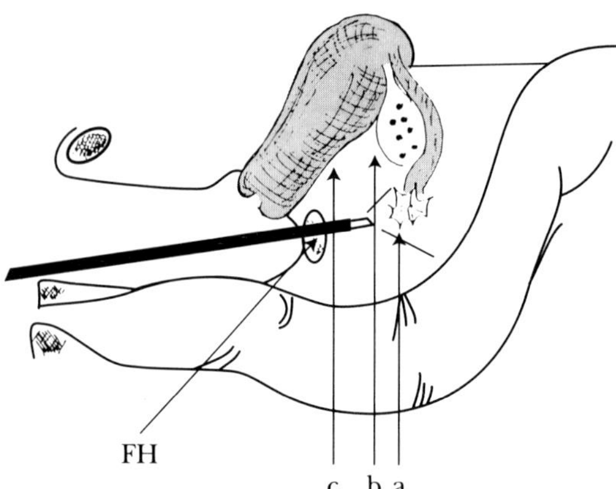

Figure 1 Schematic view of fertiloscopy. FH, balloon introducer and scope; a, b, c, cross-sections as in Figure 2

Marconi[4]. In the case of such lesions, the tube must be considered as too damaged to be repaired.

Pathological findings are the same as those encountered in laparoscopy when examination is performed under water. The only difference is that the non-mobilization of the tubo-ovarian entity allows the detection of small adhesions which would be divided by mobilization. The pathological value of such findings must be focused on in the future. Fertiloscopy seems to be pertinent to diagnose differences in pathology of the pelvis, for example in endometriosis. Various aspects can be visualized, and magnification under water allows the detection of small lesions. Post-PID lesions are often encountered, and these adhesions are well observed without mobilization of the adnexae, with its risk of rupturing some connecting adhesions.

Careful examination of the tubo-ovarian structure allows the detection of any subtle abnormalities known as hypofertility factors. Every finding is reported on a special file and every procedure is videorecorded.

Indications

Several cases can be encountered, depending on whether or not the patient has previous hysterosalpingography or any evidence of previ-ous PID (especially with a positive *Chlamydia* serology result).

In the case of previous normal hysterosalpingography with no suspicion of tubal disease, fertiloscopy takes place under local anesthesia (or sometimes under neuroleptanalgesia, if wished) before referring the patient to an *in vitro* fertilization (IVF) program if fertiloscopy is normal. In this case, it can replace laparoscopy, which, in our opinion, must be proposed before entering any assisted reproductive technology (ART) program.

If a pathology is found, surgical laparoscopy will then be performed for a second time. In the case of abnormal hysterosalpingography and/or suspicion of tubal damage, fertiloscopy is carried out under general anesthesia, so a surgical laparoscopy can be performed at the same time if it is needed. In these cases, salpingoscopy is important, to detect patients with a poor prognosis owing to intra-ampullary lesions, where IVF should be the option.

Fertiloscopy is also of interest as a second-look procedure after tubal surgery, or to control the effects of an endometriosis treatment, for example.

If fertiloscopy cannot entirely replace laparoscopy, it may avoid unnecessary laparoscopy, and can be a substitute for hysterosalpingography, which is so often imprecise.

One limitation of this technique is the impossibility to visualize the anterior part of the uterus, but this area is rarely involved in infertility except in the case of anterior myoma; however, it can be easily detected by ultrasonography. A unique endometriosis location in the vesicouterine cul-de-sac may not be detected, but once again, it is very rare to see a patient with only this localization of endometriosis.

In the case of a negative dye test, it is necessary to complete fertiloscopy by a proximal tubal method such as selective salpingography or falloposcopy (represented in our experience by 9% of cases).

Another limitation is the obliteration of the pouch of Douglas (in the case of endometriosis of the rectovaginal septum or if there is a fixed uterine retroversion). Performing fertiloscopy in this case exposes the patient to the risk of

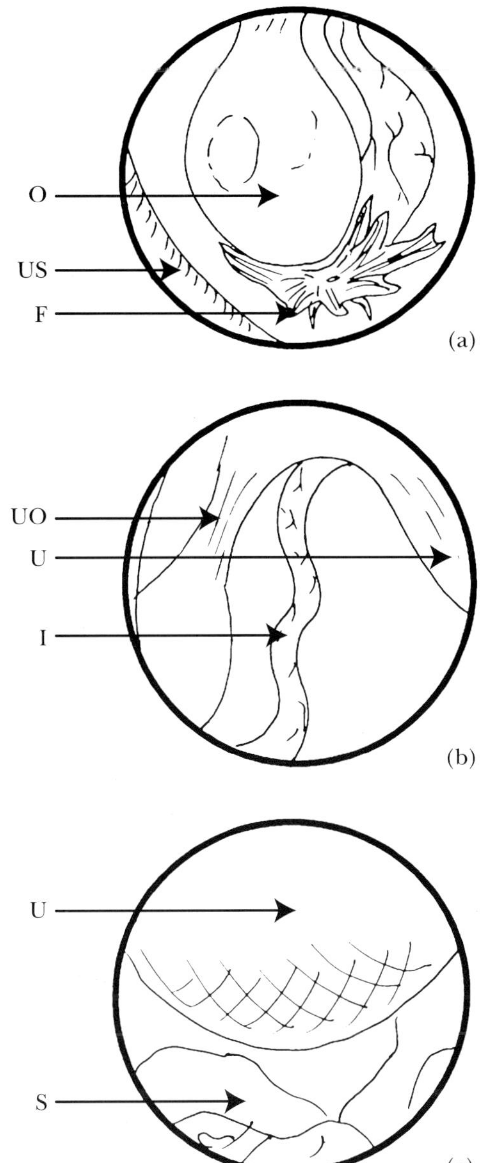

Figure 2 Fertiloscopic anatomy. O, right ovary; US, uterosacral ligament; F, fimbria; UO, utero-ovarian ligament; U, uterus; I, right isthmus; S, sigmoid

Results

Between October 1997 and January 1999, 300 fertiloscopies were performed on a routine basis. Sixty-six cases were performed under local anesthesia without any general sedation (22%).

Other cases were performed under neuroleptanalgesia, either as the patient's choice, or because it was thought that a further laparoscopy should be carried out at the same time. In six cases (2%), visualization of the pelvis was not satisfactory (three cases because of adhesions and three cases owing to a misplacement of the introducer between peritoneum and vaginal wall): in these cases, laparoscopy was added to replace the fertiloscopy. In one case (0.3%), a rectal injury occured. No treatment was applied, except antibiotics for 2 days.

All fertiloscopic parameters were considered to be completely normal in 114 cases (38%). In the remaining 180 cases, various pathological conditions were found. Endometriosis was discovered in 48 cases (16%). Post-PID lesions were found in 79 cases (26.3%). In 53 cases, subtle abnormalities were discovered according to the classification of Yablonski[6].

According to these findings, we decided not to perform a complementary laparoscopy when either visualization with fertiloscopy appeared normal or subtle abnormalities were found. So, in these 167 cases (55%), patients were referred directly to an IVF program. In 17 other cases (5.6%) of post-PID lesions, abnormal findings on salpingoscopy precluded these patients for tubal repair; therefore, IVF was also the preferred option for them. In the other 116 patients, the surgical route was chosen; this was a surgical laparoscopy at the same time of fertiloscopy in 89 patients (29.6%), and delayed laparoscopy in 24 cases (8%) who had fertiloscopy under local anesthesia. In three cases, a microsurgical laparotomy was performed to treat a proximal tubal obturation. When laparoscopy followed fertiloscopy, the findings were always confirmative in the cases of PID lesions. In cases of endometriosis, one patient classified as American Fertility Society (AFSr) stage II during the fertiloscopy was reclassified as AFSr stage III because of a deep ovarian localization not previously noted. In eight cases, additional

rectal injury, and underlines the necessity of gynecological examination and vaginal ultrasonography prior to fertiloscopy. Rectal injury must, of course, be avoided; nevertheless, if it occurs, the perforation is usually under the peritoneum and can be treated conservatively.

foci were discovered in the anterior cul-de-sac, but these did not affect the initial revised AFS score.

Conclusion

Fertiloscopy seems to be an interesting diagnostic procedure, by virtue of its unique combination of a 'one occasion' procedure of hysteroscopy, transvaginal hydropelviscopy, dye testing and salpingoscopy. A complete morphological evaluation of fertility can be made, except for the lumen of the proximal part of the tube where a falloposcopy should be added, to check this tubal portion. Falloposcopy is rather difficult, and we think that this technique should be reserved for cases with proximal pathology. Otherwise, in these cases, a selective salpingography is possibly the best option to visualize the interstitial and isthmic part of the tubes.

The consideration of contraindications and the practice of preoperative ultrasonography and clinical examination will allow the complication rate to be kept very low. We had only one rectal perforation in a patient with a deep endometriotic infiltration of the rectovaginal septum. This patient was probably poorly explored, because infiltration was clinically rather evident. Perforation was extraperitoneal and therefore treated conservatively as mentioned.

This perforation occurred early on in the work (case number 26), at a time when the trocar was directly inserted in the pouch of Douglas. Following that, we introduced the use of the Veres needle inserted before the trocar, to create a safety hydric-space, by spreading the bowel from the uterus, so creating a 'space of security'[7]. Therefore, penetration of the trocar became safer, and we had no further complications of this kind.

With fertiloscopy, the diagnostic sequence can be made under local anesthesia. However, its aim is not to replace laparoscopy, which remains indispensable. Nevertheless, fertiloscopy can avoid unnecessary laparoscopies when findings are normal or too pathological to propose tubal repair (60.6% of cases in our experience). Hence, fertiloscopy is also helpful to distinguish those patients who should undergo tubal laparoscopic repair from those who can directly enter an IVF procedure. It can also be a good survey tool after tubal surgery.

In the future, fertiloscopy could help provide a better understanding of the ovum pick-up phenomena. Operative fertiloscopy will remain reserved for small procedures such as ovarian microbiopsy, puncture-limited adhesiolysis or ovarian drilling. Of course, further studies are necessary, but fertiloscopy already appears to be a good diagnostic alternative to laparoscopy in the management of tuboperitoneal infertility.

References

1. Gordts S, Campo R, Rombauts L, Brosens I. Transvaginal hydrolaparoscopy as an outpatient procedure for infertility investigation. *Hum Reprod* 1998; 13:99–103
2. Watrelot A, Gordts S, Andine JP, Brosens I. Une nouvelle approche diagnostique: la fertiloscopie. *Endomag* 1997;21:7–8
3. Watrelot A, Dreyfus JM, Andine JP. Fertiloscopie: la culdoscopie de l'an 2000. Indications et résultats. *Endomag* 1998;23:17–28
4. Marconi G, Quintana R. Methylene blue dyeing of cellular nuclei during salpingoscopy, a new *in-vivo* method to evaluate vitality of tubal epithelium. *Hum Reprod* 1998;13:3414–17
5. Brosens IA. The value of salpingoscopy in tubal infertility. *Reprod Med Rev* 1996;5:1–11
6. Yablonski R. Subtle abnormalities of the tube. *Fertil Steril* 1990;53:515–20
7. Watrelot A, Dreyfus JM, Andine JP, Cohen M. Fertiloscopy: anatomo-technical basis and indications. *Ref Gynecol Obstet* 1999;6:47–52

Section V
Menopause

Postmenopausal genital bleeding 32

O. Rodriguez-Armas

Introduction

It has been well accepted that primates may have cyclical menstrual bleeding during their reproductive years. Before menarche and after menopause any spontaneous genital bleeding should be considered abnormal.

The endometrium is an unique kind of tissue. The evolutionary development of viviparity demands an appropiate maternal site for a limited but secure fetal interface for reproductive success. The mission of the endometrium is therefore of fundamental importance for reproduction. It initiates and maintains pregnancy as efficiently as possible.

Postmenopausal genital bleeding describes any bleeding that happens after more than 12 months of amenorrhea in a menopausal patient not on hormone replacement therapy (HRT). It is considered abnormal and must be investigated.

The endometrium is recognized as one of the most hormone-sensitive of all adult tissues. Rising levels of estrogen rapidly initiate cellular mitosis and tissue structuring, even after these processes have been dormant or atrophic for many years after the menopause.

Moreover, postmenopausal genital bleeding studies can sometimes show that atrophic endometrium with no estrogenic stimulation is responsible for the majority of cases of postmenopausal genital bleeding, perhaps up to 82% of all cases[1]. In these cases the epithelium is columnar to low cuboidal and lacks mitotic activity; it sometimes demonstrates cystic atrophy.

Endometrial polyps and submucosal fibroids may also produce postmenopausal genital bleeding. Polyps can be sessile or pedunculated and may range in size from microscopic lesions to lesions large enough to occupy the entire endometrial cavity.

Approximately less than 20% of such bleeding arises from malignant tumors[2]. Therefore, it becomes mandatory to thoroughly evaluate the pelvis, and a cervical or endometrial carcinoma must be ruled out.

Postmenopausal genital bleeding can be produced by endometrial hyperplasia, which is the result of continuously unopposed estrogen exposure. Two major categories of endometrial hyperplasia have been identified: the hyperplasia with cytologic atypia and that without atypia[3]. The classification of the International Society of Gynecological Pathologists (ISGP) and the World Health Organization, separating endometrial hyperplasia into the following four categories, is widely accepted: simple hyperplasia, complex or adenomatous, simple atypical hyperplasia and complex atypical hyperplasia[4].

The presence of cytologic atypia appears to be a more important predictor of the progression of hyperplasia to carcinoma than the architectural anomalies. One study showed that 23% of the atypical hyperplasias progressed to carcinoma, compared with 2% of the non-atypical hyperplasias which progressed to malignancy[4].

Those carcinomas that develop from endometrial hyperplasia are usually of the well-differentiated endometrioid type[5].

Postmenopausal genital bleeding is caused by endometrial carcinoma in less than 10% of cases, but accounts for more than 90% of all uterine malignancies generally observed in women over the age of 50[6].

Two types of histological endometrial carcinoma have been identified by Kurman and colleagues[5]. Type I occurs mainly among pre- and perimenopausal women, appears to be related to a history of estrogen exposure and presents as a low-grade type or endometrioid carcinoma.

Type II does not appear to be related to a history of estrogen exposure and is usually a high-grade type (serous clear cell).

The type I profile is associated to a history of endometrial hyperplasia, whereas the type II profile is not[7].

Endometrioid-type carcinoma is the most common primary epithelial endometrial malignancy. The gross appearance varies from a large mass that occupies the endometrial cavity to a diffuse process of endometrial thickening.

The International Federation of Gynecology and Obstetrics (FIGO) and the ISGP have classified the tumor according to architectural and nuclear features[8]. The well-differentiated adenocarcinoma (FIGO grade I) is characterized by a 5% or less solid pattern of tumor growth (excluding the squamous or morular solid component)[9]. If nuclear atypia is marked, despite the architectural features, the lesion is classified as a FIGO grade II lesion[8]. In this group (moderately differentiated adenocarcinoma; FIGO grade II), the solid component corresponds to 6–50% of the tumor and consists of anaplastic cells[8].

FIGO grade III lesions, poorly differentiated adenocarcinomas, are largely composed of solid areas.

In the past, endometrioid carcinomas with squamous components which appeared benign were referred to as adenocanthomas and those with malignant squamous components were known as adenosquamous carcinomas. Today, due to their similar behavior, both are designated according to the degree of squamous differentiation[6].

Serous-type endometrial carcinoma histologically resembles its ovarian counterpart. Five to 10% of all endometrial carcinomas are of the serous type[6]. These tumors have a poor prognosis.

A careful medical history, screening for risk factors, height, weight, age, gravidity, parity, age of menarche, years since menopause and documentation of hypertension, diabetes, obesity, HRT or tamoxifen therapy need to be investigated. A thorough physical and gynecological examination is mandatory in any patient who presents with postmenopausal genital bleeding.

For the patient on HRT, bleeding is normal if it follows certain patterns. For patients on a cyclical regimen with oral estrogen, the normal withdrawal bleeding starts on or after the 10th day of progestogen.

For patients on continuous combined therapy, breakthrough bleeding is acceptable for the first 3–6 months. If it persists, or if bleeding occurs after a period of amenorrhea, it must be considered abnormal and evaluated.

Evaluation of postmenopausal genital bleeding

Postmenopausal genital bleeding represents today approximately 5–10% of gynecological office visits[9]. With the aging of world population and the increasing use of HRT, the incidence of this problem is likely to grow.

Over 55% of all cases of postmenopausal genital bleeding are caused by non-organic lesions (atrophy, hormones, etc.) and they deserve observation and/or control of the dosage of hormonal regimens[9].

Ultrasound examinations (pelvic, transvaginal or sonohysterogram) are tests of paramount importance in assessing endometrial thickness and intracavitary lesions that may produce postmenopausal genital bleeding.

A transvaginal thickness of 5 mm or more for women not taking HRT and 8 mm or more for women taking HRT could represent histologically an endometrial hyperplasia or endometrial carcinoma[10].

Transvaginal sonohysterography using sterile saline solution increases detection sensitivity of intraluminal masses such as polyps and submucosal myomas. Transvaginal sonohysterography has proven to be an accurate modality for diagnosis, with a sensitivity of 86% and 100% specificity for intracavitary lesions[11].

Office endometrial biopsy is a sensitive and relatively inexpensive test for identifying endometrial hyperplasia and endometrial carcinoma, with a reported sensitivity of approximately 85–90% for the detection of endometrial carcinoma[10].

The Novak curette or Pipelle cannula are the most popular instruments used today for endometrial sampling in patients with postmenopausal genital bleeding.

Approximately 45% of postmenopausal genital bleeding originates from benign or malignant lesions[9]. Besides ultrasound examinations (vaginal, pelvic or transvaginal sonohysterography) and office endometrial biopsy, hysteroscopy and fractional curettage are very important tests in assessing the endometrial cavity to detect the source of the irregular bleeding.

Management of postmenopausal genital bleeding

Treatment of postmenopausal genital bleeding will depend on its cause. For most of the time, the management is observation when atrophic endometrium is the cause.

Stopping or modifying hormonal regimens are indicated for patients on HRT.

Endometrial ablation using electrocautery, laser or hydrothermia is used to destroy non-malignant endometrium.

Hysterectomy (either abdominal, vaginal or laparoscopic) is the treatment of choice when a benign lesion recurs after curettage or in those cases with large benign lesions or endometrial hyperplasia.

Endometrial carcinoma requires a more aggressive approach, particularly when an extensive type of tumor is encountered. Radical hysterectomy and radiation therapy are used for some advanced stages and/or poorly differentiated histological types of tumor.

References

1. Choo YC, Mac KC, Hsv C, et al. Postmenopausal uterine bleeding from atrophic endometrium. *Obstet Gynecol* 1985;66:225–8
2. Diamond MP, Osteen KG. *Endometrium and Endometriosis*. Oxford, UK: Blackwell Science, 1997
3. Bokhman JV. Two pathogenetic types of endometrial carcinoma. *Gynecol Oncol* 1983;15:10–17
4. Kurman RJ, Norris HJ. Endometrial hyperplasia and related cellular changes. In Kurman RJ, ed. *Blaustein's Pathology of the Female Genital Tract*, 5th edn. New York: Springer Verlag, 1995:411–37
5. Kurman RJ, Kaminski PF, Norris HJ. The behavior of endometrial hyperplasia: a long term study of untreated hyperplasia in 170 patients. *Cancer* 1985;96:403–12
6. Kurman RJ, Zaino RJ, Norris HJ. Endometrial carcinoma. In Kurman RJ, ed. *Blaustein's Pathology of the Female Genital Tract*, 5th edn. New York: Springer Verlag, 1995:411–37
7. Creasman WT. Announcement, FIGO stages: 1988 revisions. *Gynecol Oncol* 1989;35:125–7
8. Kazadi-Branga J, Jurado-Chacon M. Etiologic study of 275 cases of endouterine hemorrhage by uterine curettage. *Rev Fr Gynecol Obstet* 1994;89:129–33
9. Granberg S, Wikland M, Karlsson B, et al. Endometrial thickness as measured by endovaginal ultrasonography for identifying endometrial abnormalities. *Am J Obstet Gynecol* 1991;164:47–52
10. O'Connell LP, Fries MH, Zeringue E, et al. Triage of abnormal postmenopausal bleeding: a comparison of endometrial biopsy and transvaginal sonohysterography versus fractional curettage with hysteroscopy. *Am J Obstet Gynecol* 1997;178:956–61

Potential of dehydroepiandrosterone as hormone replacement therapy

33

F. Labrie

Introduction

There is no medical problem related to women's health with a higher negative impact on morbidity (and frequently mortality) than the menopause, a condition closely associated with declining sex steroid availability. The most important problems associated with the menopause are osteoporosis and atherosclerosis. It seems appropriate to recall that, in the United States alone, osteoporosis affects presently more than 25 million people, while this already serious problem grows further with the increasing life expectancy of the population. Such an incidence of osteoporosis results in approximately 300 000 hip fractures annually in the United States, with an annual increase of 10 000–20 000 owing to aging of the population. More than 50% of hip fracture patients lose their social independence permanently. Moreover, between 12 and 20% of hip fracture patients die within 1 year from complications of such a fracture. It is estimated that 1.7 million hip fractures occur annually world-wide as a complication of osteoporosis.

The most widely recognized fact concerning the menopause is that there is a progressive decrease and finally an arrest of estrogen secretion by the ovaries. The cessation of ovarian estrogen secretion is illustrated by the marked decline in circulating 17β-estradiol levels. This easily measurable change in circulating estradiol levels, coupled with the demonstrated beneficial effects of estrogens on menopausal symptoms and bone resorption[1], has concentrated most of the efforts of hormone replacement therapy on various forms of estrogen, as well as on combinations of estrogen and progestin to avoid the potentially harmful stimulatory effects of estrogens used alone on the endometrium, which can result in endometrial hyperplasia and cancer. It should be mentioned, however, that recent data suggest that progestins have a negative impact on breast cancer, with reports indicating an increased risk of this cancer[2-5].

Despite the well-known beneficial effects of estrogen therapy on menopausal symptoms[6-8] and its role in reducing bone loss and coronary heart disease[9-14], compliance is low. Women decide not to take estrogens and to stop treatment early because of the fear of breast and uterine cancer[8] and of symptoms associated with this therapy, namely intermittent bleeding, breast tenderness and fluid retention with weight gain.

We feel that the increased understanding of androgen and estrogen formation in peripheral target tissues, a new field called intracrinology[15-25], and our recent observations indicating the predominant role of androgens over that of estrogens in the prevention of bone loss after ovariectomy in the rat[26] as well as the observation of a stimulatory effect of dehydroepiandrosterone (DHEA) on bone formation in postmenopausal women[25], have paved the way for a timely and potentially highly significant progress in the field of sex steroid replacement therapy and aging. Such a possibility is well supported by our observations and those of others of a series of beneficial effects of DHEA observed in postmenopausal women[25,27,28].

Role of DHEA in peripheral sex steroid formation: intracrinology

The approach proposed is based upon the recent progress achieved in our understanding of sex steroid physiology in men and women[15-25] and the recognition that women, at menopause, are not only deprived of estrogen activity because of a declining ovarian function, but have already been submitted for a few years to a decreasing exposure to androgens as a result of the reduced secretion of DHEA by the adrenals.

Humans, with some other primates, are unique among animal species in having adrenals that secrete large amounts of the inactive precursor steroids DHEA and especially dehydroepiandrosterone sulfate (DHEA-S), which are converted into potent androgens and/or estrogens in peripheral tissues. Plasma DHEA-S levels are 5000–25 000 times higher than those of estradiol and 2000–10 000 times higher than those of testosterone, in adult women, thus providing a large supply of substrate for the formation of estrogens and/or androgens. As mentioned above, the local synthesis and action of sex steroids in peripheral target tissues has been termed intracrinology[15,29]. Recent and rapid progress in this area has been made possible following elucidation of the structure of most of the tissue-specific genes that encode the steroidogenic enzymes responsible for the transformation of DHEA-S and DHEA into androgens and/or estrogens locally in peripheral tissues[16,19,21,22,30,31].

The almost exclusive focus on the role of ovarian estrogens has removed the attention from the dramatic 70% fall in circulating DHEA which already occurs between the ages of 20–30 and 40–50 years[23,32–36]. As DHEA is transformed to both androgens and estrogens in peripheral tissues, such a fall in serum DHEA and DHEA-S explains why women at menopause, as mentioned above, are not only lacking estrogens but are also deprived of androgens.

In fact, normal women produce an amount of androgens equivalent to two-thirds of the androgens made in men[24]. The pool of androgens in women decreases progressively from the age of 30 years in parallel with the decrease in the serum concentrations of DHEA and DHEA-S[23]. Consequently, it appears logical to use both androgenic and estrogenic replacement therapy at peri- and postmenopausause, to maintain a physiological balance between these two classes of sex steroids in every cell and tissue,

a goal which can only be met by the local formation of androgens and estrogens in peripheral tissues from a precursor steroid such as DHEA.

The major importance of DHEA and DHEA-S in human sex steroid physiology is illustrated by the fact that our best estimate of the intracrine formation of estrogens in peripheral tissues accounts for 75% of total estrogen formation in women before the menopause and close to 100% after the menopause[15].

Also demonstrated in our previous studies, supplementation with physiological amounts of exogeneous DHEA permits the biosynthesis of androgens and estrogens only in the specific target tissues which contain the appropriate steroidogenic enzymes. The androgens and estrogens thus synthesized remain in the cells of origin, and very little leakage occurs into the circulation. In fact, the most striking effects of DHEA administration on serum steroid concentrations are on the circulating levels of the glucuronide derivatives of the metabolites of dihydrotestosterone (DHT), namely ADT-G, 3α-diol-G and 3β-diol-G. These metabolites are produced locally in the peripheral intracrine tissues which possess the appropriate steroidogenic enzymes to synthesize DHT from the adrenal precursors DHEA and DHEA-S and, thereafter, DHT is metabolized into the inactive glucuronide conjugates[15,21]. This local biosynthesis and action of androgens in target tissues eliminates the exposure of other tissues to androgens, and thus minimizes the risks of undesirable masculinizing or other androgen-related side-effects. The same applies to estrogens, although we feel that a reliable parameter of total estrogen secretion (comparable to the glucuronides for androgens) is not yet available.

Role of androgens in bone physiology

A predominant role of androgens in bone physiology has already been suggested[37]. In fact, both testosterone and DHT increased the transcription of α(I)-procollagen mRNA in osteoblast-like osteosarcoma cells[38]. Treatment with DHT has also been shown to stimulate endochondral bone development in the orchiectomized rat[39]. Bone mineral density measured in the lumbar spine, femoral trochanter and total body was increased more by estrogen plus testosterone implants than by estradiol alone over a 24-month treatment period in postmenopausal women[40].

In established osteoporosis, anabolic steroids have been reported to help prevent bone loss[41]. Similarly, subcutaneous estradiol and testosterone implants have been found to be more efficient than oral estrogen in preventing osteoporosis in postmenopausal women[42]. Although the difference has been attributed to the different routes of administration of the estrogen, the cause of the difference could well be the action of testosterone. Androgen therapy, as observed with nandrolone decanoate, has been found to increase vertebral bone mineral density in postmenopausal women[43]. Although androgens are gaining increasing support owing to their unique actions in postmenopausal women, virilizing effects are observed with the use of testosterone[44,45]. It should also be mentioned that the prevention of bone loss achieved with DHEA in the ovariectomized rat is mostly because of an androgenic effect[26].

Other roles of androgens in women

It is likely that the androgens produced from DHEA have other beneficial effects in postmenopausal women. The detailed benefits of androgens added to estrogen replacement therapy (ERT) or hormone replacement therapy (HRT) have been described in terms of general well-being, energy, mood and general quality of life[46, 47]. Improvements in the major psychological and psychomatic symptoms, namely irritability, nervousness, memory and insomnia have been observed following addition of androgens to ERT[48].

Loss of libido and/or sexual satisfaction are common in early postmenopause. The addition of androgens to HRT is known to have beneficial effects on these problems[46, 49, 50]. Moreover, a positive correlation has been found in postmenopausal women between sexual behavior and circulating levels of androgens. In addition, androgenic compounds have been found to be beneficial for the treatment of the mastalgia frequently caused by HRT[51]. Estrogen replacement therapy may result in severe breast pain which may lead to discontinuation of therapy.

The androgenic effect of DHEA should also be useful in reducing hot flushes. In fact, androgen therapy is successful in reducing hot flushes in hypogonadal men[52]. The addition of androgens has been found to be effective in relieving hot flushes in women who have had unsatisfactory results with estrogen alone[53].

Other potential benefits of DHEA in women

As mentioned above, the 70–95% reduction in the formation of DHEA and DHEA-S by the adrenals during aging results in a dramatic reduction in the formation of androgens and estrogens in peripheral target tissues, which could well be involved in the pathogenesis of age-related diseases such as insulin resistance[54,55] and obesity[56–58]. Low circulating levels of DHEA-S and DHEA have, in fact, been found in patients with breast cancer[59], and DHEA has been found to exert antioncogenic activity in a series of animal models[60–62]. DHEA has also been shown to have immunomodulatory effects *in vitro*[63] and *in vivo* in fungal and viral diseases[64], including human immunodeficiency virus (HIV)[65]. On the other hand, a stimulatory effect of DHEA on the immune system has been described in postmenopausal women[66].

Effects of DHEA in postmenopausal women: increased bone formation and other effects

Introduction

As mentioned above, osteoporosis is a major problem among aging women, causing morbidity and mortality, mainly through increased fracture rates[67]. To avoid the limitations of standard ERT or HRT, we have studied the effect of DHEA administration to 60– to 70-year-old women for 12 months on bone mineral density, parameters of bone formation and turnover, serum lipids, glucose and insulin, adipose tissue mass, muscular mass, energy, well-being, and vaginal and endometrial histology[25,27]. DHEA was administered percutaneously. We have thus evaluated the effect of chronic replacement therapy with a 10% DHEA cream applied once daily for 12 months in 60- to 70-year-old women ($n = 15$).

Bone mineral density

As presented in Table 1, total hip bone mineral density (BMD) increased significantly from 0.744 ± 0.021 to 0.753 ± 0.023 g/cm^2 (1.2%) after 6 months of treatment ($p < 0.05$) and to 0.759 ± 0.025 g/cm^2 (2.0%) after 12 months of DHEA administration ($p < 0.05$). On the other hand, after 12 months of DHEA treatment, the femoral Ward's triangle BMD increased from 0.486 ± 0.026 to 0.494 ± 0.026 g/cm^2 (1.6%, while the lumbar spine BMD increased from 0.829 ± 0.030 to 0.839 ± 0.033 g/cm^2 (1.2%), although these last changes did not reach the level of statistical significance.

Biochemical markers of bone physiology

The serum concentration of osteocalcin, a marker of bone formation, increased from 1.16 ± 0.30 μg/l at pretreatment to 1.95 ± 0.59 (not significant), 2.28 ± 0.53 ($p < 0.05$), 2.49 ± 0.58 ($p < 0.01$, 115% of control value) and 2.44 ± 0.47 μg/l ($p < 0.01$, 110% of control value) after 3, 6, 9 and 12 months of treatment, respectively (Figure 1). Following cessation of DHEA administration, the serum levels of osteocalcin returned to pretreatment values of 1.52 ± 0.33 and 1.14 ± 0.58 μg/l at 3 and 6

months under placebo, these values being not statistically different from pretreatment values (data not shown).

In parallel with the above-indicated effects on serum osteocalcin, the serum concentration

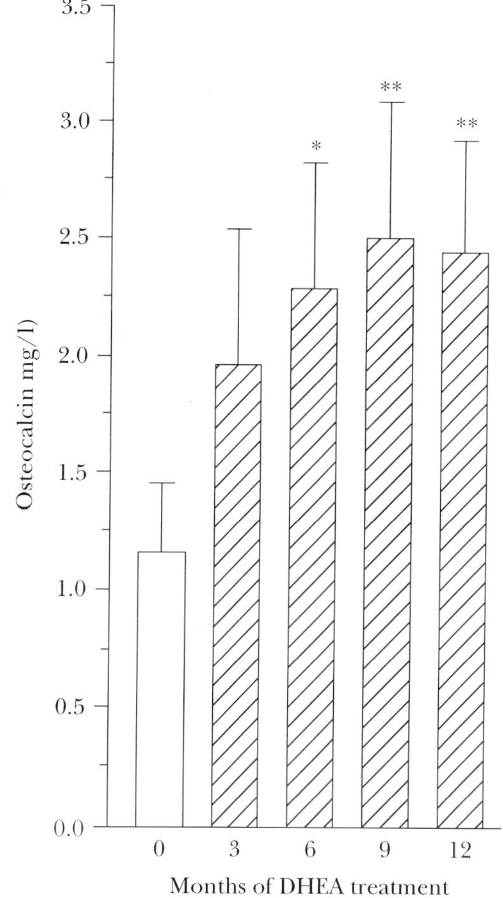

Figure 1 Effect of dehydroepiandrosterone (DHEA) administered percutaneously for up to 12 months on serum concentrations of osteocalcin[25]. *$p < 0.05$, **$p < 0.01$, vs. pretreatment value

Table 1 Effect of percutaneous administration of dehydroepiandrosterone (DHEA) for 6 and 12 months on bone mineral density (90 cm^2) in total hip, Ward's triangle and lumbar spine ($n = 14$)[25]. Values are expressed a mean $\pm$ SD

Site	Pretreatment	6 months DHEA	12 months DHEA
Total hip	0.744 ± 0.021	0.753 ± 0.023*	0.758 ± 0.025*
Ward's triangle	0.486 ± 0.026	0.500 ± 0.026	0.494 ± 0.026
Lumbar spine	0.829 ± 0.030	0.835 ± 0.032	0.839 ± 0.033

*$p < 0.05$, DHEA treatment vs. pretreatment value

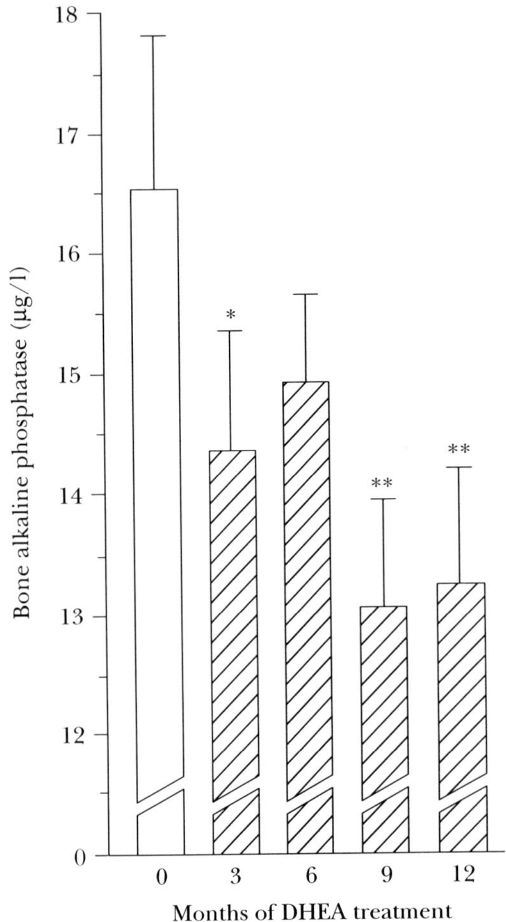

Figure 2 Effect of dehydroepiandrosterone (DHEA) administered percutaneously for up to 12 months on serum concentrations of bone alkaline phosphatase[25].*$p < 0.05$,**$p < 0.01$, vs. pretreatment value

of bone alkaline phosphatase decreased from $16.5 \pm 1.3\,\mu g/l$ (pretreatment) to 14.4 ± 0.9 ($p < 0.05$), 14.9 ± 0.7 (not significant), 13.0 ± 0.9 ($p < 0.01$) and $13.2 \pm 1.0\,\mu g/l$ ($p < 0.01$) at the same time intervals (Figure 2). The values observed 3 and 6 months after cessation of DHEA treatment were not significantly different from those measured at pretreatment or at 6 months of DHEA treatment, although they suggested a trend towards a return to pretreatment values. The urinary hydroxyproline/creatinine ratio, a marker of bone resorption, decreased from $24.0 \pm 1.7\,\mu mol/mmol$ creatinine at pretreatment to 20.6 ± 1.4 ($p < 0.05$) and $17.2 \pm 0.93\,\mu mol/mmol$ creatinine ($p < 0.01$) at 3 and 6 months of DHEA treatment, respectively. At 9 and 12 months of treatment, the urinary hydroxyproline/creatinine ratio was decreased at 18.4 ± 0.9 ($p < 0.01$) and $19.0 \pm 1.3\,\mu mol/mmol$ ($p < 0.01$), respectively (data not shown). Total serum alkaline phosphatase decreased from $92.4 \pm 6.9\,\mu/l$ at pretreatment to 84.6 ± 4.1 (not significant), 82.6 ± 4.1 ($p < 0.05$), 74.9 ± 4.1 ($p < 0.01$) and $77.1 \pm 4.8\,U/l$ ($p < 0.01$) at 3, 6, 9 and 12 months, respectively (Table 2).

Vaginal cytology

Vaginal cytology was examined as a specific parameter of the estrogenic action of DHEA. Before treatment, ten women had a completely atrophic vaginal smear exclusively composed of parabasal cells (see Figure 3a and b, as example). In eight of these ten women, under DHEA treatment, the vaginal cytology was

Table 2 Effect of 12-month percutaneous administration of dehydroepiandrosterone (DHEA) to 60–70-year-old women on plasma alkaline phosphatase, sex hormone-binding globulin (SHBG) and DHEA concentrations[25]. Values are expressed as mean $\pm$ SD

	Months of treatment				
Parameter	0	3	6	9	12
Plasma alkaline phosphatase (U/l)	92.4 ± 6.9	84.6 ± 4.1	82.6 ± 4.1*	74.9 ± 4.1**	77.1 ± 4.8**
SHBG (nmol/l)	65.0 ± 9.8	52.7 ± 5.6*	51.7 ± 5.3*	51.9 ± 7.1**	53.5 ± 6.2*
DHEA (nmol/l)	3.9 ± 0.5	31.6 ± 2.6	30.8 ± 2.4	31.5 ± 3.0	31.2 ± 3.0

*$p < 0.05$,**$p < 0.01$, vs. pretreatment value

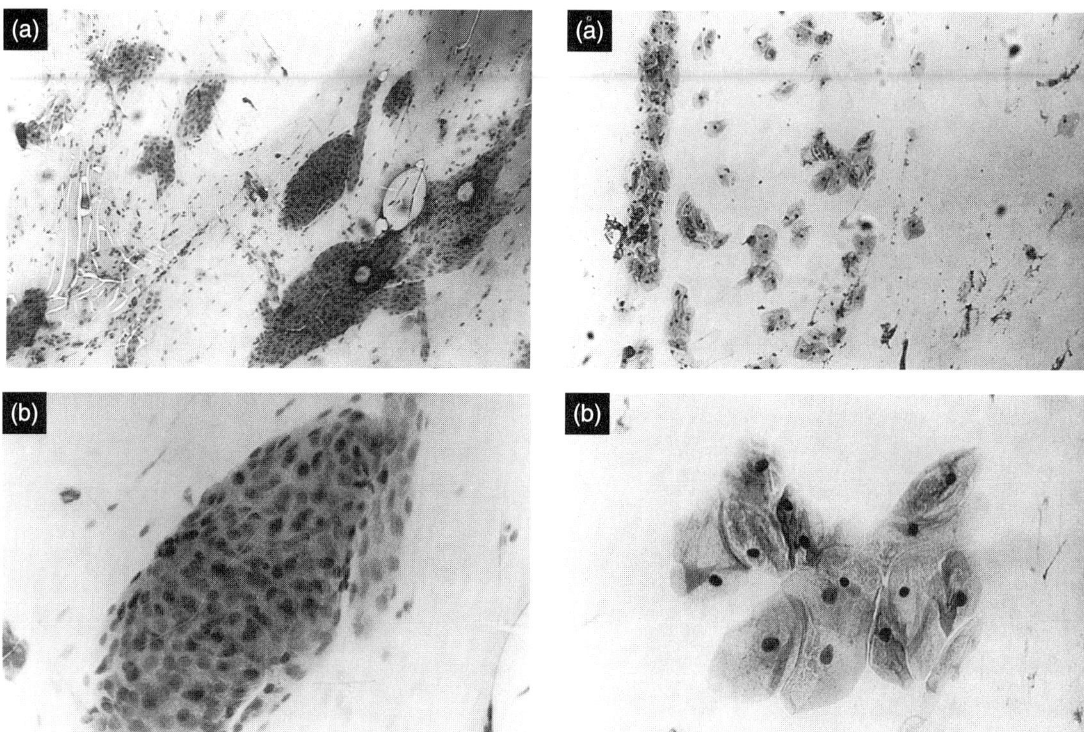

Figure 3 Atrophic vaginal smear with numerous parabasal cells in 65-year-old woman before starting treatment with dehydroepiandrosterone (DHEA) (× 100). (b) Atrophic vaginal smear with numerous parabasal cells in 65-year-old woman before starting treatment with DHEA at higher magnification (× 300)[25]

Figure 4 (a) Vaginal smear from same patient as Figure 3 after 12 months of dehydroepiandrosterone (DHEA) treatment showing superficial pyknotic cells (× 100). (b) Vaginal smear from same patient as Figure 3 after 12 months of DHEA administration showing superficial pyknotic cells at higher magnification (× 300)[25]

converted into a pattern typical of normally cycling women, showing mainly the presence of superficial pyknotic cells (see Figure 4a and b, as example). In two of the ten women having a zero maturation index value at start of treatment, no significant change in the cytological maturation value was observed at up to 12 months of treatment (data not shown). In the three women who had a maturation value between 1 and 40 at the start of treatment, stimulation was also observed, and the cytology became typical of the normal reproductive range in all of them at 3 months, the first time interval measured after the start of DHEA administration (data not shown). In the last two women, the maturation value was already in the normal range of reproductive age at pretreatment, and it remained unchanged during treatment (data not shown).

Endometrial histology

Considering the major concern in relation to the stimulatory effect of estrogens on endometrial proliferation with the associated risk of endometrial carcinoma[68,69], an endometrial biopsy was performed before starting treatment and after 12 months of DHEA administration. As can be seen in Figure 5, the endometrial atrophy seen in all women at start of treatment remained unaffected by 12 months of DHEA administration.

Sebum secretion

As skin sebaceous glands are known to contain all the steroidogenic enzymes which catalyze the transformation of DHEA into the androgen DHT[70–73] and androgens are the main

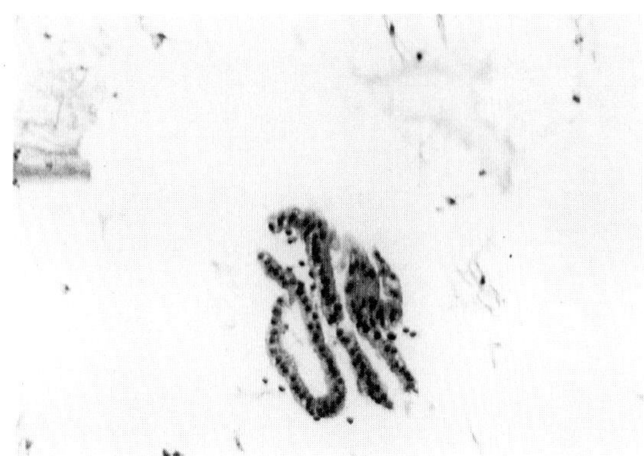

Figure 5 Atrophic endometrium after 12 months of dehydroepiandrosterone (DHEA) treatment in representative 65-year-old woman ($\times 50$)[25]

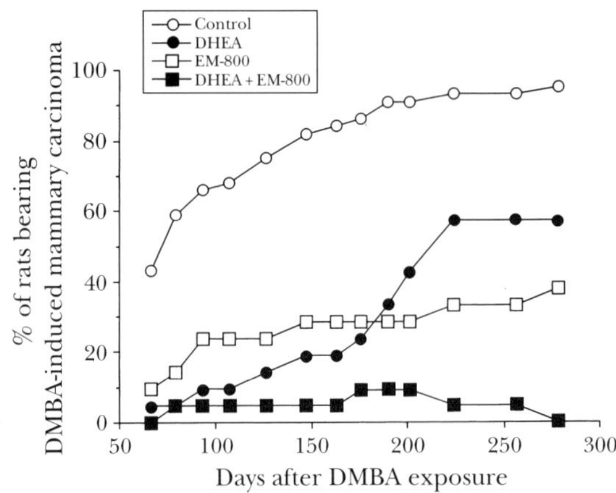

Figure 6 Effect of treatment with dehydroepiandrosterone (DHEA) (10 mg, percutaneously, once daily) or EM-800 (74 µg, orally, once daily) alone or in combination for 9 months on incidence of 2-dimethylbenz(a)anthracene (DMBA)-induced mammary carcinoma in rat throughout 279-day observation period. Data are expressed as percentage of total number of animals in each group[82]

stimulators of sebaceous gland activity[73–76], we have measured the effect of DHEA treatment on sebum secretion. As measured by the Sebutape technique on six facial sites, percutaneous administration of DHEA led to comparable 66–79% levels of stimulation ($p < 0.01$) of sebum secretion measured after 3, 6, 9 and 12 months of treatment (data not shown). Sebum secretion had already returned to pretreatment values 3 months after cessation of DHEA therapy (data not shown).

Lipids

As far as serum lipids are concerned, we have observed a small but not statistically significant decrease in serum triglycerides, cholesterol and lipoprotein components up to 12 months of percutaneous administration of DHEA[27]

Inhibition of breast cancer development and growth

Prevention of breast cancer

As antiestrogens[77–81] as well as DHEA[62], independently, can inhibit the development of 7,12-dimethylbenz(a)anthracene (DMBA)-induced mammary carcinoma, we have studied the potential benefits of combining the new pure antiestrogen EM-800 and DHEA on the development of mammary carcinoma induced

by DMBA in the rat. As the maintenance of bone density and the lipid profile are a main concern at menopause and during antiestrogen therapy, we have also investigated the effect of such a combination on bone mineral metabolism and on the serum lipid profile[82].

Although treatment with DHEA or the antiestrogen EM-800 alone decreased DMBA-induced mammary tumor incidence from 95 to 57% or 38%, respectively, at approximately 9 months after DMBA administration, only two tumors developed in the group of animals who received the combination of DHEA and EM-800, and these two tumors disappeared before the end of the experiment ($p < 0.01$ versus DHEA or EM-800 alone) (Figure 6).

Average tumor number per tumor-bearing animal as well as average tumor area per tumor-bearing animal were also further decreased in animals that received the combination therapy, compared to the effect of each treatment alone ($p < 0.01$).

DHEA induced 6.9% ($p < 0.01$), 10.6% ($p < 0.05$) and 8.2% ($p < 0.01$) increases in BMD of total skeleton, lumbar spine and femur, respectively. The addition of EM-800 to DHEA did not affect the enhancing effect of DHEA on bone mass in these intact animals. The combination of the two drugs had important inhibitory effects on the urinary excretion of calcium and phosphorus as well as on the urinary hydroxyproline/creatinine ratio. Serum total alkaline phosphatase was stimulated by DHEA[82].

Treatment with EM-800 decreased both serum triglycerides and cholesterol levels, while DHEA had an inhibitory effect on serum triglycerides (Figure 7). While treatment with EM-800 caused a marked atrophy of the mammary gland, DHEA alone reduced lobular hyperplasia seen in aged intact rats. Treatment with EM-800 caused a marked inhibition of uterine and vaginal weight[82]. The present data show the additive inhibitory effects of DHEA and EM-800 on the development of DMBA-induced mammary carcinoma in the rat, thus suggesting the potential benefits of such a combination for the prevention of breast cancer in women while preserving or even increasing bone mass and maintaining a favorable lipid profile.

Inhibition of growth of breast cancer

Since, as mentioned above, androgens inhibit breast cancer[79,83], we have studied the possibility that DHEA could inhibit the growth of the human breast cancer ZR-75-1 cell line *in vivo* in nude mice. To avoid the inhibitory effects of DHEA on gonadotropin secretion, and be able to assess the direct effects of DHEA-derived steroids on breast cancer growth, we have used ovariectomized animals supplemented with estrone.

Estrone by itself caused a 9.4-fold increase in ZR-75-1 tumor area after 9.5 months of treatment, whereas the daily oral administration of 15, 50 or 100 μg of EM-800 in estrone-supplemented mice led to inhibitions of 88%, 93% and 94%, respectively. DHEA, at the doses of 0.3 mg, 1.0 mg and 3.0 mg, inhibited tumor weight by 67%, 82% and 85%, respectively (Figure 8). Combination of a daily 15 μg oral dose of EM-800 with the three doses of topical DHEA produced 84–94% inhibitions of estrone-stimulated ZR-75-1 tumor growth, these

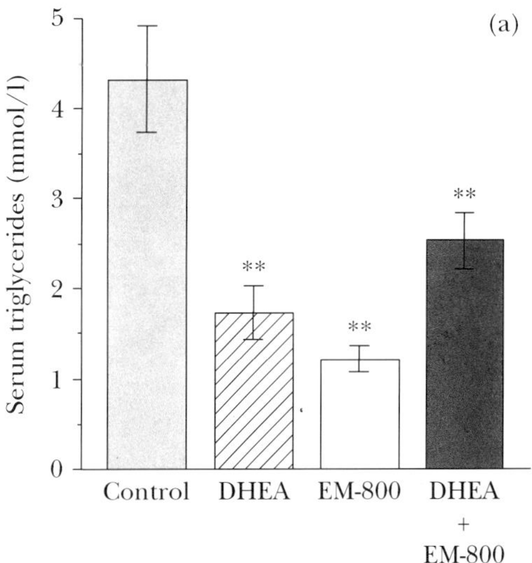

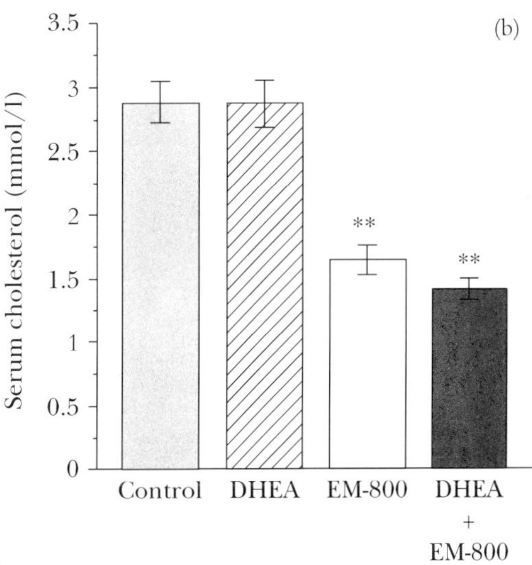

Figure 7 Effect of treatment with dehydroepiandrosterone (DHEA) (10 mg, percutaneously, once daily) or EM-800 (75 μg, orally, once daily) alone or in combination for 9 months on serum triglyceride (a) and cholesterol (b) levels in rat. Data are expressed as mean ± SEM. **$p < 0.01$, experimental vs. respective control[82]

values being not significantly different from the 88% inhibition achieved by EM-800 alone.

Discussion

The present study describes for the first time a series of medically important beneficial effects of DHEA administered for 12 months to

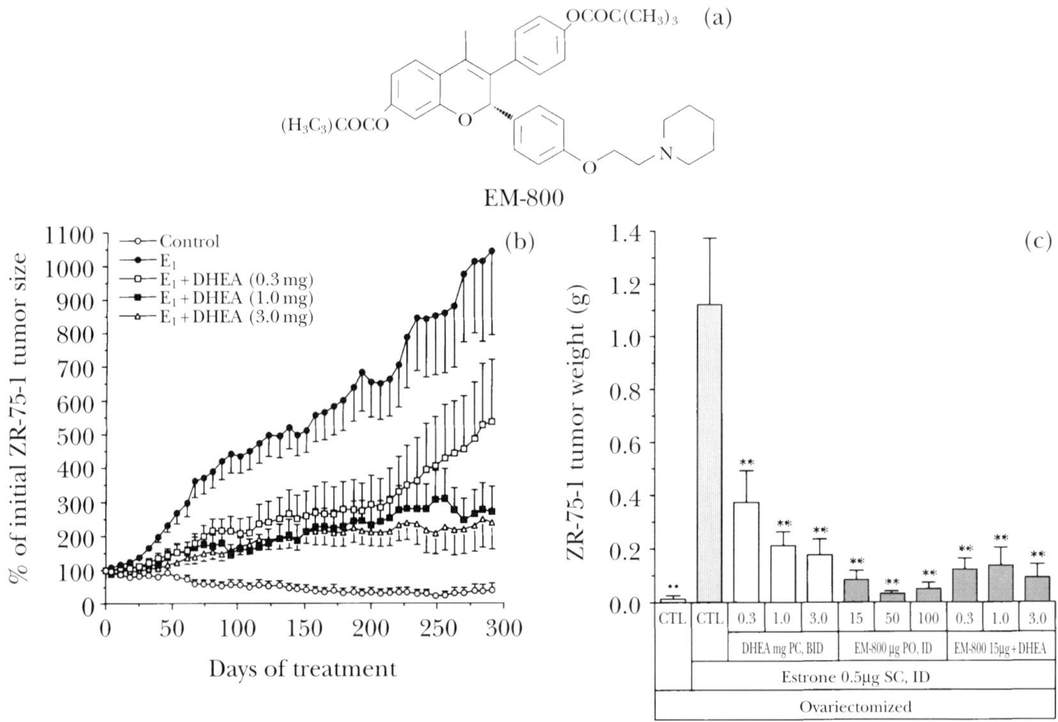

Figure 8   (a) Structure of novel antiestrogen EM-800. (b) Effect of increasing doses of dehydroepiandrosterone (DHEA) (total dose of 0.3, 1.0 or 3.0 mg) administered percutaneously in two doses daily on average ZR-75-1 tumor size in ovariectomized nude mice supplemented with 0.5 µg estrone (E₁) daily. Ovariectomized mice receiving vehicle alone were used as additional controls. Initial tumor size was taken as 100%. DHEA (0.3, 1,0 or 3.0 mg per animal per day) was administered percutaneously on dorsal skin in 0.02-ml solution of 50% ethanol–50% propylene glycol. (c) Effect of treatment with increasing doses of DHEA (0.3, 1.0 or 3.0 mg) or EM-800 (15, 50 or 100 µg) in 0.2-ml 4% ethanol–4% polyethylene glycol 600–1% gelatin–0.9% NaCl alone or in combination (EM-800 at 15 µg and DHEA at 0.3, 1.0 or 3.0 mg) for 9.5 months on ZR-75-1 tumor weight in ovariectomized nude mice supplemented with E₁. **$p < 0.01$, treated vs. control ovariectomized mice supplemented with E₁. CTL, control; PC, percutaneously; BID, twice daily; PO, by mouth; ID, once daily; SC, subcutaneously[86]

postmenopausal women. Possibly the most important effect could be the DHEA-induced stimulation of bone mineral density. The relatively rapid change in bone mineral density is accompanied by an increase in the value of a marker of bone formation, namely serum osteocalcin concentration, while a decrease in bone resorption reflected by a decrease in urinary hydroxyproline excretion was observed in parallel. In addition, the estrogenic stimulation of vaginal cytology in the absence of any stimulatory effect on the endometrium is also of major interest. Our data also confirm the beneficial effects of DHEA on well-being and energy reported previously[28].

The present data clearly suggest the interest of a new approach to hormone replacement therapy having potentially improved efficacy and tolerance. It is possible that DHEA replacement therapy (DRT) could not only correct but also prevent the multiple problems associated with the menopause, a phenomenon preceded and accompanied by a decreased formation of both androgens and estrogens during aging in women.

The present data certainly suggest that DHEA treatment has no deleterious effects but rather indicate a trend towards positive effects on the serum lipid and lipoprotein profile, although a larger cohort of subjects is needed to reach definitive conclusions. On the other hand, it should be mentioned that conjugated equine estrogens raise triglyceride levels and show a deterioration of the insulin response[84,85]. In fact, our data show an inhibitory effect of DHEA treatment on fasting blood glucose and insulin levels[27], thus suggesting an advantage over equine estrogens on glucose metabolism.

In this context, it is important to indicate that the absence of a stimulatory effect of DHEA on the human endometrium[25] eliminates the need to administer a progestin to neutralize the potential effect of estrogens on the endometrium. Concerning the breast, DHEA is known to prevent the development[82] and to inhibit the growth[62] of dimethylbenz(a)anthracene mammary tumors in the rat. DHEA, in addition, inhibits the growth of human breast cancer xenografts in nude mice[86]. Thus, in contrast to estrogens and progestins, which exert stimulatory effects, DHEA is expected to inhibit both the development and the growth of breast cancer in women.

The inhibitory effect of DHEA on the growth of human breast cancer xenografts supports the use of DHEA as hormone replacement therapy in women. Moreover, as the administration of DHEA does not interfere with the inhibitory effect of EM-800 on ZR-75-1 tumor growth, combined treatment with DHEA and EM-800 (or EM-652) could possibly be a convenient therapy in symptomatic postmenopausal women with breast cancer.

EM-652 is a third-generation selective estrogen receptor modulator (SERM), having pure and potent antiestrogenic activity in the mammary gland and endometrium while decreasing serum cholesterol and triglyceride levels and preventing bone loss. The potential benefits of such a combination can be seen in Figure 9. Most importantly, such a combination appears

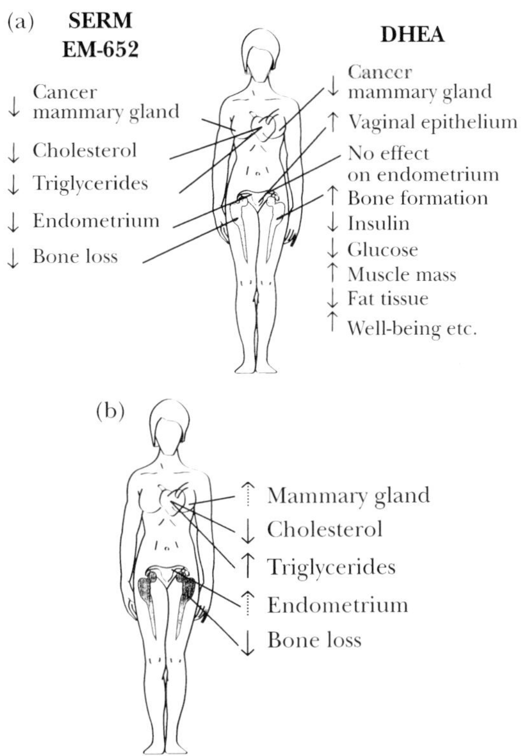

Figure 9 Comparison of potential benefits of combining dehydroepiandrosterone (DHEA) with EM-652. HCl, a selective estrogen receptor modulator (SERM) having pure antiestrogenic activity in mammary gland and endometrium (a) compared to standard hormone replacement therapy (HRT) (b). {right arrow} benefits, {right arrow} negative effects from available evidence: there are no negative effects expected from combination EM-652. HCL + DHEA while potential stimulation of breast and endometrial cancers are risks associated with estrogen therapy. Combination EM-652. HCl + DHEA has series of potential benefits not achievable with standard HRT

to possess the ideal characteristics for prevention of breast and uterine cancer while preventing bone loss, cardiovascular risks and other problems associated with the menopause.

References

1. Christiansen C, Christensen MS, Larsen NE, *et al.* Pathophysiological mechanisms of estrogen effect on bone metabolism. Dose–response relationships in early postmenopausal women. *J Clin Endocrinol Metab* 1982;55:1124–30

2. Horwitz KB. The molecular biology of RU486. Is there a role for antiprogestins in the treatment of breast cancer? *Endocr Rev* 1992;13:146–63

3. Musgrove ES, Lee CS, Sutherland RL. Progestins both stimulate and inhibit breast cancer cell cycle progression while increasing expression of transforming growth factor α, epidermal growth factor receptor, c-*fos*, and c-*myc* genes. *Mol Cell Biol* 1991;11:5032–43

4. Clarke CL, Sutherland RL. Progestin regulation of cellular proliferation. *Endocr Rev* 1990;11: 266–301

5. Colditz GA, Hankinson SE, Hunter DJ, *et al.* The use of estrogens and progestins and the risk of breast cancer in postmenopausal women. *N Engl J Med* 1995;332:1589–93

6. Lomax P, Schonbaum E. Postmenopausal hot flushes and their management. *Pharmacol Ther* 1993;57:347–58

7. Greendale GA, Judd HL. The menopause: health implications and clinical management. *J Am Geriatr Soc* 1993;41:426–36

8. Grady D, Rubin SM, Petitti DB, *et al.* Hormone therapy to prevent disease and prolong life in postmenopausal women. *Ann Intern Med* 1992; 117:1016–37

9. Lobo RA. Clinical review 27: Effects of hormonal replacement on lipids and lipoproteins in post-menopausal women. *J Clin Endocrinol Metab* 1991; 73:925–30

10. Harris ST, Genant HK, Baylink DJ, *et al.* The effects of estrone (Ogen) on spinal bone density of postmenopausal women. *Arch Intern Med* 1991; 151:1980–4

11. Stampfer MJ, Colditz GA, Willett WC, *et al.* Postmenopausal estrogen therapy and cardio-vascular disease. Ten year follow up from the nurses' health study [Comments]. *N Engl J Med* 1991;325:756–62

12. Barrett-Connor E, Bush TL. Estrogen and coronary heart disease in women [Comments]. *J Am Med Assoc* 1991;265:1861–7

13. Lindsay R. Hormone replacement therapy for prevention and treatment of osteoporosis. *Am J Med* 1993;95:37s–9s

14. Field CS, Ory SJ, Wahner HW, *et al.* Preventive effects of transdermal 17β-estradiol on osteo-porotic changes after surgical menopause: a two year placebo controlled trial. *Am J Obstet Gynecol* 1993;168:114–21

15. Labrie F. Intracrinology. *Mol Cell Endocrinol* 1991; 78:C113–18

16. Labrie F, Simard J, Luu-The V, *et al.* Structure, function and tissue-specific gene expression of 3 β-hydroxysteroid dehydrogenase/5-ene-4-ene isomerase enzymes in classical and peripheral intracrine steroidogenic tissues. *J Steroid Biochem Mol Biol* 1992;43:805–26

17. Labrie F, Simard J, Luu-The V, *et al.* Structure and tissue-specific expression of 3b-hydroxysteroid dehydrogenase/5-ene-4-ene isomerase genes in human and rat classical and peripheral steroidogenic tissues. *J Steroid Biochem Mol Biol* 1992;41: 421–35

18. Labrie F, Simard J, Luu-The V, *et al.* Structure, regulation and role of 3β-hydroxysteroid dehydrogenase, 17β-hydroxysteroid dehydro-genase and aromatase enzymes in formation of sex steroids in classical and peripheral intracrine tissues. In Sheppard MC, Stewart PM, eds. *Hormone, Enzymes and Receptors.* London: Baillière Tindall 1994;451–74

19. Labrie Y, Durocher F, Lachance Y, *et al.* The human type II 17β-hydroxysteroid dehydro-genase gene encodes two alternatively-spliced messenger RNA species. *DNA Cell Biol* 1995;14: 849–61

20. Luu-The V, Dufort I, Paquet N, *et al.* Structural characterization and expression of the human dehydroepiandrosterone sulfotransferase gene. *DNA Cell Biol* 1995;14:511–18

21. Labrie F, Simard J, Luu-The V, *et al.* The 3β-hydroxysteroid dehydrogenase/isomerase gene family: lessons from type II 3β-HSD congenital deficiency. In Hansson V, Levy FO, Taskén K, eds. *Signal Transduction in Testicular Cells. Ernst Schering Research Foundation Workshop.* Berlin, Heidelberg, New York: Springer-Verlag, 1996: 185–218

22. Labrie F, Luu-The V, Lin SX, *et al.* The key role of 17β-HSDs in sex steroid biology. *Steroids* 1997; 62:148–58

23. Labrie F, Bélanger A, Cusan L, *et al.* Marked decline in serum concentrations of adrenal C19 sex steroid precursors and conjugated androgen metabolites during aging. *J Clin Endocrinol Metab* 1997;82:2396–402

24. Labrie F, Bélanger A, Cusan L, *et al.* Physiological changes in DHEA are not reflected by the serum levels of active androgens and estrogens but of their metabolites: intracrinology. *J Clin Endocrinol Metab* 1997;82:2403–9

25. Labrie F, Diamond P, Cusan L, *et al.* Effect of 12-month DHEA replacement therapy on bone,

vaginum, and endometrium in postmenopausal women. *J Clin Endocrinol Metab* 1997;82:3498–505

26. Martel C, Labrie F. Important androgenic component in the stimulatory effect of dehydroepiandrosterone (DHEA) on bone density in the rat. *Presented at the 8th International Congress on the Menopause*, Sydney, Australia, 1996: abstr

27. Diamond P, Cusan L, Gomez JL, *et al*. Metabolic effects of 12-month percutaneous DHEA replacement therapy in postmenopausal women. *J Endocrinol* 1996;150:S43–50

28. Morales AJ, Nolan JJ, Nelson JC, *et al*. Effects of replacement dose of dehydroepiandrosterone in men and women of advancing age. *J Clin Endocrinol Metab* 1994;78:1360–7

29. Labrie C, Bélanger A, Labrie F. Androgenic activity of dehydroepiandrosterone and androstenedione in the rat ventral prostate. *Endocrinology* 1988;123:1412–17

30. Labrie F, Sugimoto Y, Luu-The V, *et al*. Structure of human type II 5α-reductase. *Endocrinology* 1992;131:1571–3

31. Luu-The V, Zhang Y, Poirier D, *et al*. Characteristics of human types 1, 2 and 3 17β-hydroxysteroid dehydrogenase activities: oxidation–reduction and inhibition. *J Steroid Biochem Mol Biol* 1995;55:581–7

32. Vermeulen A, Deslypene JP, Schelfhout W, *et al*. Adrenocortical function in old age: response to acute adrenocorticotropin stimulation. *J Clin Endocrinol Metab* 1982;54:187–91

33. Vermeulen A, Verdonck L. Radioimmunoassays of 17β-hydroxy-5α-androstan-3-one, 4-androstene-3,17-dione, dehydroepiandrosterone, 17β-hydroxyprogesterone and progesterone and its application to human male plasma. *J Steroid Biochem* 1976;7:1–10

34. Orentreich N, Brind JL, Rizer RL, *et al*. Age changes and sex differences in serum dehydroepiandrosterone sulfate concentrations throughout adulthood. *J Clin Endocrinol Metab* 1984;59:551–5

35. Bélanger A, Candas B, Dupont A, *et al*. Changes in serum concentrations of conjugated and unconjugated steroids in 40- to 80-year-old men. *J Clin Endocrinol Metab* 1994;79:1086–90

36. Migeon CJ, Keller AR, Lawrence B, *et al*. Dehydroepiandrosterone and androsterone levels in human placenta. Effect of age and sex: day-to-day and diurnal variations. *J Clin Endocrinol Metab* 1957;17:1051–62

37. Chesnut CH, Ivey JL, Gruber HE, *et al*. Stanozolol in postmenopausal osteoporosis: therapeutic efficacy and possible mechanisms of action. *Metabolism* 1983;32:571–80

38. Benz DJ, Haussler MR, Thomas MA, *et al*. High-affinity androgen binding and androgenic regulation of α1(I)-procollagen and transforming growth factor-β steady state messenger ribonucleic acid levels in human osteoblast-like osteosarcoma cells. *Endocrinology* 1991;128:2723–30

39. Kapur SP, Reddi AH. Influence of testosterone and dihydrotestosterone on bone-matrix induced endochondral bone formation. *Calcif Tissue Int* 1989;44:108–13

40. Davis SR, McCloud P, Strauss BJ, *et al*. Testosterone enhances estradiol's effects on postmenopausal density and sexuality. *Maturitas* 1995;21:227–36

41. Hennernan PM, Wallach S. The role of androgens and estrogens and their metabolic effects. A review of the prolonged use of estrogens and androgens in postmenopausal and senile osteoporosis. *AMA: Arch Int Med* 1957;100:715–23

42. Savvas M, Studd JWW, Fogelman I, *et al*. Skeletal effects of oral oestrogen compared with subcutaneous oestrogen and testosterone in postmenopausal women. *Br Med J* 1988;297:331–3

43. Need AG, Horowitz M, Bridges A, *et al*. Effects of nandrolone decanoate and antiresorptive therapy on vertebral density in osteoporotic postmenopausal women. *Arch Intern Med* 1989;149:57–60

44. Studd JW, Collins WP, Chakravarti S *et al*. Estradiol and testosterone implants in treatment of psychosexual problems in postmenopausal woman. *Br J Obstet Gynaecol* 1987;84:314–15

45. Burger HG, Hailes J, Menelaus M, *et al*. The management of persistent menopausal symptoms with oestradiol–testosterone implants: clinical, lipid and hormonal results. *Maturitas* 1984;6:351–8

46. Sherwin BB. Affective changes with estrogen and androgen replacement therapy in surgically menopausal women. *J Affect Disord* 1988;14:177–87

47. Sherwin BB, Gelfand MM. Differential symptom response to parenteral estrogen and/or androgen administration in the surgical menopause. *Am J Obstet Gynecol* 1985;151:153–60

48. Notelovitz M, Watts N, Timmons C, *et al*. Effects of estrogen plus low dose androgen vs estrogen alone on menopausal symptoms in oophorectomized/hysterectomized women. *Presented at meeting of the North American Menopause Society*, Montreal, 1991:101

49. Leiblum S, Bachmann G, Kemmann E, *et al*. Vaginal atrophy in the postmenopausal woman. The importance of sexual activity and hormones. *J Am Med Assoc* 1983;249:2195–8

50. Sherwin BB, Gelfand MM. The role of androgen in the maintenance of sexual functioning in oophorectomized women. *Psychosom Med* 1987;49:397–409

51. Pye JK, Mansel RE, Hughes LE. Clinical experience of drug treatments for mastalgia. *Lancet* 1985;2:373–7

52. De Fazio J, Meldrum DR, Winer JH, *et al.* Direct action of androgen on hot flushes in the human male. *Maturitas* 1984;6:3–8

53. Sherwin BB, Gelfand MM. Effects of parenteral administration of estrogen and androgen on plasma hormone levels and hot flushes in the surgical menopause. *Am J Obstet Gynecol* 1984; 148:552–7

54. Schriock ED, Buffington CK, Hubert GD, *et al.* Divergent correlations of circulating dehydro-epiandrosterone sulfate and testosterone with insulin levels and insulin receptor binding. *J Clin Endocrinol Metab* 1988;66:1329–31

55. Coleman DL, Leiter EH, Schwizer RW. Therapeutic effects of dehydroepiandrosterone (DHEA) in diabetic mice. *Diabetes* 1982;31:830–3

56. Nestler JE, Barlascini CO, Clore JN, *et al.* Dehydroepiandrosterone reduces serum low density lipoprotein levels and body fat but does not alter insulin sensitivity in normal men. *J Clin Endocrinol Metab* 1988;66:57–61

57. MacEwen EG, Kurzman ID. Obesity in the dog: role of the adrenal steroid dehydroepiandrosterone (DHEA). *J Nutr* 1991;121:S51–5

58. Tchernof A, Després JP, Bélanger A, *et al.* Reduced testosterone and adrenal C19 steroid levels in obese men. *Metabolism* 1995;44:513–19

59. Zumoff B, Levin J, Rosenfeld RS, *et al.* Abnormal 24-hr mean plasma concentrations of dehydro-epiandrosterone and dehydroisoandrosterone sulfate in women with primary operable breast cancer. *Cancer Res* 1981;41:3360–3

60. Schwartz AG, Pashko L, Whitcomb JM. Inhibition of tumor development by dehydroepiandro-sterone and related steroids. *Toxicol Pathol* 1986; 14:357–62

61. Gordon GB, Shantz LM, Talalay P. Modulation of growth, differentiation and carcinogenesis by dehydroepiandrosterone. *Adv Enzyme Regul* 1987;26:355–82

62. Li S, Yan X, Bélanger A, *et al.* Prevention by dehydroepiandrosterone of the development of mammary carcinoma induced by 7,12-dimethyl-benz(a)anthracene (DMBA) in the rat. *Breast Cancer Res Treat* 1993;29:203–17

63. Suzuki T, Suzuki N, Daynes RA, *et al.* Dehydro-epiandrosterone enhances IL2 production and cytotoxic effector function of human T cells. *Clin Immunol Immunopathol* 1991;61:202–11

64. Rasmussen KR, Arrowood MJ, Healey MC. Effectiveness of dehydroepiandrosterone in reduction of cryptosporidial activity in immuno-suppressed rats. *Antimicrob Agents Chemother* 1992; 36:220–2

65. Henderson E, Yang JY, Schwartz A. Dehydro-epiandrosterone (DHEA) and sysnthetic DHEA analogs are modest inhibitors of HIV-1 IIIB replication. *Aids Res Hum Retroviruses* 1992;8:625–31

66. Casson PR, Andersen RN, Herrod HG, *et al.* Oral dehydroepiandrosterone in physiologic doses modulates immune function in postmenopausal women. *Am J Obstet Gynecol* 1993;169:1536–9

67. Johnston CC Jr, Epstein S. Clinical, biochemical, radiographic, epidemiologic, and economic features of osteoporosis. *Orthop Clin North Am* 1981;12:559–69

68. Franceschi S. The epidemiology of endometrial cancer. *Gynecol Oncol* 1991;41:1–16

69. Friedl A, Jordan VC. What do we know and what don't we know about tamoxifen in the human uterus. *Breast Cancer Res Treat* 1994;31:27–39

70. Pochi PE, Strauss JS. Sebaceous gland response in man to the administration of testosterone, Δ4-androstenedione and dehydroisoandro-sterone. *J Invest Dermatol* 1969;52:32–6

71. Dumont M, Luu-The V, Dupont E, *et al.* Characterization, expression and immunohisto-chemical localization of 3β-hydroxysteroid de-hydrogenase/ Δ^5–Δ^4 isomerase in human skin. *J Invest Dermatol* 1992;99:415–21

72. Luu-The V, Sugimoto Y, Puy L, *et al.* Characterization, expression and immunohistochemical localization of 5α-reductase in human skin. *J Invest Dermatol* 1994;102:221–6

73. Chen C, Bélanger A, Labrie F. Adrenal steroid precursors exert potent androgenic action in the hamster sebaceous glands of flank organs and ears. *Endocrinology* 1996;137:1752–7

74. Baillie AH, Thomson J, Milne JA. The distribution of hydroxysteroid dehydrogenase in human sebaceous glands. *Br J Dermatol* 1966;78:451–7

75. Cusan L, Dupont A, Bélanger A, *et al.* Treatment of hirsutism with the pure antiandrogen fluta-mide. *J Am Acad Dermatol* 1990;23:462–9

76. Cusan L, Dupont A, Gomez JL, *et al.* Comparison of flutamide and spironolactone in the treatment of hirsutism: a randomized controlled trial. *Fertil Steril* 1994;61:281–7

77. Jordan VC. Effect of tamoxifen (ICI 46 474) on initiation and growth of DMBA-induced rat mammary carcinoma. *Eur J Cancer* 1976;12: 419–24

78. Jordan VC, Rowsby L, Dix CJ, *et al.* Dose-related effects of non-steroidal antioestrogens and oestrogens on the measurement of cytoplasmic oestrogen receptors in the rat and mouse uterus. *J Endocrinol* 1978;78:71–81

79. Dauvois S, Geng CS, Lévesque C, *et al.* Additive inhibitory effects of an androgen and the anti-estrogen EM-170 on estradiol-stimulated growth of human ZR-75–1 breast tumors in athymic mice. *Cancer Res* 1991;51:3131–5

80. Kawamura I, Mizota T, Kondo N, *et al.* Antitumor effects of droloxifene, a new antiestrogen drug, against 7,12-dimethylbenz(a)anthracene-induced mammary tumors in rats. *Jpn J Pharmacol* 1991;57:215–24

81. Labrie F, Li S, Labrie C, *et al.* Inhibitory effect of a steroidal antiestrogen (EM-170) on estrone-stimulated growth of 7,12-dimethylbenz(a) anthracene (DMBA)-induced mammary carcinoma in the rat. *Breast Cancer Res Treat* 1995; 33:237–44

82. Luo S, Sourla A, Labrie C, *et al.* Combined effects of dehydroepiandrosterone and EM-800 on bone mass, serum lipids, and the development of dimethylbenz(a)anthracene (DMBA)-induced mammary carcinoma in the rat. *Endocrinology* 1997;138:4435–44

83. Kennedy BJ. Fluxymesterone therapy in treatment of advanced breast cancer. *N Engl J Med* 1958;259:673–5

84. Mashchak CA, Lobo RA, Dozono-Takano R, *et al.* Comparison of pharmacodynamic properties of various estrogen formulations. *Am J Obstet Gynecol* 1982;144:511–18

85. Lobo RA. Absorption and metabolic effects of different types of estrogens and progestogens. *Obstet Gynecol Clin North Am* 1987;14:143–67

86. Couillard S, Labrie C, Bélanger A, *et al.* Effect of dehydroepiandrosterone and the antiestrogen EM-800 on the growth of human ZR-75-1 breast cancer xenografts. *J Natl Cancer Inst* 1998;90: 772–8

Selective estrogen receptor modulators: new option for postmenopausal women

34

A. R. Genazzani and M. Gambacciani

Introduction

The menopause represents a critical event in a woman's life. At this time, a series of biological transformations take place, and each of these can interfere with the woman's well-being and quality of life. In developed countries, with an increase of life-expectancy for women, physicians are facing new problems occurring in the postmenopausal period. Thus, management of the climacteric period has become one of the major issues for the gynecologist.

After the menopause, the endocrine and metabolic consequences of ovarian failure can affect a woman's health and quality of life[1–16]. Vasomotor and sleep disturbances, psychological and emotional stress, and genitourinary and sexual complaints can really jeopardize a woman's well-being (Table 1). In addition, a series of metabolic changes related to hypoestrogenism can cause an increase in body weight with an android body fat distribution that provokes profound changes in body image. Estrogen deprivation leads to a decreased collagen content in both skin and mucosae, with degenerative changes in elastic fibers. These changes cause a reduction in epidermal and mucosal thickness which, in addition to a reduction of vascularization of these areas, contributes to the postmenopausal urogenital and sexual complaints. Clinical and epidemiological studies have clearly shown that the postmenopausal condition is an important risk factor for chronic disorders such as cardiovascular disease and osteoporosis, which are major causes of morbidity, disability and mortality in the aging population. A critical increase in osteoporosis and related fractures, as well as an increase in cardiovascular diseases and events, represents the long-term consequences of chronic hypoestrogenism during the postmenopausal years. The possible relationship between estrogen deprivation and Alzheimer's disease remains to be clarified. Clinical evidence demonstrates that estrogen deprivation can increase the risk and the severity of senile dementia. In some studies, a lower incidence of senile dementia and a better mental performance has been observed in estrogen users, in comparison with untreated women[17–19]. Today, there is a large body of evidence that estrogen replacement therapy can rapidly cure and even prevent all the symptoms related to estrogen deficiency. However, in women with an intact uterus, the use of progestin is mandatory to prevent endometrial hyperstimulation. Therefore, estrogen is associated with progestin prescription in the majority of women, in various schedules of estroprogestin therapy or hormone replacement therapy (HRT). Unfortunately, progestin administration is often associated with unwanted clinical and metabolic side-effects (Table 2).

Hormone replacement therapy is currently required and prescribed for the control of

Table 1 Menopausal factors affecting quality of life

Vasomotor and sleep disturbances
Psychological and emotional stress
Genitourinary and sexual complaints
Changes in body image
Osteoporosis: backache, fractures
Cardiovascular disease: angina
Alzheimer's disease

climacteric symptoms. These are short-term objectives ('today's goals'), related to the reduction of symptoms and the cure of dystrophic processes. In addition, there are 'tomorrow's goals' for HRT: the prevention of osteoporosis[1-7] and cardiovascular disease[8-16], and possibly Alzheimer's disease[17-19] (Table 3). These are the long-term goals that physicians want to achieve for ameliorating women's health and quality of life in the future. However, long-term compliance is not satisfactory. The current use of HRT is little and often short-lasting. The vast majority of postmenopausal women use HRT for relieving subjective symptoms, especially in the first period after the menopause in which the greatest problems are related to vasomotor symptoms. Long-term compliance, the most important for prevention, is highly unsatisfactory, jeopardized by bleedings, apprehension of side-effects, weight gain and primarily fear of cancer, particularly breast cancer. Postmenopausal women face a difficult dilemma: whether they should or should not take HRT. In fact, HRT may protect against osteoporosis and heart disease, but may increase the risk of breast and endometrial cancer[20]. Thus, there could be serious consequences in the decision whether or not to take estrogen. The possible increased breast cancer risk associated with long-term HRT use makes it a less desirable option for many women. We have to consider that nearly half of the postmenopausal women who begin hormone treatment discontinue use within 1 year[21]. From this aspect, many women may benefit from the introduction of a new class of drugs, the selective estrogen receptor modulators (SERMs). The SERMs act as estrogen agonists on bone and the cardiovascular system, while they act as estrogen antagonists on endometrium and breast tissues. In this regard, SERMs may represent an alternative approach of a safe, long-term HRT for decreasing postmenopausal osteoporosis and cardiovascular risk in the postmenopausal female population[22].

SERMS: a new class of drug

Long-term HRT, for some women, is clearly not an ideal treatment. Therefore, other compounds have been sought as an ideal preparation, with estrogenic effects in some tissues, as bone and the cardiovascular system, but not in others, as breast and endometrium (Table 4). The SERMs are drugs that have all these tissue-specific effects. Therefore, in the continuous search for an 'ideal estrogen', a SERM is defined as a compound that produces estrogen agonism in one or more desired target tissues (such as bone, cardiovascular system, liver, etc.) together with estrogen antagonism and/or

Table 2 Unwanted effects of progestins

Somatic symptoms
Breast tenderness
Edema
Abdominal cramping

Psychic symptoms
Depression
Anxiety
Irritability

Androgenic action
Raised insulin levels
Unfavorable lipid profile

Table 3 Postmenopausal hormone replacement therapy

Today's goals (short-term)
Therapeutic effects on symptoms:
   neurovegetative, cosmetic
   psychological
   genitourinary

Tomorrow's goals (long-term)
Prevention of:
   osteoporosis
   cardiovascular disease
   depression
   Alzheimer's disease

Table 4 Characteristics of ideal hormone replacement therapy preparation

Eliminates climacteric symptoms
Low cost
High acceptability
Low complications and side-effects
Prevents osteoporosis
Reduces cardiovascular disease risk
Breast safety

minimal agonism in reproductive tissue such as the breast or uterus. SERMs bind with high affinity to the estrogen receptor, and evoke either an agonist or an antagonist response in a tissue-selective manner. The great advantage of these new molecules is that they have favorable effects on the skeletal and cardiovascular systems while lacking the undesirable effects of estrogen on reproductive tissue. Potentially, with these new drugs, the benefits of estrogen may be derived without the accompanying risks. Tamoxifen, a first-generation SERM, has been used to prevent the recurrence of breast cancer, and in addition caused considerable excitement when it was found to protect against osteoporosis[23] and cardiovascular disease[24,25]. Unfortunately, it was later found to increase the incidence of endometrial hyperplasia and cancer[26]. The new-generation SERMs, such as raloxifene, have a different and more selective profile[27–40]. The SERMs' molecular mechanism of action involves high-affinity binding with the ligand-binding domain of the estrogen receptor, evoking a conformation change in receptor structure, dimerization of the receptor, and association of the receptor dimer with DNA-response elements and one or more receptor-associated proteins. The capacity of SERMs to discriminate tissue-selective response is probably correlated to the diversity of receptor-associated proteins in different tissues, the different distributions of estrogen receptor subtypes (ERα and ERβ) and the activation of multiple-response elements in different genes[28]. Some SERMs (such as raloxifene) exert their actions on different metabolic processes secondary to postmenopausal hypoestrogenism. Raloxifene lowers serum cholesterol after ovariectomy in rats, inhibits low-density lipoprotein (LDL) oxidation and exerts other cardiovascular protective actions in rats[29]. However, raloxifene does not induce estrogenic action on the endometrium. In a recent study, endometrial morphological changes were evaluated in postmenopausal women assigned to placebo, raloxifene hydrochloride 200 or 600 mg/day, or conjugated estrogens (0.625 mg/day)[27]. After 8 weeks of treatment, statistically significant estrogenic effects were

noted in 77% of estrogen-treated women versus 15% of placebo-treated women versus 0% of raloxifene-treated women[27]. Therefore, as expected, estrogen treatment stimulated the postmenopausal endometrium. In contrast, raloxifene did not induce histopathological evidence of endometrial stimulation in healthy postmenopausal women. Further studies confirmed that the long-term administration of raloxifene is unable to induce endometrial proliferation[30,31]. In addition, the analysis of data from over 12 000 postmenopausal women enrolled in osteoporosis studies provided evidence that raloxifene administration induces a significant ($p < 0.001$) reduction in risk of breast cancer, with the relative risk of 0.42[40]. In other words, from these preliminary data, raloxifene seems to be able to reduce by 60% the incidence of breast cancer in postmenopausal women.

As for cardiovascular disease, recently reported are the results of a large study designed to identify the effects of raloxifene on surrogate end-points of cardiovascular risk in postmenopausal women, and to compare them with those induced by HRT[32]. In a double-blind, randomized, parallel trial conducted in the United States, 390 healthy postmenopausal women were recruited and randomized to receive one of four treatments: raloxifene 60 mg/day, raloxifene 120 mg/day, HRT (conjugated equine estrogen 0.625 mg/day and medroxyprogesterone acetate 2.5 mg/day) or placebo[32]. The main outcome measures were the change from baseline of lipid levels and coagulation parameters after 3 and 6 months of treatment. Compared to placebo, both dosages of raloxifene significantly lowered LDL cholesterol by 12% ($p < 0.001$), similar to the 14% reduction with HRT ($p < 0.001$). Both dosages of raloxifene significantly lowered lipoprotein(a) by 7% to 8% ($p < 0.001$), less than the 19% decrease with HRT ($p < 0.001$). Raloxifene increased high-density lipoprotein-2 (HDL2) cholesterol by 15% to 17% ($p < 0.05$), less than the 33% increase with HRT ($p < 0.001$). Raloxifene did not significantly change levels of high-density lipoprotein (HDL) cholesterol, triglycerides or plasminogen activator inhibitor-1 (PAI-1), whereas HRT increased HDL cholesterol by 11% and triglycerides by 20%, and decreased PAI-1 by 29% (for all, $p < 0.001$). Raloxifene significantly lowered fibrinogen by 12% to 14% ($p < 0.001$), unlike HRT, which had no effect. Neither treatment changed fibrinopeptide A or prothrombin fragments 1 and 2. From these data, it is clear that raloxifene favorably alters biochemical markers of cardiovascular risk by decreasing LDL cholesterol, fibrinogen and lipoprotein(a), and by increasing HDL2 cholesterol without raising triglycerides. In contrast to HRT, raloxifene had no effect on HDL cholesterol and PAI-1, and a lesser effect on HDL2 cholesterol and lipoprotein(a)[32].

The effects of raloxifene on bone mineral density, along with the actions on serum lipid concentrations and endometrial thickness, were studied in 601 postmenopausal women in a multicentric European study[32]. The women were randomly assigned to receive 30, 60 or 150 mg of raloxifene or placebo daily for 24 months. The women receiving each dose of raloxifene had significant increases from baseline values in bone mineral density of the lumbar spine, hip and total body, whereas those receiving placebo had decreases in bone mineral density[33]. After 24 months, the difference in the change in bone mineral density between the women receiving 60 mg of raloxifene per day and those receiving placebo was $2.4 \pm 0.4\%$ for the lumbar spine, 2.4% for the total hip and 2.0% for the total body ($p < 0.001$ for all comparisons)[33]. Serum concentrations of total cholesterol and LDL cholesterol decreased in all the raloxifene groups, whereas serum concentrations of HDL cholesterol and triglycerides did not change[33]. Endometrial thickness measured by vaginal ultrasound was similar in the raloxifene and placebo groups at all times during the study[33]. The proportion of women receiving raloxifene who reported hot flushes or vaginal bleeding was not different from that of women receiving placebo. The results of this study show that daily therapy with raloxifene increases bone mineral density, lowers serum concentrations of total and LDL cholesterol, and does not stimulate the endometrium[33].

As for the treatment of established osteoporosis, results have recently been published from a 1-year prospective, randomized, double-blind trial conducted in 143 postmenopausal osteoporotic women (aged 68.4 ± 5.0 years) with at least one prevalent vertebral fracture and low bone mineral density (BMD), comparing groups receiving raloxifene at 60 or 120 mg/day and a control group receiving supplements of 750 mg/day of calcium and 400 IU/day of vitamin D[34]. There were no differences among groups in the occurrence of uterine bleeding, thrombophlebitis, breast abnormalities or increased endometrial thickness (assessed by ultrasonography)[34]. Compared to controls, the changes in values over 1 year for raloxifene at each dose, respectively, were significant for serum bone alkaline phosphatase (–14.9%, –8.87%), serum osteocalcin (–20.7%, –17.0%) and urinary C-telopeptide fragment of type I collagen/creatinine (–24.9%, –30.8%), markers of bone turnover; significant changes were also found for serum total cholesterol (–7.0%) and LDL cholesterol (–11.4%), and for the LDL/HDL cholesterol ratio (–13.2%)[34]. BMD increased significantly in the total hip (1.66%) and ultradistal radius (2.92%)[34].

As discussed above, the total available data seem to suggest that raloxifene exerts estrogen agonist actions on bone and the cardiovascular system, determining positive effects on cardiovascular and osteoporotic risks. No significant differences in the severity of subjective climacteric complaints have been observed in raloxifene- and placebo-treated subjects[38,39]. Moreover, there is an increased interest in the interaction of SERMs with neuronal plasticity and brain functions. A dramatic increase in neurite growth was evidenced *in vitro* with raloxifene[35]. Furthermore, when co-administered with estradiol, the increased neurite growth persisted or perhaps even accelerated[35]. These observations have raised the possibility of protective or therapeutic effects of raloxifene on cognitive functions and brain degenerative diseases such as Alzheimer's dementia[35]. These *in vitro* data on neurite growth in response to raloxifene[35] are encouraging, and clinical trials are needed to determine whether similar effects can be detected *in vivo*. If so, it may be possible to exploit raloxifene for the prevention of postmenopausal cognitive defects associated with Alzheimer's disease, in addition to its beneficial effects on bone loss and lipids.

Future challenges and opportunities

Short-term HRT is required for the treatment of subjective postmenopausal complaints. On the other hand, 5–10 years of HRT is important for a woman's well-being, and the risk/benefit ratio is good enough to suggest widespread use of HRT in the vast majority of postmenopausal women. Today, the outlook for chronic pharmacotherapy in the postmenopausal condition is promising. Randomized, ongoing clinical trials will provide greater understanding of the benefits and liabilities of chronic HRT over the next 5–10 years. Depending on the outcome of these trials, overall HRT use and compliance may improve as both patient and physician better understand the risk/benefit ratio of HRT. However, the challenge of women who cannot or do not want to take HRT is compelling. The need of a safe, effective therapy alternative to HRT started the research into improved hormones with a refined profile, which would obviate the possible risks of long-term estrogen therapy.

A novel class of compound, the SERM, appears to hold promise in this regard. With raloxifene as the first example of a SERM displaying appropriate selectivity for bone and cholesterol metabolism in extensive preclinical and clinical trials, alternatives to the use of traditional, non-selective estrogens in postmenopausal therapy become a real possibility.

In conclusion, the favorable effect of raloxifene on osteoporosis and cardiovascular disease risks, without any detectable side-effects on other estrogen-response tissues, such as the uterus and breast, are quite encouraging. The particular action of raloxifene on breast tissue and the preliminary data on breast cancer incidence are of paramount importance. As these data continue to be confirmed in other clinical trials, raloxifene will become a new important therapeutic choice for women who have a positive personal or familiar history of breast cancer. Today, we can maintain that raloxifene is the choice for postmenopausal women who cannot, or do not, want to take HRT. In addition, raloxifene is indicated for postmenopausal women who do not accept long-term HRT on account of the possible risk correlated with chronic hormone administration. The absence of estrogen-related adverse effects with raloxifene should improve the long-term compliance. Chronic raloxifene administration can really decrease the incidence of fractures and possibly cardiovascular events without increasing the incidence of breast cancer. These particular characteristics can make raloxifene an ideal drug for the long-term therapy of postmenopausal women.

References

1. Riggs BL, Wahner HW, Dunn WL, Mazess RB, Offord KP, Melton LJ III. Differential changes in bone mineral density of the appendicular and axial skeleton with aging. *J Clin Invest* 1981;67:328–35
2. Gambacciani M, Spinetti A, De Simone L, *et al.* The relative contribution of menopause and aging to postmenopausal vertebral osteopenia. *J Clin Endocrinol Metab* 1993;77:1148–52
3. Nilas L, Christiansen C. The pathophysiology of peri- and postmenopausal bone loss. *Br J Obstet Gynaecol* 1989;96:580–7
4. Wallach S, Henneman P. Prolonged estrogen therapy in postmenopausal women. *J Am Med Assoc* 1959;171:1637
5. Lindsay R. Estrogen therapy in the prevention and management of osteoporosis. *Am J Obstet Gynecol* 1987;156:1347

6. Gambacciani M, Spinetti A, Taponeco F, *et al.* Longitudinal evaluation of premenopausal vertebral bone loss: effects of a low dose oral contraceptive preparation on bone mineral density and metabolism. *Obstet Gynecol* 1994;8:392–4

7. Noteloviz M. Osteoporosis: screening, prevention, and management. *Fertil Steril* 1993;59:707–25

8. Bush TL, Barrett-Connor E. Noncontraceptive estrogen use and cardiovascular disease. *Epidemiol Rev* 1985;7:80–104

9. Rosenberg L, Armstrong B, Jick H. Myocardial infarction and estrogen therapy in postmenopausal women. *N Engl J Med* 1976;294:1256–9

10. Ross RK, Paganini-Hill A, Mack TM, *et al.* Menopausal oestrogen therapy and protection from death from ischaemic heart disease. *Lancet* 1981;18:858–62

11. Henderson BE, Ross RK, Paganini-Hill A, Mack TM. Estrogen use and cardiovascular disease. *Am J Obstet Gynecol* 1986;154:1181–6

12. Henderson BE, Paganini-Hill A, Ross RK. Estrogen replacement therapy and protection from acute myocardial infarction. *Am J Obstet Gynecol* 1988;159:312–17

13. Stampfer MJ, Colditz GA, Willet WC, *et al.* Postmenopausal estrogen therapy and cardiovascular disease: ten-year follow-up from the Nurses' Health Study. *N Engl J Med* 1991;325:756–62

14. Session DR, Kelly AC, Jewelewicz R. Current concepts in estrogen replacement therapy in the menopause. *Fertil Steril* 1993;2:277–84

15. Mason CA. Primary care for postreproductive women: further thoughts concerning steroid replacement. *Am J Obstet Gynecol* 1994;170:936–66

16. Lobo RA, Speroff L. International consensus conference on postmenopausal hormone therapy and the cardiovascular system. *Fertil Steril* 1994;61:592–5

17. Ming-Xin T, Jacobs Y, Marder K, *et al.* Effect of oestrogen during menopause on risk and age at onset of Alzheimer's disease. *Lancet* 1996;348:429–32

18. Takeyoshi O, Kunihiro I, Kenji A, *et al.* Low-dose estrogen replacement therapy for Alzheimer disease in women. *Menopause* 1994;3:125–30

19. Paganini-Hill A, Henderson VW. Estrogen replacement therapy and risk of Alzheimer disease. *Arch Intern Med* 1996;156:2213–17

20. Col NF, Eckman MH, Kars RH, *et al.* Patient-specific decision about hormonal replacement therapy in postmenopausal women. *J Am Med Assoc* 1997;277:1140–7

21. Johannes CB, Crawford SL, Posner JG, *et al.* Longitudinal patterns and correlates of hormonal replacement therapy use in middle-age women. *Am J Epidemiol* 1994;140:439–52

22. Hol T, Cox MB, Bryant HU, *et al.* Selective estrogen receptor modulators and postmenopausal women's health. *J Women's Health* 1997;6:523–31

23. Love RR, Mazess RB, Barden HS, *et al.* Effects of tamoxifene on bone mineral density in postmenopausal women with breast cancer. *N Engl J Med* 1992;326:852–6

24. MacDonald CC, Stewart HJ, for the Scottish Breast Cancer Committee. Fatal myocardial infarction in the Scottish adjuvant tamoxifen trial. *Br Med J* 1991;303:435–7

25. Rutqvist LE, Mattsson A, for the Stockholm Breast Cancer Committee Study Group. Cardiac and thromboembolic morbidity among postmenopausal women with early stage breast cancer in a randomized trial of adjuvant tamoxifen. *J Natl Cancer Inst* 1993;85:1398–406

26. Van Leeuwen FE, Benraadt J, Coebergh JWW, *et al.* Risk of endometrial cancer after tamoxifen treatment of breast cancer. *Lancet* 1994;343:448–52

27. Boss SM, Huster WJ, Neild JA, Glant MD, Eisenhut CC, Draper MW. Effects of raloxifene hydrochloride on the endometrium of postmenopausal women. *Am J Obstet Gynecol* 1997;177:1458–64

28. Paech K, Webb P, Kuiper GGJM, *et al.* Differential ligand activation of estrogen receptors ERα and ERβ at AP1 sites. *Science* 1997;277:1508–10

29. Black LJ, Stato M, Rowley ER, *et al.* Raloxifene (LYI39481 HCl) prevents bone loss and reduces serum cholesterol without causing uterine hypertrophy in ovariectomized rats. *J Clin Invest* 1994;93:63–9

30. Goldstein S, Srikanth R, Parson A, *et al.* Effects of raloxifene on the endometrium in healthy postmenopausal women. *Menopause* 1998;5:277–8

31. Graham CD, William JH, Wei S, *et al.* Endometrial effects of raloxifene assessed by bleeding rate, ultrasonography, and biopsy. *Menopause* 1998;5:282–3

32. Walsh BW, Kuller LH, Wild RA, et al. Effects of raloxifene on serum lipids and coagulation factors in healthy postmenopausal women. *J Am Med Assoc* 1998;279:1445–51

33. Delmas PD, Bjarnason NH, Mitlak BH, *et al.* Effects of raloxifene on bone mineral density, serum cholesterol concentrations, and uterine endometrium in postmenopausal women. *N Engl J Med* 1997;337:1641–7

34. Lufkin EG, Whitaker MD, Nickelsen T, *et al.* Treatment of established postmenopausal osteoporosis with raloxifene: a randomized trial. *J Bone Miner Res* 1998;13:1747–54

35. Nilsen J, Mor G, Naftolin F. Raloxifene induces neurite outgrowth in estrogen receptor positive PC12 cells. *Menopause* 1998;5:211–16

36. Fuchs-Young R, Glasebrook AL, Short LL, *et al.* Raloxifene is a tissue-selective agonist/

antagonist that functions through the estrogen receptor. *Ann NY Acad Sci* 1995;761:355–60

37. Ettinger B, Black D, Cummings S, *et al.*, for MORE Study Group. Raloxifene reduces the risk of incident vertebral fractures: 24-month interim analysis. *Menopause* 1998;5:248–9

38. Lu Y, Cohen F, Lakshmanan M. Characterization of hot flushes during raloxifene therapy: analyses of adverse event reports from an integrated placebo-controlled clinical trial database. *Menopause* 1998;5:282–3

39. Cohen F, Watts S, Beymer K. Vaginal complaints in healthy postmenopausal women: data from 3-years comparing raloxifene with conjugated estrogens or placebo. *Menopause* 1998;5:283

40. Jordan ASC, *et al.* Incidents of primary breast cancer are reduced by raloxifene: integrated data from multicenter double-blind, randomized trials in 12 000 postmenopausal women. *ASCO Proc* 1998;17:466

Vaginal progesterone in the menopause: cyclical and constant combined regimens for new physiological options in hormone replacement therapy

35

D. de Ziegler, R. Ferriani and C. Bulletti

Introduction

Hormone replacement therapy (HRT) is in essence a long-term treatment. Hence, one may rightfully wonder whether vaginal treatments are compatible with long-term therapies. Is there not a simpler way to administer progesterone? Is it not the simplest of all treatments that will offer the best chances for long-term compliance? It is because long-term treatment with vaginal progesterone may appear odd at first glance that we are addressing this issue here. Particularly, many of the clinical motivations for prescribing vaginal progesterone in HRT are counterintuitive and ought to be reviewed. The rationale and our past experience with such treatments will be presented. The reader will see that vaginal administration is the best possible option if physiological replacement of progesterone, the actual hormone produced by the corpus luteum, is preferred.

Physiological replacement is primarily indicated when potential adverse effects of synthetic progestins or massive exposure to progesterone metabolites, as seen after oral ingestion of progesterone, are to be avoided. However, physiological replacement may also be favored for reasons of personal preference by women for whom any form of HRT would otherwise be medically acceptable. Here, physiological replacement with natural progesterone follows a line of personal preference rather than medical need. This is not less important, however, because treatment forms that gain patient preference, and not necessarily the simplest ones, are the most likely to secure long-term compliance.

Results reported in this paper show that the lack of side-effects encountered with vaginal progesterone is the best possible guarantee for long-term compliance in women who have experienced side-effects with oral progestins in the past. Non-oral administration of the natural ovarian hormone is also most reassuring for women who fear unwanted consequences from synthetic molecules, however often these concerns are medically proven unfounded. Finally, other women simply express a lingering preference for natural products.

The recent development of a sustained-release vaginal gel of progesterone, Crinone® 4% (Wyeth), offers new prospects for long-term use of vaginal progesterone in the menopause. Because of its bioadhesive properties, this progesterone gel has sustained effects which limit the number of daily applications needed. Two primary options exist for using Crinone in the menopause. The first of these is in a cyclical association with estrogen therapy; daily administration of Crinone 4% for 10 days per month offers few side-effects and highly predictable monthly withdrawal bleeding. The second option is twice-weekly administration in constant combined association with estrogen replacement therapy, achieving constant exposure of the uterus to progesterone. In our studies, this latter regimen resulted in a high rate of complete and persistent amenorrhea. In the following sections, we will review the theoretical advantages of vaginal progesterone in HRT and discuss the clinical experience achieved with these two regimens.

Routes of administration for natural hormone replacement

Natural progesterone is absorbed when ingested orally in micronized form. However, oral progesterone is almost entirely metabolized during the first liver pass[1,2]. This explains why oral progesterone induces unphysiologically high levels of progesterone metabolites and notably 5α-reduced metabolites[1,2]. Figure 1 depicts progesterone and progesterone metabolites measured after oral or vaginal administration of 100 mg of micronized progesterone. After oral administration, less than 10% of the dose ingested is found as unchanged progesterone in the peripheral circulation. The high degree of liver metabolism of natural progesterone has led to the development of synthetic derivatives of progesterone, or 'synthetic progestins'. These products are designed to duplicate progesterone action on the endometrium (genomic effects) while remaining active when administered orally due to their resistance to enzymatic degradation.

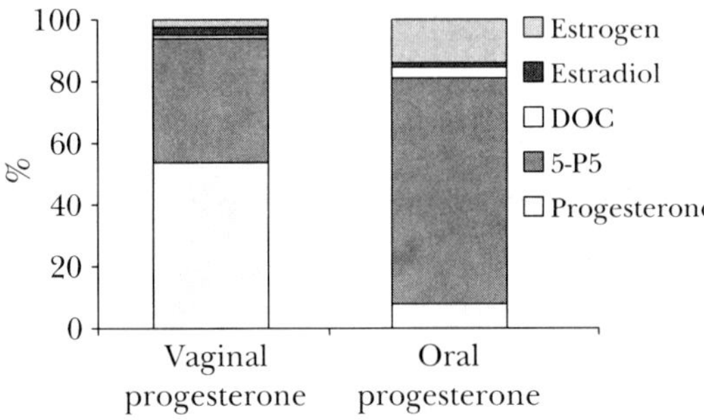

Figure 1 Progesterone metabolites after oral or vaginal administration of 100 mg of micronized progesterone. The intense progesterone metabolism during the first liver pass results in unphysiologically high levels of progesterone metabolites, particularly 5α-reduced metabolites, after oral ingestion of micronized progesterone[2]. DOC, desoxycortisone; 5-P5, 5α-dehydroprogesterone

Transdermal administration of progesterone is not and will not be feasible in the foreseeable future for the following three reasons. First, the amounts of progesterone needed to duplicate endogenous production are two orders of magnitude larger than those given in estrogen therapy. During the early follicular phase, the ovary produces 0.05 mg of estrogen per 24 h (i.e. the amount replaced in HRT). This increases to 0.4–0.6 mg per 24 h at mid-cycle during the preovulatory peak in estrogen production. Contrasting with those relatively small amounts, the high point of mid-luteal production of progesterone by the corpus luteum is approximately 25 mg per 24 h. Secondly, the skin is poorly permeable to progesterone. Thirdly, the skin is rich in 5α-reductase which inactivates a large fraction of the small amount of progesterone absorbed through the skin. Hence, the concept that transdermal progesterone creams can safely and effectively be used in the menopause is erroneous. Cooper and colleagues have clearly demonstrated that regular administration of the highly publicized transdermal cream Progest® failed to raise plasma progesterone to therapeutic levels[3]. This finding is in agreement with the lack of endometrial effects of this product[3]. One propounder of transdermal progesterone treatment, apparently aware of the lack of efficacy of this product, also recommends that women avoid the use of estrogens. Considering the lack of efficacy of transdermal progesterone, the concomitant ban on estrogen use is probably well inspired. Indeed, if estrogens are avoided, Progest becomes a harmless, albeit expensive, inactive placebo. On the contrary, if transdermal progesterone creams such as Progest are used in conjunction with conventional estrogen therapy (at bone-sparing doses), the inefficacy of progesterone skin creams would rapidly become overt and lead to a high incidence of endometrial hyperplasia and/or cancer.

Other non-oral routes that have been tested for administering progesterone include nasal, rectal and vaginal administration[4–7]. While nasal administration elevates plasma levels, it is insufficient to trigger complete predecidual transformation of the endometrial stroma[7].

Moreover, the nasal route suffers from the cumbersome requirement of multiple (≥ 3) daily administrations. Hence, early investigators have converged toward vaginal administration as the best practical non-oral option available[5,8]. We will see in the following sections of this chapter how we later discovered that vaginal administration is more than a mere form of non-oral administration. While not truly anticipated at first, there is now a wealth of information suggesting that vaginal progesterone offers targeted delivery to the uterus, the primary end organ where progesterone effects are sought.

Vaginal progesterone: direct access to the uterus

It has been more than 12 years since vaginal progesterone was first used for priming endometrial receptivity in recipients of donor egg *in vitro* fertilization and frozen embryo transfers[5]. Since then, investigators have been swayed by the unexpectedly high predictability of this form of treatment when assessed on end organ efficacy (endometrial histology). Evidence for the putative phenomenon of direct vagina-to-uterus transport had already been gained by researchers using progesterone preparations not originally designed for vaginal administration[9,10]. However, it is only with the advent of the sustained release vaginal gel of progesterone, Crinone 4%, that the discrepancy between the marginal plasma progesterone levels achieved and full endometrial efficacy became truly overt[11]. This new hypothesis of a functional 'portal' system[12] has since survived various methodological challenges of its veracity and clinical significance.

The sustained release vaginal gel of progesterone, Crinone 4%, has permitted a reduction in the number of vaginal applications. In a dose-ranging study, the capability of this delivery system was stressed. In one of the study groups, Crinone 4% containing 45 mg progesterone was administered every 48 h from the 15th day of estrogen replacement cycles onward. Plasma progesterone levels were determined every 6 h for the first 6 days of Crinone treatment (Figure 2). Peaks of plasma proges-

terone levels were under 5 ng/ml, while minimum levels were at or near 1 ng/ml. Despite these progesterone levels, that were in the luteal phase defect range, morphological changes of endometrial glands (Figure 3) and stroma (Figure 4) were similar to findings with higher doses of vaginal progesterone[13] or intramuscular progesterone[14,15], or in the menstrual cycle[16]. The discrepancy observed in this study between low peripheral levels and high endometrial efficacy has been the basis of the 'first uterine pass effect' hypothesis.

Supporting the paradigm of direct vagina-to-uterus transport of vaginally-administered progesterone, endometrial tissue concentrations of progesterone have been found markedly

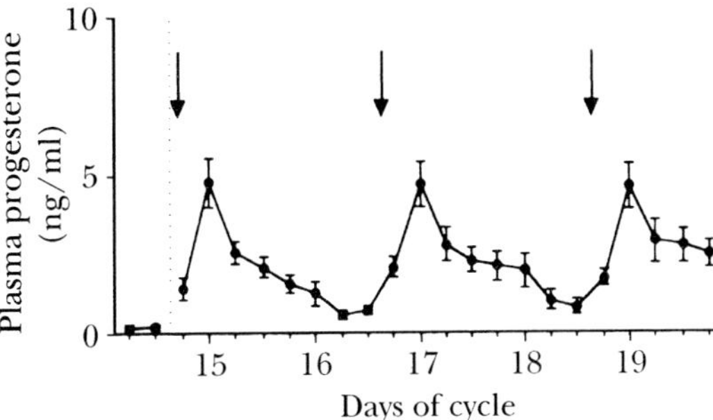

Figure 2 Plasma progesterone after Crinone® 4% administration. Every second day administration of Crinone 4% (45 mg) (marked by arrows) resulted in plasma progesterone levels between 5 ng/ml and 1 ng/ml. Despite these low levels, endometrial biopsies showed full secretory transformation of endometrial glands (day 20) and stroma (day 24)[11]

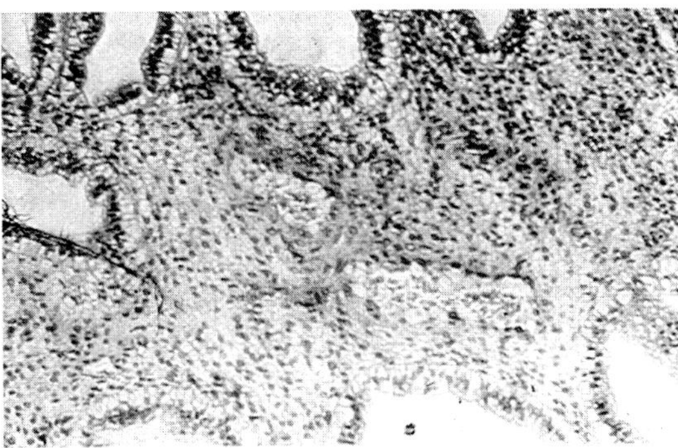

Figure 3 Endometrial histology on day 20 in women receiving Crinone 4% every other day. Results are characterized by the secretory transformation of endometrial glands with a characteristic upward displacement of the nuclei by glycogen-filled vacuoles[11]

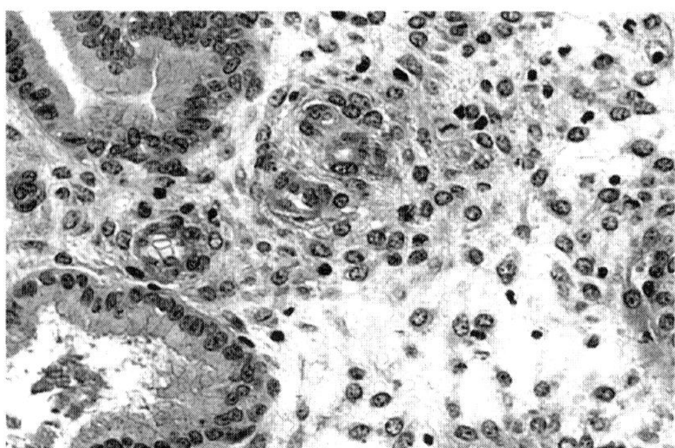

Figure 4 Endometrial histology on day 24 in women receiving Crinone 4% every other day. Results are characterized by the secretory transformation of the endometrial stroma. The late luteal phase is characterized by the predecidual transformation of stromal cells. While stained estrogen and progesterone receptors remain present in the nuclei of stromal cells, they have disappeared from glandular cells[11]

higher after vaginal rather than intramuscular administration[9]. In this study, endometrial tissue samples were obtained by transvaginal–transcervical aspiration. In order to rule out the possibility of contamination of tissue samples by progesterone still present in the vagina, the study was repeated on endometrial tissue obtained at the time of abdominal hysterectomies[17]. In this study, endometrial progesterone was approximately seven times higher after the vaginal gel Crinone as compared to after intramuscular administration of similar amounts of progesterone. Further emphasizing the vaginal route paradox, peripheral levels of progesterone were markedly higher after intramuscular rather than vaginal administration of progesterone[17].

Evidence supporting the 'first uterine pass effect' and clues for possible mechanisms were sought using an extensively documented human *ex vivo* uterine perfusion model[18]. Bulletti and associates[18] documented that tritiated progesterone applied to the rim of vaginal tissue removed with the hysterectomy specimen traveled directly to the uterine fundus in approximately 5 h (Figure 5). In distinct experiments, it was demonstrated that prior sealing of the cervical canal with latex failed to affect the direct transport of tritiated progesterone[17].

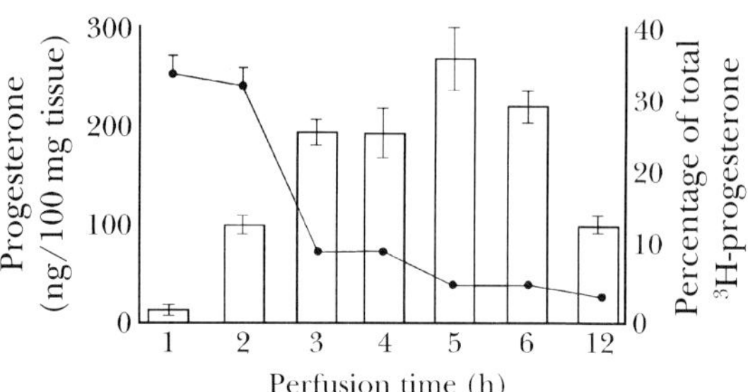

Figure 5 The first uterine pass effect. Venous absorption and uterine diffusion following vaginal placement of tritiated progesterone provide experimental validation of direct vagina-to-uterus transport of progesterone, or the 'first uterine pass effect'. Venous absorption peaks after approximately 2 h while uterine diffusion is at a maximum after 5 to 6 h. To take full benefit of the first uterine pass effect, progesterone must remain in the vagina over time. This can be achieved by repeating vaginal administrations (capsules, suppositories, etc.) or using a sustained-release system such as the vaginal gel Crinone 4%[18]. The columns denote data obtained by endometrial extraction of progesterone, while the line represents data obtained on the output of ^{3}H-progesterone from the veins

The mechanism responsible for direct uterine transport of progesterone administered vaginally has not been entirely elucidated as yet. Circumstantial evidence supports the existence of a countercurrent exchange mechanism with vein-to-artery diffusion of progesterone absorbed through the vaginal mucosa. Studying women who underwent abdominal hysterectomy after receiving vaginal progesterone, Cicinelli and colleagues[10] observed that progesterone concentration was higher in uterine than in peripheral arteries (Figure 6). The fact that the progesterone concentration in the uterine artery exceeded that in the peripheral circulation strongly supports the theory that vagina-to-uterus transport follows a countercurrent vein-to-artery exchange mechanism (Figure 7). The principles and physiological examples of countercurrent exchange were recently reviewed[19]. This publication also reviewed non-human data supportive of direct vagina-to-uterus transport.

The direct transport to the uterus of substances placed in the vagina is convenient for delivering certain substances targeted at the uterus. However, it is appropriate to query the physiological significance of this newly unveiled

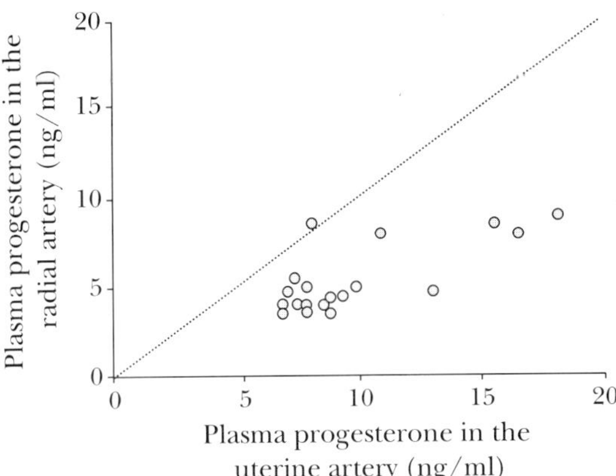

Figure 6 Countercurrent distribution of progesterone from the vagina to the uterus. After vaginal administration of progesterone, hormone concentrations in the uterine artery are approximately twice those seen in the brachial artery. This finding suggests that direct vagina-to-uterus transport results from countercurrent exchange with vein-to-artery diffusion[10]

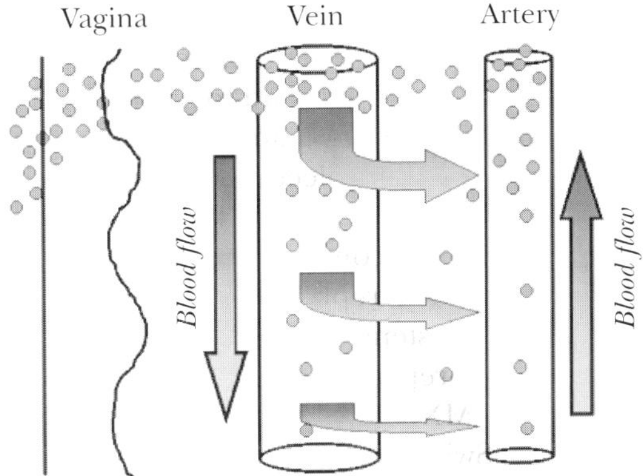

Figure 7 The countercurrent exchange system. While substances are normally transported from arteries to veins, countercurrent exchanges from veins to arteries can also take place if the following conditions are satisfied: (1) proximity with the exchange surface; (2) a higher concentration in the venous flow; and (3) flow in the opposite direction. Countercurrent exchanges are directly related to the exchange surface size and the vein-to-artery gradient and inversely related to the velocity of vascular flux[19]

functional 'portal' system. Why would nature have developed a mechanism that favors transport from the vagina to the uterus? The role of prostaglandins in uterine contractility and particularly for stimulating retrograde propulsion of sperm from the cervix to the distal end of the tubes may provide interesting clues. In the light of our prior work, we hypothesized that prostaglandins introduced vaginally through intercourse travel directly to the uterus (and possibly tubes) where they activate contractility. Thus prostaglandins from sperm would be the primary beneficiary of this local transport system. This would permit prostaglandins to enhance sperm transport without raising prostaglandins in the peripheral circulation. Hence, vaginal administration of substances such as progesterone is most likely an indirect benefit of a local countercurrent exchange system normally involved in the transport of sperm prostaglandins.

Vaginal progesterone in the menopause: clinical experience with Crinone

It has now been amply documented that hormone replacement therapy (HRT) prevents postmenopausal bone loss[20,21]. Furthermore, epidemiological data suggest that HRT may also prevent the increase in cardiovascular morbidity and mortality described after menopause[22,23]. However, despite these highly encouraging results, long-term compliance to HRT remains notoriously low[24]. Aside from the fear of breast cancer, which is highly emotional, two factors are most commonly incriminated by women who discontinue HRT: (1) uterine bleeding; and (2) treatment-induced side-effects (mainly psychological). Here we describe how natural progesterone administered vaginally can provide new therapeutic options for better control of uterine bleeding with fewer side-effects.

In infertility patients, vaginal progesterone succeeds in triggering predecidual changes, but oral progesterone does not[6,9,13,25,26]. In HRT, a different situation prevails. Here the primary objective of progestagen treatments is to prevent the risk of endometrial hyperplasia seen with estrogen-only treatments[27]. However, while full secretory transformation of the endometrium is not strictly necessary, it may be the key to improved control of menstrual bleeding. The recent availability of Crinone has opened new therapeutic possibilities. Indeed, the novelty of the product, particularly its sustained-release properties, allows a reduction in the number of daily applications needed. Furthermore, Crinone is an emulsion rather than a lipid-based preparation. This endows the gel with very stable pharmacokinetic properties, keeping drug delivery and absorption from being influenced by the degree of local moisture[11]. It was a logical clinical extension of the infertility experience with Crinone to test the feasibility and possible advantages of using this new vaginal progesterone gel in HRT. Knowing that vaginal progesterone reliably induces withdrawal bleeding without triggering the subjective side-effects characteristic of synthetic progestagens[9,13,28,29], we were confident that vaginal progesterone would be effective in HRT. Patient acceptance of long-term treatment with a vaginal product was, however, unknown and needed testing.

We recently reported primary data on using the vaginal progesterone gel in HRT[30]. In our study, two regimens using vaginal progesterone have been tested in HRT. First, in a cyclical regimen the vaginal progesterone gel was used daily for 10 consecutive days every month in conjunction with continuous estrogen therapy. The objective of the cyclical regimen was to achieve predictable withdrawal bleeding upon discontinuation of vaginal progesterone treatment. Second, we tested whether the sustained-release properties of the vaginal progesterone gel permitted sufficient uterine exposure to progesterone with limited applications in order to achieve a 'no bleed' HRT regimen. Practical considerations limited the number of Crinone administrations to twice a week. The objective here was to maintain amenorrhea in the largest possible fraction of women. In this study, 136 menopausal women received vaginal progesterone as part of their HRT regimen[30]. All participants had > 6 months of amenorrhea or had received HRT for over 2 years without interruption. Participants were treated with cyclical and/or constant combined regimens, depending on their personal preferences or prevailing clinical conditions. The cyclical regimen was recommended for women who were less than 3 years into the menopause. Conversely, women more than 3 years into the menopause and/or ≥ 53 years of age were offered the constant combined regimen as the primary option.

In the cyclical regimen, women received the estrogen preparation of their choice at doses commonly prescribed for the prevention of osteoporosis. Moreover, from the 1st to the 10th day of each calendar month women also used one daily application of the vaginal gel progesterone, Crinone 4%, containing 45 mg progesterone per 1.125 g gel administered as previously described by Warren and colleagues[31]. Morning application of the gel was preferred by most patients and appears to provide better dispersion of the gel with a lower risk of accumulating gel residues. Participating women were told to expect withdrawal bleeding for 1 to 6 days after discontinuing Crinone treatment. Bleeding was reviewed at each clinical visit (every 6 months). Taking advantage of the recent improvements in endometrial visualization on ultrasound[32], an endometrial biopsy was performed only in those cases where endometrial thickness was > 10 mm and/or abnormal in aspect or echogenicity, and in all cases of dysfunctional uterine bleeding (bleeding other than withdrawal).

In the constant combined regimen, women received estrogen replacement therapy from transdermal systems or oral preparations. Transdermal preparations most often used were Estraderm® MX 0.05 (Novartis Pharmaceuticals, Basle, Switzerland), delivering 0.05 mg of estrogen per 24 h or oral conjugated equine estrogens (Premarin® 0.625 mg/day). In all cases, estrogen treatment was pursued continuously. Moreover, patients self-administered one application of the vaginal gel Crinone 4% twice weekly. Crinone was administered on the days transdermal systems were changed or on two set days of the week. Women were told to expect to remain amenorrheic after starting their treatment but that unscheduled spotting or bleeding might occur. Light sporadic and/or intermittent spotting was described as potentially acceptable to the patient. However, women were told to report at once if heavy/persistent and/or abnormal bleeding occurred. Participants were evaluated every 6 months.

All clinical evaluations included ultrasound at baseline and during treatment. Patients on both treatment arms were evaluated at 6-month intervals. In women receiving the cyclical regimen, endometrial thickness ≤ 10 mm was acceptable provided that no irregularities in shape and/or echogenicity were seen. In the constant combined regimen, the endometrial thickness needed to be ≤ 5 mm or an endometrial biopsy was performed. All women with dysfunctional uterine bleeding underwent biopsies irrespective of the endometrial thickness and treatment regimen received.

The bleeding patterns observed in Groups I (cyclical) and II (constant) are described in Table I. In women receiving vaginal progesterone cyclically, 91.3% experienced the expected withdrawal bleeding pattern exclusive of any other form of bleeding. Of them, 58 (92%) elected to stay on vaginal progesterone for HRT beyond 6 months, while two opted for other treatment options and three discontinued hormone therapy altogether. Breakthrough and/or other forms of abnormal bleeding affected six women. No endometrial sampling (endometrial aspiration and/or hysteroscopy) showed evidence of endometrial hyperplasia or cancer. In Group II the vast majority of women remained amenorrheic throughout the entire treatment period. At 6 months, 80.6% of women who were amenorrheic at inclusion had remained so throughout treatment. Data on a subset of 14 women who were followed for 18 months indicted that 12 (86%) remained amenorrheic throughout that period. Bleeding was mild and/or isolated and spontaneously resolved in 9/67 (13.4%) women. Four women (6%) had heavy bleeding and discontinued treatment. Ultrasound data are illustrated in Table 2. None of the endometrial samplings motivated by bleeding and endometrial thickness > 5 mm showed hyperplasia and/or cancer. At 6 months, a vast majority of women elected to remain on treatment.

Progesterone and synthetic progestins

While the actions of progesterone and synthetic progestins on endometrial tissue are similar (genomic effects), notorious differences in side-effects are encountered between the man-made products and natural hormone. These may reflect diverging non-genomic effects.

In a study looking at vaginal progesterone in conjunction with estrogen therapy, Warren and associates[31] observed less psychological side-effects when women were taking estrogen and progesterone than when women were receiving estrogen alone (Figure 8). This is drastically different from findings commonly seen with synthetic progestins. No definitive explanation exists for this difference between synthetic progestins and natural progesterone. It can be hypothesized, however, that the explanation lies in intrinsic differences in the non-genomic effects of these products.

Besides its genomic action through binding the progesterone receptor, progesterone also acts at the cell membrane level. There, it decreases excitability either directly or through

Table 1 Bleeding patterns observed in women receiving the vaginal progesterone gel cyclically (Group I) for 10 consecutive days of each month or continuously (Group II) with applications twice-weekly[30]

	Group I ($n = 69$)	Group II ($n = 67$)
Mean age (years)	50 ± 1.5	58 ± 5.3
Expected outcome (%): withdrawal bleeding (Group I) or amenorrhea (Group II)	63 (91.3)	54 (80.6)
Acceptable mild bleeding (%)	—	9 (13.4)
Abnormal/heavy bleeding (%)	6 (8.7)	4 (6.0)

Table 2 Endometrial thickness (mm) at baseline and during treatment in women receiving the vaginal gel of progesterone cyclically (Group I) or continuously (Group II)[30]

	Group I	Group II
Baseline	4.1 ± 1.5	
with HRT		6.7 ± 1.5
without HRT		3.7 ± 0.7
During treatment	4.9 ± 0.9	
with bleeding		3.8 ± 1.8
no bleeding		3.9 ± 1.2

its 5α-reduced 3α-OH metabolite, allopregnanolone. The latter product has known efficacy for the γ-aminobutyric acid ($GABA_A$) receptor complex where it exerts an allosteric activation of the GABA-ergic Cl^- pump. This raises the resting potential and decreases excitability. One of the major synthetic progestins, medroxyprogesterone acetate, undergoes similar metabolic changes to progesterone on 17 cycle end of the molecule. However, the metabolite of medroxyprogesterone acetate that is symmetrical to allopregnanolone fails to bind and activate the $GABA_A$ complex (Figure 9)[33].

The fact that synthetic progestins often induce unpleasant psychological side-effects is possibly due to non-genomic properties differing from those of progesterone. This may also explain other idiosyncrasies of synthetic progestins. While natural progesterone does not antagonize the beneficial effects of estrogen in a non-human primate model, medroxyprogesterone acetate does. Here again, progesterone and progestins may have different effects on the smooth muscles of vascular walls. The same discrepancy between the negative effects of medroxyprogesterone acetate and the

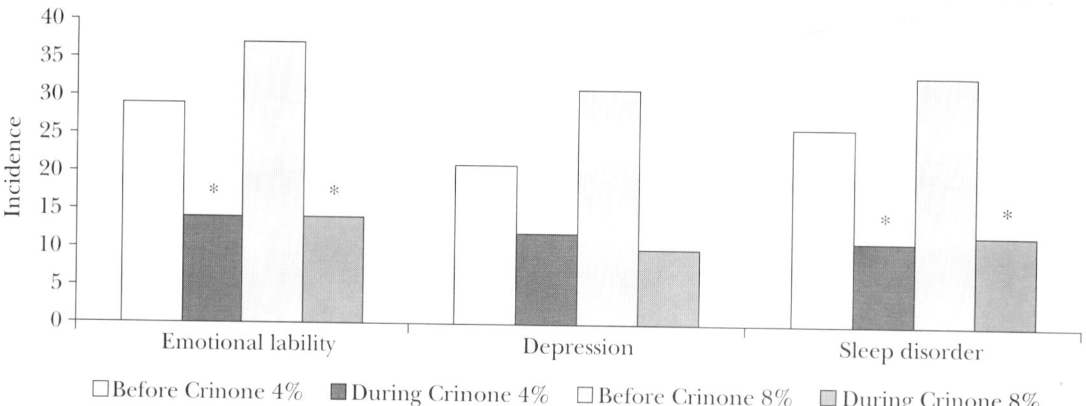

Figure 8 Psychological symptoms before or during treatment with progesterone gel. Psychological symptoms decreased while patients received either Crinone 4% or 8% as compared to estrogen alone. These findings are dramatically different from observations commonly made with synthetic progestins[31].*$p < 0.05$ compared with before treatment

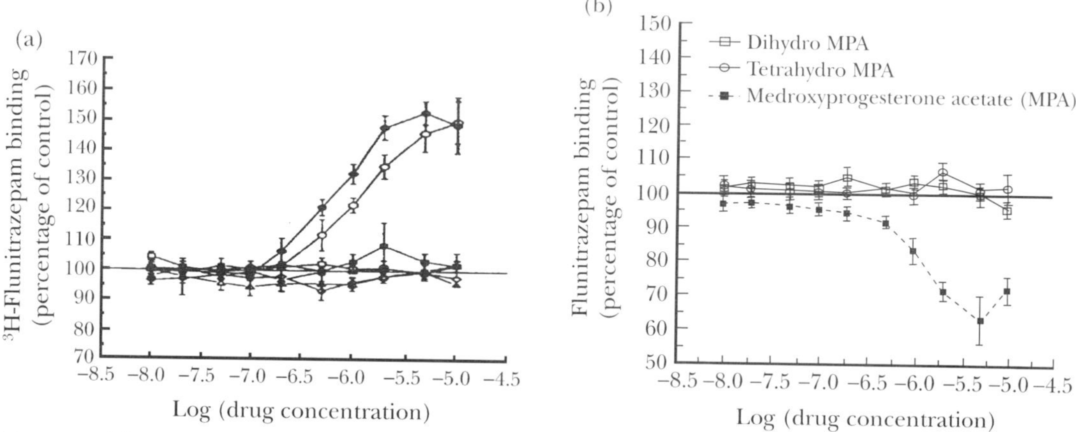

Figure 9 Allosteric activation of the γ-aminobutyric acid (GABAA) receptor. (a) Metabolites of progesterone: 5α dihydroprogesterone (DHP), and its 3αOH derivative (THP) exert allosteric activation of GABAA. (b) Metabolites of medroxyprogesterone acetate fail to exert similar effects. It is likely that the acetate radical added in the 17 position alters the spatial configuration of the molecule and its ability to bind to GABAA[33]

beneficial action of progesterone has been observed in the human coronary artery[34]. Rosano and colleagues[34] showed that medroxyprogesterone acetate entirely antagonized the beneficial effects of estrogen therapy on coronary ischemia. In contrast, the vaginal progesterone gel induced further beneficial effects beyond those seen with estrogen only.

In conclusion, progesterone and synthetic progestins exert different side-effects, namely psychological and cardiovascular effects. Different non-genomic properties of progesterone and synthetic progestins are the probable explanation for the divergent findings. Hence, whenever side-effects or unwanted cardiovascular consequences of synthetic progestins are feared, clinicians should revert to a physiological approach, using non-oral estradiol and vaginal progesterone.

Summary

The data available with vaginal progesterone speak for the safety and efficacy of the vaginal progesterone gel Crinone 4% in hormone replacement therapy. The cyclical regimen with daily administration for 10 days/month provides improved predictability of withdrawal bleeding. The constant combined regimen with twice-weekly administration provides a higher rate of amenorrhea than seen with other existing regimens. With either regimen, however, all the data indicate that vaginal progesterone will find its place among hormone replacement therapy options. Most importantly, the lack of side-effects is likely to improve long-term compliance of hormone replacement therapy regimens and largely make up for the inconvenience of vaginal administration.

References

1. Nahoul K, Dehennin L, Scholler R. Radioimmunoassay of plasma progesterone after oral administration of micronized progesterone. *J Steroid Biochem* 1987;26:241–9

2. Nahoul K, Dehennin L, Jondet M, *et al.* Profiles of plasma estrogens, progesterone and their metabolites after oral or vaginal administration of estradiol or progesterone. *Maturitas* 1993;16:185–202

3. Cooper A, Spencer C, Whitehead MI, *et al.* Systemic absorption of progesterone from Progest cream in postmenopausal women. *Lancet* 1998;351:1255–6

4. Nillius SJ, Johansson EDB. Plasma levels of progesterone after vaginal, rectal or intramuscular administration of progesterone. *Am J Obstet Gynecol* 1971;110:470–7

5. Schmidt CL, De Ziegler D, Gagliardi CL, *et al.* Transfer of cryopreserved–thawed embryos: the natural cycle versus controlled preparation of the endometrium with gonadotropin-releasing hormone agonist and exogenous estradiol and progesterone (GEEP). *Fertil Steril* 1988;49:609–16

6. Bourgain C, Devroey P, Van Waesberghe L, *et al.* Effects of natural progesterone on the morphology of the endometrium in patients with primary ovarian failure. *Hum Reprod* 1990;5:537–43

7. Cicinelli E, Savino F, Cagnazzo I, *et al.* Comparative study of progesterone plasma levels after nasal spray and intramuscular administration of natural progesterone in menopausal women. *Gynecol Obstet Invest* 1993;35:172–4

8. Steingold K, Stumpf P, Kreiner D, *et al.* Estradiol and progesterone replacement regimens for the induction of endometrial receptivity. *Fertil Steril* 1989;52:756–60

9. Miles RA, Paulson RJ, Lobo RA, *et al.* Pharmacokinetics and endometrial tissue levels of progesterone after administration by intramuscular and vaginal routes: a comparative study. *Fertil Steril* 1994;62:485–90

10. Cicinelli E, Cignarelli M, Sabatelli S, *et al.* Plasma concentrations of progesterone are higher in the uterine artery than in the radial artery after vaginal administration of micronized progesterone in an oil-based solution to postmenopausal women. *Fertil Steril* 1998;69:471–3

11. Fanchin R, De Ziegler D, Bergeron C, *et al.* Transvaginal administration of progesterone: dose–response data support a first uterine pass effect. *Obstet Gynecol* 1997;90:396–401

12. De Ziegler D. Hormonal control of endometrial receptivity. *Hum Reprod* 1995;10:4–7

13. De Ziegler D, Bergeron C, Cornel C, *et al.* Effects of luteal estradiol on the secretory transformation of human endometrium and plasma gonadotropins. *J Clin Endocrinol Metab* 1992;74:322–31

14. Navot D, Anderson TL, Droesch K, *et al.* Hormonal manipulation of endometrial maturation. *J Clin Endocrinol Metab* 1989;68:801–7

15. Navot D, Bergh PA, Williams M, *et al.* An insight into early reproductive processes through the *in vivo* model of ovum donation. *J Clin Endocrinol Metab* 1991;72:408–14

16. Noyes RW, Hertig AT, Rock J. Dating the endometrial biopsy. *Fertil Steril* 1950;1:3–25

17. de Ziegler D, Cicinelli E, Bulletti C. Vaginal progesterone gel: evidence of a direct vagina-to-uterus transport. Wyeth-Ayerst Laboratories Sponsored Symposium: Vaginal Progesterone in Assisted Fertility: New Data on Implantation and Pregnancy Rates. Presented at the *54th Annual Meeting of ASRM* San Francisco, 1998

18. Bulletti C, De Ziegler D, Flamigni C, *et al.* Targeted drug delivery in gynecology: the first uterine pass effect. *Hum Reprod* 1997;12:1073–9

19. Cicinelli E, de Ziegler D. Selective distribution to the uterus of progesterone administered per vaginam: an overview on possible mechanisms. *Hum Reprod* 1999;in press

20. Lindsay R, Bush TL, Grady D, *et al.* Therapeutic controversy. Estrogen replacement in menopause. *J Clin Endocrinol Metab* 1996;81:3829–38

21. Nilas L, Christiansen C. The pathophysiology of peri- and postmenopausal bone loss. *Br J Obstet Gynaecol* 1996;96:580–7

22. Barret-Connor E. The menopause, hormone replacement, and cardiovascular disease: the epidemiologic evidence. *Maturitas* 1996;23:227–34

23. Grodstein F, Stampfer MJ, Manson JE, *et al.* Postmenopausal estrogen and progestin use and the risk of cardiovascular disease. *N Engl J Med* 1996;335:453–61

24. Ravnikar VA. Compliance with hormone therapy. *Am J Obstet Gynecol* 1987;156:1332–4

25. Toner JP, Gibbons WE. Crinone 8% used once a day for replacement in donor egg recipients: a status report. Presented at the *54th Annual Meeting of the American Society for Reproductive Medicine,* San Francisco, 1998

26. Simon JA, Robinson DE, Andrews MC, *et al.* The absorption of oral micronized progesterone: the effect of food, dose proportionality, and comparison with intramuscular progesterone. *Fertil Steril* 1993;60:26–33

27. Lobo RA. The role of progestins in hormone replacement therapy. *Am J Obstet Gynecol* 1992;166:1997–2004

28. Hahn RG. Compliance considerations with estrogen replacement: withdrawal bleeding and other factors. *Am J Obstet Gynecol* 1989;161:1854–8

29. Panay N, Studd J. Progestogen intolerance and compliance with hormone replacement therapy in menopausal women. *Hum Reprod* 1997;3:159–71

30. de Ziegler D, Ferriani R, Moraes LAM, *et al.* Vaginal progesterone in menopause: experience with a sustained- and controlled-release gel of progesterone, Crinone® 4%, in cyclical and constant combined regimens. In *Proceedings of Progesterone: A Natural Life-supporting Hormone,* Montegridolfo, July 12–14, 1998

31. Warren MA, Biller BMK, Shangold MM. Transvaginal administration of a new polycarbophil-based progesterone gel for hormone replacement therapy in women with secondary amenorrhea. *Am J Obstet Gynecol* 1999;in press

32. Archer DF, Pickar JH, Bottiglioni F. Bleeding patterns in postmenopausal women taking continuous combined or sequential regimens of conjugated estrogens with medroxyprogesterone acetate. *Obstet Gynecol* 1994;83:686–92

33. McAuley JW, Kroboth PD, Stiff DD, *et al.* Modulation of (3H) flunitrazepam binding by natural and synthetic progestational agents. *Pharmacol Biochem Behav* 1993;45:77–83

34. Rosano GMC, Sarrel PM, Chierchia SL, *et al.* Medroxyprogesterone acetate (MPA) but not natural progesterone (P) reverses the effect of estradiol-17β (E2) upon exercise-induced myocardial ischemia. A double-blind cross-over study. Presented at the *American Heart Association (AHA) Meeting,* New Orleans, November 1996. *Circulation* 1996;94(Suppl):abstr 0104

36

Postmenopausal hormone therapy and breast cancer

L. Speroff

Introduction

Sufficient evidence exists to indicate the possibility of a slightly increased risk of breast cancer associated with long durations (5 or more years) of postmenopausal estrogen use. However, the epidemiologic data on this relationship are by no means consistent and uniform. A review of the epidemiologic studies on postmenopausal hormone therapy and the risk of breast cancer fails to provide definitive evidence regarding this issue.

Recent studies

The latest reports from the Nurses' Health Study represent 16 years of follow-up (1976–1992)[1,2]. During that period, 1935 cases of breast cancer were identified among more than 69 000 postmenopausal women. The analysis revealed that women who had used estrogen in the past (even for 10 or more years) were not at increased risk of breast cancer. However, the relative risk for current users was 1.46 (confidence interval 1.22–1.74) for 5–9 years of use, and 1.46 (1.20–1.76) for 10 or more years of use.

By virtue of the large numbers in the Nurses' Health Study and the careful analyses by the investigators, reports from this study must be given great credibility. The 16-year follow-up report is disturbing with its finding of an increased risk in current users. Because estrogen users may be examined more frequently, detection bias is a major concern. It is noteworthy that current users had a 14% higher prevalence of mammography compared to never users. Current users were different when compared to never users (history of benign breast disease, childbirth only once or twice, menarche at age 13 or less, body mass index of

21–23). Another important consideration is the need to adjust for alcohol consumption, an accepted risk factor for breast cancer. In the Iowa Women's Health Study, an increased risk of breast cancer was observed only in those women who consumed one drink or more of alcohol daily[3]. The concern is that alcohol consumption raises estrogen levels in hormone users to very high concentrations[4,5]. Although each of these factors standing alone would not explain the observed outcome in the Nurses' Health Study, what is the additive effect of all factors? Thus, the finding of an increased relative risk in long-term current users is not definitive and not free of all confounding variables. The size of the statistical risk is not outside the range of influence by biases.

Based on 359 deaths due to breast cancer, the risk of dying of breast cancer in the Nurses' Health Study was 0.80 (0.60–1.07) for past users, 0.99 (0.66–1.48) for current users with less than 5 years of use, and 1.45 (1.01–2.09) with 5 or more years of use. These mortality data raise a question of 'prevalence bias', also called interdependence between the probabilities of disease incidence in a population (an issue of competing risks)[6]. Is it possible that the protection against cardiovascular disease is so great with long durations of estrogen use that the long-term current users develop a problem that is prevalent with aging, namely breast cancer? The never users, deprived of the cardiovascular benefit of estrogen, may develop cardiovascular disease before living long enough to experience breast cancer.

In a study of 1686 cases and 2077 controls in the Eastern USA, the relative risk for current users was 1.1 (0.7–1.6), and for a duration of use of 15 or more years the relative risk was 0.9 (0.4–1.9)[7]. As in the Eastern USA, a study from Toronto found no evidence for an increased risk in either current or recent users or in users for up to 15 years[8]. A case–control study from Washington found no increased risk of breast cancer with past or long-term current use of estrogen alone or with estrogen–progestin[9]. These large case–control studies failed to support the conclusion of the Nurses' Health Study that current users are associated with an increased risk, even with long durations of use. On the other hand, other studies (of smaller size and limited statistical power) have found an increased risk of breast cancer in current users and long-term users[10,11]. A prospective study from the National Cancer Institute could document only an increase in the risk of *in situ* breast cancer (not invasive disease), possibly reflecting surveillance bias in women taking either estrogen alone or a combination of estrogen and progestin[12].

The Iowa Women's Health Study, like the Nurses' Health Study, is prospectively following a cohort of women (selected in 1985). After 6 years of follow-up, a statistically significant increase in the risk of breast cancer could not be detected in ever users or current users of hormone therapy[13]. A report through 8 years of follow-up focused on whether postmenopausal hormone therapy increased the risks for breast cancer and mortality in women with a family history of breast cancer[14]. Even in women with a positive family history of breast cancer who were current users of hormone therapy for more than 5 years, there was no significant increase in the rate of breast cancer. A very large case–control study found no increased risk of breast cancer associated with the ever use of estrogen alone or estrogen and progestin combinations, and when long-term use for 15 years or more was examined, again no increase in risk was detected[15].

Meta-analyses

An Australian meta-analysis of 23 studies of estrogen use and breast cancer concluded 'un-equivocally' that estrogen use did not alter the risk of breast cancer[16]. In the meta-analysis by Dupont and Page[17], the authors concluded that 'considerable and consistent' evidence exists that a daily dose of 0.625 mg conjugated estrogens taken for several years does not appreciably increase the risk of breast cancer[17]. They found no evidence of an association between the duration of treatment and the risk of breast cancer at this dosage.

A third meta-analysis was from the Centers for Disease Control[18]. This meta-analysis was conducted using what the authors called a 'dose–response curve' for duration of use. The curve for each study analyzed was calculated by plotting breast cancer risk against duration of estrogen use. The combined dose–response slope represented the average change in risk associated with estrogen use over time. The analysis concluded that duration of estrogen use was associated with an increased risk of breast cancer, regardless of whether menopause was natural or surgical. No increase in risk was noted in the first 5 years of use, but after 15 years of use the risk was increased by 30%.

A fourth meta-analysis, from Spain, concluded that estrogen is associated with a very small, but statistically significant, increased relative risk of breast cancer and that the increased risk is higher among current users[19]. Confining their analysis to a dose of 0.625 mg conjugated estrogens, however, the Spanish epidemiologists could not detect a statistically significant increased risk. Indeed, this meta-analysis concluded that an estrogen dose of 0.625 mg conjugated estrogens is safe.

A fifth meta-analysis from the epidemiologists associated with the Nurses' Health Study concluded (based on 25 case–control and six cohort studies) that there is no increased risk of breast cancer in ever users of estrogen[20]. Current use was associated with an increased risk (which was lost 2 years after using estrogen), and there was a slight increase with more than 10 years of use (but there was no linear trend with increasing duration of use). This observation in long-term users could be influenced by an increased proportion of current users in this group, and the increased risk in current users could be a consequence of detection bias.

Reanalysis of the literature

A team of epidemiologists invited all investigators who had previously studied the association of postmenopausal hormone use and the risk of breast cancer (51 studies) to submit their original data for a collaborative combined reanalysis, an undertaking more rigorous than a standard meta-analysis. This analysis reached the following conclusions[21]:

(1) Ever users of postmenopausal hormones had an overall increased relative risk of breast cancer of 1.14;

(2) Current users for 5 or more years had a relative risk of 1.35 (confidence interval 1.21–1.49), and the risk increased with increasing duration of use;

(3) Current and recent users had evidence of having only localized disease (no metastatic disease) and ever users had less metastatic disease;

(4) There was no effect of a family history of breast cancer;

(5) There was no increase in relative risk in past users; and

(6) The increase in relative risk in current and recent users was greatest in women with lower body weights.

The most compelling reason to believe that long-term use of postmenopausal estrogen increases the risk of breast cancer is the inherent biologic plausibility. Factors known to increase a woman's exposure to estrogen are known to increase the risk of breast cancer, e.g. age of menarche and age of menopause. Indeed, in this report, the authors make a point of demonstrating that the quantitative effect of their conclusion is similar to extending the age of menopause. According to their calculations, current and recent hormone use was associated with a 2.3% increase in breast cancer risk per year and the effect of the age of menopause was

equivalent to a 2.8% increase in risk per year of delay. Many clinicians are attracted by the logic in this comparison; however, the steady exposure to postmenopausal estrogen is not exactly the same as extended exposure to cyclic ovarian function.

A strong indication that the conclusion of the reanalysis is subject to bias is the finding that current and recent hormone users had evidence only of localized disease. This is consistent with surveillance bias and hormone acceleration of tumors already present and thus detection at an early, less aggressive stage.

The influence of detection/surveillance bias

It is relevant to note that all of the studies that have examined the mortality rates of women who were taking estrogen at the time of breast cancer diagnosis have documented improved survival rates. This undoubtedly reflects earlier diagnosis in users because the greater survival rate in current users is associated with a lower frequency of late-stage disease[22–25]. There is also evidence to suggest that estrogen users develop better differentiated tumors, and that surveillance/detection bias is not the only explanation for better survival[24,26]. This implies that hormone treatment accelerates the growth of a malignant locus already in place, and it presents clinically at a less virulent and aggressive stage.

Increased utilization of mammography by hormone users is a well-recognized phenomenon. Indeed, when corrected for use of mammography, an apparent increase in breast cancer in long-term estrogen users in a retrospective cohort study lost its statistical significance[27].

If the conclusions of the reanalysis of the literature[21] were correct, it would mean that there would be a detectable increase in deaths from breast cancer due to hormone use. However, studies have indicated a *decreased* risk of breast cancer mortality in postmenopausal hormone users. For example, the American Cancer Society 9-year prospective follow-up documented a 16% reduced risk of fatal breast cancer[28]. The mortality data support the contention that accelerated tumor growth and detection/surveillance bias are influencing the results of observational studies.

Why is there no definitive answer?

The lack of a definitive answer to the question of postmenopausal hormone therapy and breast cancer, despite approximately 50 observational studies, can be attributed to the following:

(1) Individual studies lack the statistical power to overcome recognized and unrecognized biases. A large effect yields uniformity and consistency of results with case–control and cohort studies (good examples are the benefits of a reduction in the risks of endometrial and ovarian cancer with the use of oral contraception). Therefore any impact of postmenopausal hormone therapy on the risk of breast cancer is unlikely to be great, otherwise the observational studies would have achieved uniformity and consistency of results.

(2) Most of the available data are derived from a time when hormone dosages and schedules (higher doses and shorter durations) were different compared to current methods – the problem of heterogeneity. In addition to different doses and durations of exposure, heterogeneity is the result of different study designs, different sources for controls, different geographic locations, different populations, and different drugs.

(3) The method of meta-analysis was developed to combine the results of small, randomized trials[29]. Rapidly (perhaps too rapidly) the method has been extended to observational studies, especially when the results of the individual studies are contradictory. Combining the results of contradictory studies, rather than the results of small (randomized) studies, is precisely when meta-analysis is weakest. Statistical analysis is not an appropriate method to address contradictory results. Even when the technique of meta-analysis is restricted to small randomized trials, because of various subjective and objective problems, the outcomes of subsequent large randomized, controlled trials were not predicted accurately 35% of the time by the previous meta-analyses[30]. The method of meta-analysis is not infallible and does not always yield the truth.

The method of meta-analysis has not overcome the problem of achieving sufficient statistical power. The conclusions of meta-analysis of observational studies are not free of selection bias, detection bias, and the problem of a positive result emerging just by chance when multiple subgroup analyses are performed. Meta-analysis is further limited, not only when the data base is subject to biases as is the case with observational studies, but also when there is heterogeneity among the studies (different drugs, doses, durations of exposures, and populations). A meta-analysis can make the problem of bias worse by magnifying the significance level of erroneous results; a meta-analysis does not correct for design flaws in individual studies.

Our uncertainty will not be resolved by more case–control studies, more cohort studies, or more meta-analyses. Only a properly performed randomized clinical trial will provide us with definitive information.

Implications for clinicians and patients

The lack of agreement, uniformity and consistency in approximately 50 case–control and cohort studies indicates that the use of postmenopausal hormone therapy cannot be associated with a major impact on the risk of breast cancer, otherwise there would be agreement among the studies. It is helpful to compare this situation with three other conditions: the protection against ovarian cancer by oral contraceptives, the protection against coronary heart disease by postmenopausal estrogen use, and the increase in lung cancer due to cigarette smoking. Clinicians believe each of these three epidemiologic associations, despite the lack of a single randomized clinical trial, because all of the studies say the same thing, an impressive agreement and uniformity among observational studies. The results on postmenopausal hormone therapy and the risk of breast cancer indicate either a small impact of estrogen use or the effect of biases that can only be eliminated by a large, randomized trial such as the on-going Women's Health Initiative.

The comfort found in large numbers with epidemiologic research is lost to us when we must make clinical decisions with individual patients. If we wish to minimize the uncertainty from imprecise measurements, we will adopt an appropriate strategy. If we wish to emphasize the possibility or probability of an outcome, we will adopt another. It is appropriate to emphasize the benefits of postmenopausal hormone therapy, point out the continuing concern regarding the relationship between estrogen use and breast cancer (particularly long-term use), and to emphasize the absence of definitive evidence linking such therapy to an increased risk of breast cancer.

The risk of breast cancer with estrogen–progestin therapy

Only two reports have claimed that the addition of a progestational agent protects against breast cancer[31,32]. The first was limited by bias in treatment selection (the breast cancer risk factor profiles were not matched in the treated and untreated groups)[31]. The second study, although it is the only randomized, placebo-controlled trial, was hampered by small numbers[32].

At the present time, the available epidemiologic evidence on the impact of combined estrogen–progestin treatment indicates neither a protective nor a detrimental effect. Recent studies find that the addition of a progestin does not change the findings with estrogen alone[2,9–12]. Balancing the information available involving all of the health issues affected by hormone therapy, a combined estrogen–progestin program in appropriate doses continues to offer significant benefits for postmenopausal women. As time goes on, more studies and greater duration of use should provide us with better answers to many of our questions. By virtue of the magnitude of the postmenopausal female population,

these questions deserve continuing biologic and epidemiologic research from both the public health and individual points of view.

Summary

(1) Some epidemiologic case–control and cohort studies conclude that long-term (5 or more years) or current use of postmenopausal hormone therapy is associated with a slight increase in the risk of breast cancer. This conclusion might be due to confounding biases, particularly detection/surveillance bias.

(2) All epidemiologic studies fail to find an increased risk of breast cancer associated with short-term (less than 5 years) use or past use of postmenopausal hormone therapy.

(3) The epidemiologic data agree that the addition of a progestin to the treatment regimen neither increases nor decreases the risk observed in individual studies.

(4) The epidemiologic data indicate that a positive family history of breast cancer should not be a contraindication to the use of postmenopausal hormone therapy.

(5) Women who develop breast cancer while using postmenopausal hormone therapy have a reduced risk of dying from breast cancer. This is because of two factors: increased surveillance and early detection, and acceleration of tumor growth so that tumors appear at a less virulent and aggressive stage.

Should a woman who has had breast cancer use postmenopausal hormones?

The increasing incidence of breast cancer, together with earlier detection and treatment, is producing a growing pool of patients for whom the question of estrogen treatment is important and at the same time difficult. The problem is easy to articulate: we have no data. There are absolutely no published clinical trials of sufficient size and scope in which the impact of estrogen treatment has been documented when given to women with previously treated breast cancer.

Because there is good reason to believe that breast cancer is hormonally influenced, it is not hard to understand the breast surgeon or medical oncologist who believes that estrogen treatment is foolish and dangerous. Yet that position is just as unencumbered by data as the position of the gynecologist who believes that appropriate patients stand to benefit more from estrogen compared to the unknown risk of breast cancer recurrence.

The argument that postmenopausal hormone therapy should not be given to women who have had breast cancer is a reasonable one. It is based on the recognition of a large body of evidence that indicates that breast cancer is a hormone-responsive tumor. The overriding fear of many clinicians (and patients) is that metastatic cells are present (perhaps being controlled by various host defense factors) that will be susceptible to stimulation by exogenous hormones[33]. However, many women who have had breast cancer are aware of the benefits of postmenopausal hormone treatment (especially protection against cardiovascular disease and osteoporosis) and are asking clinicians to help make this risk–benefit decision. In addition, some women suffer from such severe hot flushing and vaginal dryness that they are willing to consider hormonal treatment.

On the other side of this debate is the clinician who has been impressed by the breast cancer studies with positive results reviewed in this chapter. Because of the current lack of epidemiologic data, both sides of this debate are strongly influenced by theoretical considerations and clinical experiences, which unfortunately often become an obstacle to the patient's own informed choice.

There is one small series in which a combination of 0.625 mg conjugated estrogens and 0.15 mg norgestrel was given continuously for a short period of time (a maximum of 6 months) to women who had been previously treated for breast cancer[34]. Over the next 2 years, no patients developed recurrence. Another small series (25 and then 77 women with breast cancer ranging from *in situ* to stage III disease) received estrogen–progestin therapy for 24 to 82 months; the recurrence rate was not greater than that expected[35,36]. From this group of patients, 41 breast cancer survivors receiving hormone therapy had the same outcomes when compared to 82 women selected from a cancer registry and not taking hormones[37]. In a report from Australia, 90 women with a history of breast cancer who were given a combination of estrogen and progestin had lower mortality and recurrence rates; however, the dose of progestin was very high (which in itself can be therapeutic) and treatment was not randomized[38]. In a follow-up of 49 women treated with estrogen after treatment for localized breast cancer, only one patient developed recurrent disease[39]. In another series of 114 women, hormone treatment of disease-free patients was associated with a low rate of recurrence[40]. These patients had both positive and negative nodes and estrogen-receptor status. While the results conform to an incidence of recurrent disease no greater than expected, the outcomes may reflect biases in clinician and patient decision-making that can only be overcome with a proper long-term, randomized clinical trial.

Because of better treatment and earlier diagnosis, 50–75% of women diagnosed with breast cancer are now cured[41]. Of 100 patients with breast cancer, about 60 will be cured by mastectomy or breast-conserving surgery with radiotherapy, and would receive no benefit from adjuvant treatment. Is this group safe for hormone therapy? Of the remaining 40, some will live longer (an average of 2–3 years) because of adjuvant treatment, but only a few. Is the unknown risk with exogenous hormone treatment worth it in this group? Although intuitively it seems that the risk : benefit ratio would be more favorable in the presence of negative nodes, negative receptors, and small tumors, are negative estrogen and progesterone receptor assessments sufficient to conclude that the cancer is not sensitive to hormones? If the patient is in the high-cure category, does it make any difference what the receptor status is? Receptor status is not absolute; it is always a relative measure. The answers to all of these questions are not known.

Patients and clinicians have to incorporate all of the above considerations into the medical decision. However, patients have to take an unknown risk if they want the benefits of estrogen treatment, and clinicians have to take an unknown medical–legal risk. Some patients will choose to take estrogen, judging the benefits to be worth the unknown risk. Physicians should support patients in this decision. Other patients will prefer to avoid any unknown risks. These patients, too, deserve support in their decision.

References

1. Colditz GA, Stampfer MJ, Willett WC, *et al.* Type of postmenopausal hormone use and risk of breast cancer: 12-year follow-up from the Nurses' Health Study. *Cancer Causes Control* 1992;3:433

2. Colditz GA, Hankinson SE, Hunter DJ, *et al.* The use of estrogens and progestins and the risk of breast cancer in postmenopausal women. *N Engl J Med* 1995;332:1589

3. Gapstur SM, Potter JD, Sellers TA, *et al.* Increased risk of breast cancer with alcohol consumption in postmenopausal women. *Am J Epidemiol* 1992; 136:1221–31

4. Gavaler JS, Van Thiel DH. The association between moderate alcoholic beverage consumption and serum estradiol and testosterone levels in normal postmenopausal women: relationship to the literature. *Alcohol Clin Exp Res* 1992;16: 87–92

5. Ginsburg EL, Mello NK, Mendelson JH, *et al.* Effects of alcohol ingestion on estrogens in postmenopausal women. *J Am Med Assoc* 1996;276: 1747–51

6. Vrieze OJ, Kuipers J, Boes G. Scenario analysis in public health and competing risks. *Stat Appl* 1990;1:371

7. Kaufman DW, Palmer JR, De Mouzon J, *et al.* Estrogen replacement therapy and the risk of breast cancer: results from the case–control surveillance study. *Am J Epidemiol* 1991;134:1375–85

8. Palmer JR, Rosenberg L, Clarke EA, *et al.* Breast cancer risk after estrogen replacement therapy: results from the Toronto Breast Cancer Study. *Am J Epidemiol* 1991;134:1386–95

9. Stanford JL, Weiss NS, Voigt LF, *et al.* Combined estrogen and progestin hormone replacement therapy in relation to risk of breast cancer in middle-aged women. *J Am Med Assoc* 1995;274: 137

10. Yang CP, Daling JR, Band PR, *et al.* Non-contraceptive hormone use and risk of breast cancer. *Cancer Causes Control* 1992;3:475

11. Risch HA, Howe GR. Menopausal hormone usage and breast cancer in Saskatchewan: a record-linkage cohort study. *Am J Epidemiol* 1994;139:670–83

12. Schairer C, Byrne C, Keyl PM, *et al.* Menopausal estrogen and estrogen–progestin replacement therapy and risk of breast cancer (United States). *Cancer Causes Control* 1994;5:491–500

13. Folsom AR, Mink PJ, Sellers TA, *et al.* Hormonal replacement therapy and morbidity and mortality in a prospective study of postmenopausal women. *Am J Public Health* 1995;85:1128–32

14. Sellers TA, Mink PJ, Cerhan JR, *et al.* The role of hormone replacement therapy in the risk for breast cancer and total mortality in women with a family history of breast cancer. *Ann Intern Med* 1997;127:973–80

15. Newcomb PA, Longnecker MP, Storer BE, *et al.* Long-term hormone replacement therapy and risk of breast cancer in postmenopausal women. *Am J Epidemiol* 1995;142:788–95

16. Armstrong BK. Oestrogen therapy after the menopause – boon or bane? *Med J Aust* 1988;148:213

17. Dupont WD, Page DL. Menopausal estrogen replacement therapy and breast cancer. *Arch Intern Med* 1991;151:67–72

18. Steinberg KK, Thacker SB, Smith SJ, *et al.* A meta-analysis of the effect of estrogen replacement therapy on the risk of breast cancer. *J Am Med Assoc* 1991;265:1985

19. Sillero-Arenas M, Delgado-Rodriguez M, Rodigues-Canteras R, *et al.* Menopausal hormone replacement therapy and breast cancer: a meta-analysis. *Obstet Gynecol* 1992;79:286

20. Colditz GA, Egan KM, Stampfer MJ. Hormone replacement therapy and risk of breast cancer: results from epidemiologic studies. *Am J Obstet Gynecol* 1993;168:1473

21. Collaborative Group on Hormonal Factors in Breast Cancer. Breast cancer and hormone

replacement therapy: collaborative reanalysis of data from 51 epidemiological studies of 52 705 women with breast cancer and 108 411 women without breast cancer. *Lancet* 1997;350:1047–59

22. Hunt K, Vessey M, McPherson K. Mortality in a cohort of long-term users of hormone replacement therapy: an updated analysis. *Br J Obstet Gynaecol* 1990;97:1080

23. Strickland DM, Gambrell Jr RD, Butzin CA, *et al.* The relationship between breast cancer survival and prior postmenopausal estrogen use. *Obstet Gynecol* 1992;80:400

24. Bonnier P, Romain S, Giacalone PL, *et al.* Clinical and biologic prognostic factors in breast cancer diagnosed during postmenopausal hormone replacement therapy. *Obstet Gynecol* 1995;85:11

25. Grodstein F, Stampfer MJ, Colditz GA, *et al.* Postmenopausal hormone therapy and mortality. *N Engl J Med* 1997;336:1769–75

26. Magnusson C, Holmberg L, Norden T, *et al.* Prognostic characteristics in breast cancers after hormone replacement therapy. *Breast Cancer Res Treat* 1996;38:325–34

27. Ettinger B, Quesenberry C, Schroeder DA, *et al.* Long-term postmenopausal estrogen therapy may be associated with increased risk of breast cancer: a cohort study. *Menopause* 1997;4:125–9

28. Willis DB, Calle EE, Miracle-McMahill HL, *et al.* Estrogen replacement therapy and risk of fatal breast cancer in a prospective cohort of post-menopausal women in the United States. *Cancer Causes Control* 1996;7:449–57

29. Petitti DB. *Meta-analysis, Decision Analysis, and Cost-effectiveness Analysis: Methods for Quantitative Synthesis in Medicine.* New York: Oxford University Press, 1994

30. LeLorier J, Grégoire G, Benhaddad A, *et al.* Discrepancies between meta-analyses and subse-quent large randomized, controlled trials. *N Engl J Med* 1997;337:536–42

31. Gambrell Jr RD, Maier RC, Sanders BI. Decreased incidence of breast cancer in postmenopausal estrogen–progestogen users. *Obstet Gynecol* 1983;62:435

32. Nachtigall MJ, Smilen SW, Nachtigall RAD, *et al.* Incidence of breast cancer in a 22-year study of women receiving estrogen–progestin replacement therapy. *Obstet Gynecol* 1992;80:827–30

33. Spicer D, Pike MC, Henderson BE. The question of estrogen replacement therapy in patients with a prior diagnosis of breast cancer. *Oncology* 1990;4:49

34. Stoll BA, Parbhoo S. Treatment of menopausal symptoms in breast cancer patients. *Lancet* 1988;1:1278–9

35. Wile AG, Opfell RW, Margileth DA. Hormone replacement therapy in previously treated breast cancer patients. *Am J Surg* 1993;165:372–5

36. DiSaia PJ, Odicino F, Grosen EA, *et al.* Hormone replacement therapy in breast cancer (Letter). *Lancet* 1993;342:1232

37. DiSaia PJ, Grosen EA, Kurosaki T, *et al.* Hormone replacement therapy in breast cancer survivors: a cohort study. *Am J Obstet Gynecol* 1996;174:1494–8

38. Dew J, Eden JA, Beller E, *et al.* A cohort study of hormone replacement therapy given to women previously treated for breast cancer. *Climacteric* 1998;1:137–42

39. Vassilopoulou-Sellin R, Theriault R, Klein MJ. Estrogen replacement therapy in women with prior diagnosis and treatment for breast cancer. *Gynecol Oncol* 1997;65:89–93

40. Decker DA, Pettinga JE, Cox TC, *et al.* Hormone replacement therapy in breast cancer survivors. *Breast J* 1997;3:63–8

41. Henderson IC. Breast cancer therapy – the price of success. *N Engl J Med* 1992;326:1774

Section VI
Sexuality/sexually transmitted diseases/AIDS

The benefits and risks involved in treating impotence

J. Frick and A. Jungwirth

Introduction

Kinsey already reported in 1948 an epidemiological study of the sexual behavior of a male population in the United States. This study included 12 000 males from representative samples of the general population, stratified for age, education and occupation. Data were based on detailed and structured interviews. Kinsey reported in this first comprehensive study that the incidence of impotence increased with age, with up to 1% prior to 19 years, less than 3% between the ages of 19 and 45, 6.7% between 45 and 55 years and 25% at 75 years[1].

A recent, large epidemiological study on sexual dysfunction in a general population is the Massachusetts male aging study. This large examination provided additional data on male sexual dysfunction, defining its prevalence and identifying physiological and psychological correlates. The study included a population of 1709 non-institutional men aged between 40 and 70. The study population originated from the Boston area, and the examination included a detailed questionnaire, blood sampling and a complete analysis. The overall incidence of some degree of impotence was 52%, and complete erectile dysfunction increased from 5% at the age of 40 to 15% at the age of 70. After adjusting for age, impotence was correlated with heart disease (39%), diabetes (28%) and hypertension (15%), as well as other vascular risk factors, such as cigarette smoking. Correlations were also found with untreated medical conditions, such as ulcers (18%), arthritis (15%) and allergies (12%). In addition to all these factors, depression was the psychological variable most linked with impotence[2].

During recent years, there have been many other epidemiological studies performed regarding the incidence of erectile dysfunction. One of these is the Baltimore longitudinal study of aging, which reported a male sexual dysfunction in 8% of otherwise healthy men at the age of 55, 25% at the age of 65, 55% at the age of 75 and 75% at the age of 80[3].

Causes of male sexual dysfunction and risk factors

Recent advances in both basic science and clinical research have led to an improved understanding of the pathophysiology and treatment options of sexual dysfunction[4]. It is apparent that male sexual dysfunction does not necessarily accompany aging. Sexual dysfuncton, however, is augmented significantly by vascular risk factors, concomitant diseases, the use of medications, postoperative complications and blunt pelvic and/or perineal trauma. Further intensive research will allow a better understanding of male sexual dysfunction. This will provide the clinician with an opportunity to improve diagnostic skills and the patient with a therapeutic option, associated with minimal morbidity.

Endocrine disorders commonly associated with erectile dysfunction include hypopituitarism, non-functioning pituitary tumors, prolactin-secreting pituitary tumors or hypothyroidism. Hypogonadism as a cause of erectile dysfunction has been reported in as many as 30% of males of more than 50 years of age. In another study, decreased Leydig-cell function was reported in 83% of impotent men who presented with erectile dysfunction and type II diabetes mellitus[5].

Male sexual dysfunction was reported in 39% based on low plasma testosterone levels.

Testicular histology of impotent men has revealed some specific features of the testicular structures. Findings in these subjects have included an increase in interstitial tissue, peritubular and intratubular fibrosis connected with tubular sclerosis. At present, androgen substitution therapy is correctly indicated only for men with hypogonadism. Before initiation of therapy, a careful evaluation is required to identify the etiology of hypogonadism and the possible link with sexual or erectile dysfunction.

It is important to mention that, before treatment of erectile dysfunction, all eligible patients should be carefully counselled regarding the expected benefits and risks of all the possible treatment forms.

Treatment of erectile dysfunction

Some compounds initiate erections by virtue of their neural actions or because they are placed directely into penile smooth muscle. Some compounds support and enhance processes that are already under way. Further compounds may be directed to the central nervous system or designed to work through systemic or local action in the periphery[6]. Compounds that show a central action in treating erectile dysfunction are apomorphines, melanocyte-stimulating hormone analogs and androgens. Compounds with a peripheral action in treating impotence are prostaglandins, administered by the intracavernous and/or transurethral route, vasoactive intestinal polypeptides, sildenafil and phentolamine. There are also some additional therapeutic forms such as vacuum-erection devices. For some types of erectile dysfunction, such as priapism, Peyronie's disease and traumatic blockage of the penile artery, a carefully indicated surgical management is still fashionable[7-9]. The most evident benefit for patients suffering from sexual dysfunction will come when the medical community integrates the organic and psychogenic components of specific disorders into a holistic approach. This management will involve both members of a sexually functioning unit, but must overcome the taboos which now exist in the evaluation and basic recognition of sexual disorders.

Benefits of treating impotence

Patients have the choice of a number of therapeutic modalities, usually guided by personal preference, confidence, effectiveness regarding the degree and type of erectile dysfunction, and the level of invasiveness which the patient is willing to tolerate. The options are oral medications including hormonal therapy, vacuum-erection devices, intracavernosal injection of alprostadil or other formulations, transurethral delivery of alprostadil, implantation of a penile prosthesis, and vascular and/or penile surgery.

The introduction of all the recent new oral compounds for the treatment of erectile dysfunction will represent a revolutionary change in the management of this disease[10,11].

The benefits in treating erectile dysfunction are manifold, independent of the age of the patient, as the disorder may be a complex problem for each individual patient. As the number of therapeutic modalities has increased during the past 20 years, the patient's choice has also increased. Of importance now and in the future is to choose the most suitable modality, which guarantees the highest success with no, or a minimum of tolerable, side-effects.

We know from some studies that there is a relationship between declining testosterone levels and sexual activity and sexual desire, especially in older men, but there is little relation to erectile dysfunction. Testosterone replacement studies in older sexually dysfunctional men have shown that, sometimes, such therapy improves low libido, but very rarely does it improve erectile dysfunction. However, any improvement of sexual behavior is to be regarded as a benefit in the entire logistic approach to sexual dysfunction[12].

Basically, pharmacological treatment will expand to include more specific and effective oral compounds, with action directed both to the end-organ cavernosal tissue and to the more central areas of the brain responsible for sexual function. The development of agents that are directly injected or transported into the cavernosal tissue rather than via the peripheral blood stream will continue. This development will have advantages for all patients suffering from erectile dysfunction.

In summary, the greatest good to come from all the available therapeutic modalities for the patient suffering from sexual dysfunction might be a substantial improvement in level of disease and, therefore, a substantial improvement in the quality of life. If this goal can be reached with a minimal range of side-effects, effort must be directed to achieve this solution.

With the appearance of an effective oral therapy, pharmacological treatment of erectile dysfunction could be implemented in a sequential manner. Initially, oral therapy would be tried, followed by transurethral delivery of vasoactive compounds, and finally intracavernosal injection of agents.

Risks involved in treatment of impotence

The risks of treatment might vary, depending on the mode of administration of effective compounds, the mode of action, and the number and severity of side-effects.

Regarding hormonal treatment, consideration must always be given to the possible influence of such replacement therapy (with androgens) on the function and probable changes of the prostate. The risk of enhancing the development of prostate cancer during replacement therapy with androgens is not fully evaluated and, therefore, caution is indicated.

The major complications of intracavernous injection therapy are drug-induced prolonged erections, penile pain and fibrotic reactions. Although injection therapy has proved effective and safe for approximately 15 years, there are a significant number of patients who discontinue therapy for periods of time or stop it completely. These facts might represent real risks and disadvantages for this kind of therapy. The transurethral administration of alprostadil is a new therapy in the management of impotence. One has to consider that this mode of administration is far less effective than the intracavernous injection of vasoactive substances, and this fact might also be a disadvantage in the therapeutic approach. Regarding the oral administration of drugs for the treatment of erectile dysfunction, there are still variations in the mechanisms of action of these first-generation oral compounds. It seems likely that no single compound will manage all erectile dysfunction, and it seems that the demand for new oral compounds continues.

References

1. Kinsey AC, Pomeroy WB, Martin CE. *Sexual Behavior in the Human Male*. Philadelphia: WB Saunders, 1948:236–7
2. Feldman HA, Goldstein I, Hatzichristou DG. Impotence and its medical and psychosocial correlates: results of the Massachusetts male aging study. *J Urol* 1994;151:54
3. Diokno AC, Brown MB, Herzog AR. Sexual function in the elderly. *Arch Intern Med* 1990;150:197
4. Morley JE. Impotence. *Am J Med* 1986;80:897
5. Kaiser FE, Viosca SP, Mooradian AD. Impotence and aging: alterations in hormonal secretory patterns. *Endocr Soc* 1988;abstr 77A
6. Heaton JPW, Adams MA, Morales A. A therapeutic taxonomy for treatments for erectile dysfunction: an evolutionary imperative. *Int J Impotence Res* 1997;9:115
7. Hauri D. A new operative technique in vasculogenic erectile dysfunction. *World J Urol* 1986;4:237
8. Hatzichristou DG, Goldstein I. Arterial bypass surgery for impotence. *Curr Opin Urol* 1991;1:14
9. Zorgniotti AW, Lizza EF. Complications of penile revascularization. In Zorgniotti AW, Lizza EF, eds. *Diagnosis and Management of Impotence*. Philadelphia: BC Decker, 1991:126–30
10. Goldstein I, Lue TF, Padma-Nathan H, Rosen RC, Steers WD, Wicker PA. Oral sildenafil in the treatment of erectile dysfunction. Sildenafil study group. *N Engl J Med* 1998;338:1397
11. Porst H, Derouet H, Idzikowski M, *et al.* Oral phentolamine (Vasomax) in erectile dysfunction – results of a German multicenter-study in 177 patients. *Int J Impotence Res* 1996;8:117
12. Tenover JL. Androgen administration to aging men. *Endocrinol Metab Clin North Am* 1994;23:877

Section VII
Miscellaneous

38

Institutional role in women's health issues: role of FIGO

M. Seppälä and G. Benagiano

Introduction

The International Federation of Gynecologists and Obstetricians (FIGO) is an international organization by definition, as it represents more than 100 national societies of obstetricians and gynecologists. As such, it considers a close relationship with academic institutions and the private sector as paramount to achieve its objectives.

Traditionally, FIGO started as an international professional and scientific society of specialists in women's diseases, to provide a common forum to debate problems shared by those in the profession, as well as to gather the scientific knowledge that forms the basis of progress for those practicing obstetrics and gynecology. In recent years, however, FIGO has begun to transform itself to embrace a broader brief, and encompass the promotion of women's health in its mission. The Federation is now becoming an international advocacy forum to promote the health, as well as the status and the rights of women, to protect motherhood, to improve the ethical standards of the profession, to educate new generations of physicians to care for the health of women, and to protect the life of the new-born.

Through its national member societies, FIGO has close contacts with the specialty at the grass-roots level, allowing access to new developments that take place in prevention and treatment of diseases and disorders involving women's health. Aware of its practical limitations, the Federation, during the triennium 1994–97, addressed the broad problem of reforming its committees, redefining their mandates and identifying priority functions. As a result, the structure of committees and working groups was radically revised in 1997.

Advocacy of women's health issues

In collaboration with the World Health Organization (WHO), the United Nations Population Fund (UNFPA), the United Nations International Children's Emergency Fund (UNICEF), the World Bank and the International Planned Parenthood Federation (IPPF), a WHO/FIGO Alliance for Women's Health has been formed to exchange information on strategies aimed at implementing programs on women's health issues and at taking forward the recommendations on reproductive health made by the UN conferences on Population and Development (Cairo 1994) and on Women (Beijing 1995). Examples of the issues addressed by the Alliance are violence against women, female genital mutilation, equity of services, and women's education and empowerment to improve the health services women need. The Alliance also serves as an advisory body to FIGO's Save the Mothers Project and to the publication *World Report on Women's Health, 2000*. These and other FIGO activities are regularly reported to the member societies through the *FIGO Newsletter*, Internet Website (HTTP://www.figo.org) and the FIGO journal, *International Journal of Gynecology and Obstetrics*.

Committees

During the 3-year period of 1997–2000, FIGO will implement its specific activities through three committees working on special aspects of obstetrics and gynecology, namely oncology, perinatal health and ethics.

FIGO is well known through its staging of gynecological cancer, which needs to be kept abreast with advances in diagnosis and treatment. The staging of gynecological cancer is increasingly based on findings in surgery, yet in those cases in which surgery is not possible, staging needs to be accomplished through purely clinical means. In addition to this classic duty, the Committee of Gynecologic Oncology is also establishing educational and training activities, formulating good practice guidelines for gynecological oncology and establishing a working group to examine strategies to combat breast cancer. This committee has also the mandate to draft and supervise the publication of periodical reports on gynecological cancer, and to liaise with international cancer organizations and bodies with a view to discuss issues of mutual concern.

In view of the progress made by neonatologists in assuring the survival of very small babies, the Committee of Perinatal Health is advancing and encouraging uniform reporting of perinatal mortality in collaboration with WHO and other organizations, with the aim to disseminate this information to FIGO-affiliated societies. To decrease perinatal morbidity and mortality, the committee addresses factors that may increase fetal and neonatal morbidity and mortality, especially in developing countries, and recommends strategies for improvement. One such factor, typical of the industrialized world, is the rising number of multiple pregnancies brought about by assisted reproduction technologies, specifically addressed by the committee.

The FIGO Committee for Ethical Aspects of Reproduction and Women's Health has continued to review medical ethics relating to the specialty of obstetrics and gynecology and reproductive medicine, and is issuing guidelines on ethical problems in training, education, science and practice. The committee is a great advocate for the practice of the highest standards in ethical behavior in obstetrics and gynecology, and publishes periodically recommendations on ethical issues in obstetrics and gynecology. Periodically, the committee deliberations are published in the 'FIGO News' section of the *International Journal of Gynecology and Obstetrics*[1].

Save the Mothers Project

In 1997, FIGO launched the Save the Mothers Project, funded by UNFPA and Pharmacia and Upjohn. The project was created in the hope of mobilizing the obstetric community in developed and developing countries to work in partnership with other professionals to identify cost-effective ways to save mothers' lives in countries with particularly high mortality, by making emergency obstetric care more accessible. FIGO feels obligated to do its best to fight the tragedy of some 600 000 women who die every year of pregnancy-related complications, 99% of them in the developing countries[2]. Until recently, obstetricians have been singularly absent in safe motherhood initiatives, mostly because it was felt that women die because they have no access to an obstetrician, and therefore the problem is of logistical, not medical nature.

FIGO is trying to fight the widespread belief that obstetricians can play only a very limited role in the world battle against maternal mortality. FIGO believes that the obstetrician is in fact central in this battle: in some countries (namely Central and Latin America), obstetricians exist, but are often reluctant to be placed in remote areas; in other countries, their number is too small to cover the needs, but they can play an important role in training paramedics in the basic interventions needed for emergency obstetric care.

With this in mind, FIGO selected an initial group of five developing and five developed country societies and asked them to work in tandem. In these pilot intervention projects, FIGO member societies from the USA, Canada, the UK, Sweden and Italy will work in partnership with the obstetricians in Central America, Uganda, Pakistan, Ethiopia and Mozambique, respectively, to increase availability of emergency obstetric services in a given region, in a sustainable way. Results obtained from the various projects will be reported at the FIGO 2000 World Congress (see below).

Congresses and workshops

The FIGO World Congresses are organized every 3 years. The next FIGO World Congress of

Gynecology and Obstetrics will be held in Washington, DC, 3–8 September 2000. This will be the major congress of the specialty, attracting over 5000 professionals world-wide.

In collaboration with other international organizations, FIGO periodically organizes workshops and regional meetings. One important workshop will be organized before the World Congresses to take forward the recommendations on reproductive health made by the UN conferences in Cairo and Beijing.

Visiting professorships and fellowships

FIGO identifies and sponsors visiting professors to lecture around the world, and a fellowship program is organized in connection with every World Congress, allowing young obstetricians/gynecologists to visit hospitals in the host country.

FIGO publications

The *International Journal of Gynecology and Obstetrics* is a monthly peer-reviewed journal which publishes basic and clinical research in the fields of obstetrics and gynecology and related subjects with an emphasis on matters with world-wide interest.

The *FIGO Newsletter* provides information on current FIGO activities and appears three times a year in English, French and Spanish.

The *FIGO Report on Gynecologic Cancer* is published every 3 years to provide statistics of treatment of gynecological cancer world-wide.

The *FIGO Manual of Human Reproduction* is a survey of the major principles of physiological function, of the indications for and techniques of family planning and the demographic, economic and health consequences of population change.

World Report on Women's Health is a special issue published at the time of the FIGO World Congress. The first appeared in Montreal 1994[3] and the second in Copenhagen 1997[4]. The *World Report on Women's Health, 2000* is scheduled to appear at the time of FIGO 2000, Washington, DC.

References

1. Schenker JG. Report of the Committee for the Study of Ethical Aspects of Human Reproduction. *Int J Gynecol Obstet* 1997;59:165–8
2. World Health Organization and United Nations International Children's Emergency Fund. *Revised 1990 estimate of maternal mortality*. DOC WHO/FRM/MSM/96.11. Geneva: WHO, 1996
3. Fathalla M, ed. World Report on Women's Health. *Int J Gynecol Obstet* 1994;46:101–258
4. Seppälä M, ed. Second World Report on Women's Health. *Int J Gynecol Obstet* 1997;58:1–188

Regulation of proliferation and apoptosis of uterine myometria and leiomyomas by sex steroid hormones

39

T. Maruo, H. Matsuo, T. Samoto, Y. Shimomura, O. Kurachi, S. Mochizuki, Y. Wang and Z. Gao

Introduction

Homeostatic control of the net growth of tumors is the result of the dynamic balance between cell proliferation and cell death, and too much growth can come from too little death as well as from too much proliferation[1]. Only several years ago, many researchers trying to understand what causes the growth of tumors focused their attention on the pathways within cells that tell them when to divide. However, recent work is showing that cells also have internal pathways that tell them when to die[2]. It is possible that in tumors the death pathway may be suppressed, extending the lives of the cells[3,4].

Uterine leiomyoma is the most common smooth muscle cell tumor of the myometrium[5], and is thought to be clonal, arising from a single initiated smooth muscle cell[6]. Although the nature of the initial event is unknown, a role for ovarian steroid hormones in the growth of uterine leiomyomas is likely, because these tumors grow during the reproductive years, increase in size during pregnancy, and regress after menopause[7,8]. Furthermore, treatment with gonadotropin-releasing hormone (GnRH) analogs, which reduces ovarian steroid hormone concentrations, leads to a reduction in the size of leiomyomas; however, re-enlargement of leiomyomas occurs after therapy with GnRH analogs is discontinued[9]. These findings suggest that leiomyoma growth is dependent on ovarian steroids. On the other hand, a growing body of evidence suggests that the action of estrogen may be mediated in part by local growth factors, such as epidermal growth factor (EGF) and insulin-like growth factor-1 (IGF-1), produced by the target cells[10-12]. The mechanisms of action of ovarian steroid hormones in the regulation of leiomyoma growth and apoptosis, however, are not well defined.

We conducted the present study first to determine the proliferative activity of leiomyoma cells compared with that of adjacent normal myometrial cells throughout the menstrual cycle by immunohistochemical analysis with a monoclonal antibody to proliferating cell nuclear antigen (PCNA)[13,14]. Furthermore, to understand the role of ovarian steroids in regulating proliferative activity of leiomyoma cells, we examined whether ovarian steroid hormones could influence PCNA expression in leiomyoma cells cultured under serum-free, phenol red-free conditions. As EGF has been demonstrated to play a crucial role as a local factor in regulating leiomyoma growth[15-18], possible effects of ovarian steroid hormones on the expression of EGF and EGF receptor in the cultured leiomyoma cells were also investigated.

Recent research efforts have focused on the function of proto-oncogene and tumor suppressor gene products in directing cell fate. In particular, an explosion of research interest has centered around the role of Bcl-2 in controlling the survival and death of cells. It is now evident that the *bcl*-2 proto-oncogene encodes a 26-kDa protein, localized to mitochondrial and perinuclear membranes[19]. The product of the *bcl*-2 gene, when elevated in cells either *in vivo* or *in vitro*, prevents the normal course of apoptotic cell death in a variety of cells induced by tropic factor deprivation or other stimuli without altering proliferation[20,21]. It seems, therefore, that Bcl-2 protein may play an important role in the growth of tumors. However, to date, no information is available on the expression of Bcl-2 protein in uterine myometria and leiomyomas. We therefore also conducted the study to determine the expression of Bcl-2 protein in leiomyomas in comparison with that in the normal myometrium. Furthermore, to understand the role of ovarian steroid hormones in regulating the expression of Bcl-2 protein in uterine leiomyomas, we examined whether ovarian steroids could influence the levels of Bcl-2 protein expression in leiomyoma cells cultured *in vitro*.

Proliferative potential of uterine myometria and leiomyomas throughout the menstrual cycle

Immunohistochemical examinations of leiomyoma tissues and the adjacent normal myometrial tissues in the proliferative phase of the menstrual cycle demonstrated that PCNA label was positive only in a few normal myometrial cells (Figure 1a), whereas it was present in a somewhat greater number of leiomyoma cells (Figure 1b). Immunohistochemical staining for PCNA in those tissues in the secretory phase showed that only a few normal myometrial cell nuclei were positive for PCNA label (Figure 1c), whereas a large number of the leiomyoma cell nuclei were positive for PCNA label (Figure 1d).

Determination of the mean percentage of PCNA-positive nuclei in leiomyoma and the adjacent normal myometrial tissue sections revealed that the PCNA-positive rate was higher in leiomyoma cells than in normal myometrial cells throughout the menstrual cycle ($p < 0.01$) and that the PCNA-positive rate of leiomyoma cells was higher in the secretory, progesterone-dominated, phase than in the proliferative phase ($p < 0.01$). There were, however, no differences in the PCNA-positive rate in normal

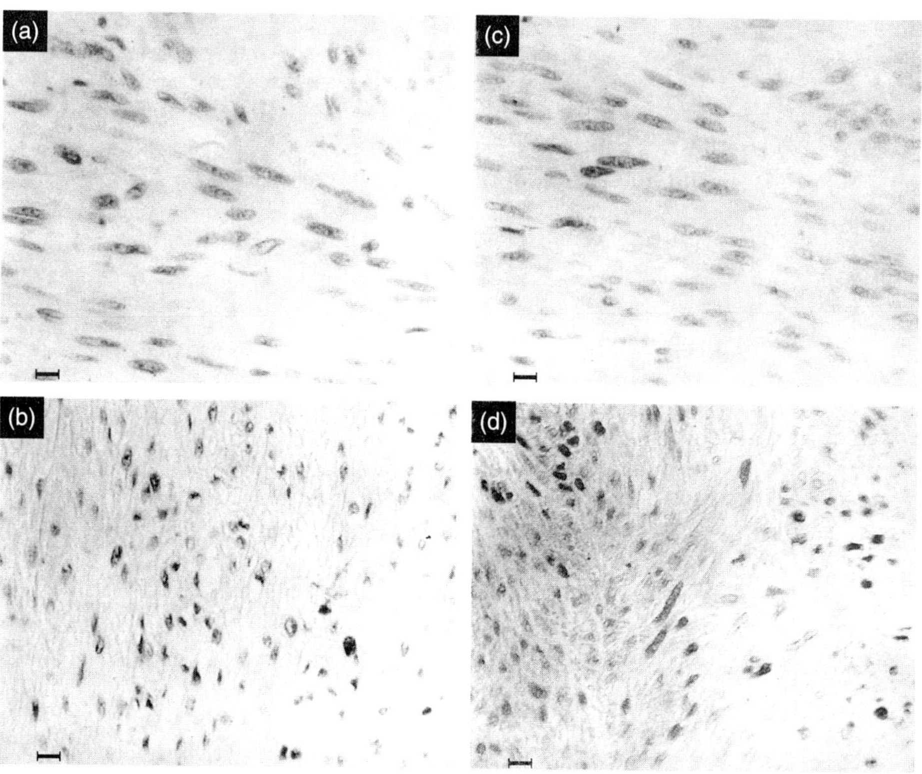

Figure 1 Immunohistochemical staining of proliferating cell nuclear antigen (PCNA) in sections of normal myometrium (a) and leiomyoma (b) in the proliferative phase, and normal myometrium (c) and leiomyoma (d) in the secretory phase of the menstrual cycle. The bars are 5 μm in length. Original magnification × 400

myometrial cells between the proliferative phase and the secretory phase (Figure 2).

The higher PCNA labeling index in leiomyoma tissues relative to the adjacent normal myometrial tissues throughout the menstrual cycle may permit the enhanced growth of leiomyomas over the adjacent normal myometria in the same uterus. With respect to the participation of progesterone in the proliferation of leiomyoma cells, Kawaguchi and colleagues[22,23] reported that the mitotic count in uterine leiomyomas is higher in the secretory phase of the menstrual cycle than in the proliferative phase and suggested that the growth of leiomyoma cells might be dependent not only on the presence of estrogen, but also on the presence of progesterone.

Regulation of proliferative potential

Because leiomyoma growth is closely associated with the reproductive years, and since the vital role of estrogen in uterine growth has been established[24], estrogen has received much attention as the major factor responsible for leiomyoma development. The mechanism underlying the stimulatory effects of ovarian steroids on leiomyoma growth, however, has not been defined. To investigate the mitogenic effects of sex steroids on uterine myometria and leiomyomas, an *in vitro* culture system of normal myometria and leiomyoma cells was established. Collagenase treatment of normal myometria and leiomyoma tissues provided a pure population of isolated cells with smooth muscle cell characteristics without either stromal or glandular epithelial cell contamination. Immunohistochemical examination of cultured cells revealed that these cells were immunostained with a monoclonal antibody directed toward the muscle-specific protein desmin, but not immunostained with antibodies to either cytokeratin 19, a cytoskeletal protein specific for epithelial cells, or vimentin, a class of intermediate filament protein present in fibroblasts.

Western immunoblot analysis showed that both cultured normal myometrial cells and leiomyoma cells contained immunoreactive PCNA with a molecular mass of approximately 36 kDa,

and the 36-kDa PCNA expression in leiomyoma cells was more abundant than that in normal myometrial cells in untreated control cultures (Figure 3). In cultures of normal myometrial cells, the addition of 17β-estradiol (10 ng/ml) remarkably increased 36-kDa PCNA expression

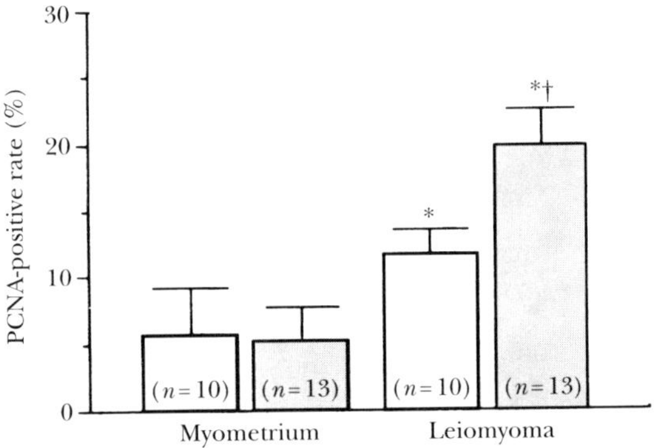

Figure 2 The mean percentage of proliferating cell nuclear antigen (PCNA)-positive nuclei in leiomyomas and the adjacent normal myometria as assessed by immunohistochemical analysis. Blank columns, proliferative phase; shaded columns, secretory phase; $*p < 0.01$ compared with myometrium; $†p < 0.01$ compared with proliferative phase

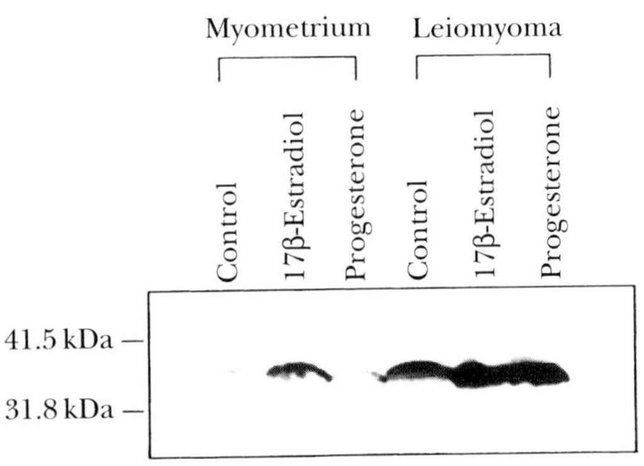

Figure 3 Effects of estradiol and progesterone on proliferating cell nuclear antigen (PCNA) protein expression in cultured normal myometrial cells and leiomyoma cells as assessed by Western immunoblot analysis. The 36-kDa PCNA protein was overexpressed in leiomyoma cells compared to normal myometrial cells. In normal myometrial cells, estradiol increased the 36-kDa PCNA protein expression, but progesterone did not. In leiomyoma cells, not only estradiol but also progesterone increased the PCNA protein expression in the cells

in the cells compared to that in control cultures, whereas such a remarkable increase in PCNA expression was not noted with the addition of progesterone (100 ng/ml). By contrast, in cultures of leiomyoma cells, treatment with either estradiol (10 ng/ml) or progesterone (100 ng/ml) increased the 36-kDa PCNA expression in the cells relative to that in control cultures (Figure 3).

Furthermore, Western immunoblot analysis with a monoclonal antibody to EGF revealed that the cultured leiomyoma cells contained immunoreactive EGF with a molecular mass of approximately 133 kDa and that the addition of progesterone (100 ng/ml) to the serum-free medium resulted in a remarkable increase in the level of expression of 133-kDa immunoreactive EGF together with the appearance of immunoreactive EGF with a molecular mass of approximately 71 kDa in the cells compared to that in control cultures (Figure 4). By contrast, the addition of estradiol (10 ng/ml) resulted in a somewhat lower expression of 133-kDa immunoreactive EGF in the cells relative to that in control cultures.

EGF receptor expression in the cultured leiomyoma cells assessed by immunocytochemical analysis with a monoclonal antibody to EGF receptor was remarkably augmented by the addition of estradiol (10 ng/ml) relative to that in control cultures, whereas the addition of progesterone (100 ng/ml) did not affect EGF expression in those cells (Figure 5).

The present study demonstrates the individual effect of ovarian steroids on the proliferative activity of leiomyoma cells cultured *in vitro* on the basis of PCNA expression. PCNA is a cell cycle-related non-histone nuclear protein with a molecular mass of 36 kDa. Elevated levels of PCNA appear in late G1 phase and become maximal during the S phase of proliferating cells, but are not detectable in resting cells[13]. Immunohistochemical PCNA labeling has been proven useful in evaluating the proportions of proliferating cells in normal and neoplastic cell populations[14]. In addition to an essential role of PCNA in DNA replication, recent studies suggested an involvement of PCNA in DNA excision repair[25]. However, because of the lack of

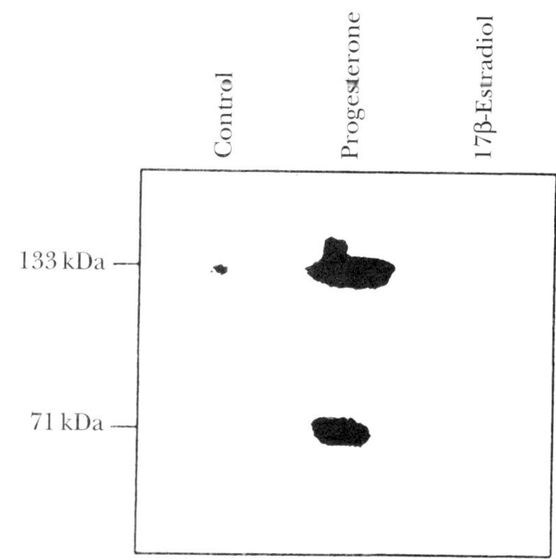

Figure 4 Effects of estradiol and progesterone on epidermal growth factor (EGF)-like protein expression in cultured leiomyoma cells as assessed by Western immunoblot analysis. The addition of progesterone (100 ng/ml) resulted in a remarkable increase in 133-kDa immunoreactive EGF expression together with the appearance of 71-kDa immunoreactive EGF, whereas the addition of estradiol (10 ng/ml) resulted in a somewhat lower expression of 133-kDa immunoreactive EGF relative to control cultures

genetic evidence, it is not clear which of the DNA repair processes is affected by PCNA.

The data in the present study demonstrate that in leiomyoma cells both estradiol and progesterone up-regulate the cell proliferating activity, whereas in normal myometrial smooth muscle cells, only estradiol up-regulates the cell proliferating activity[26]. As Eiletz and associates[27] reported that progesterone levels in human normal myometria and leiomyoma tissues were as high as 10–70 ng/g protein, whereas estradiol levels in human normal myometria and leiomyoma tissues ranged from 4–10 ng/g protein, the concentrations of sex steroids (estradiol 10 ng/ml; progesterone 100 ng/ml) that were found to be effective in the present study appear to be within the physiological tissue concentration range. The fact that cultured leiomyoma cells had an increased response to progesterone compared to cultured normal myometrial cells is consistent with the reports of Brandon and colleagues[28] showing

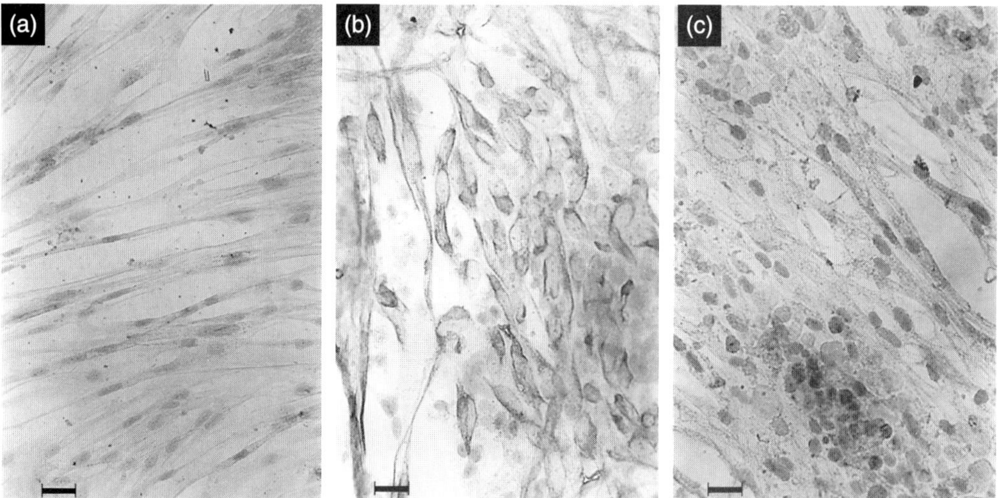

Figure 5 Effects of estradiol and progesterone on epidermal growth factor (EGF) receptor expression in cultured leiomyoma cells as assessed by immunohistochemical analysis. Compared to untreated leiomyoma cells (a), immunostaining for EGF receptor was remarkably augmented by treatment with estradiol (b), but not by the treatment with progesterone (c). The bars are 5 μm in length. Original magnification × 400

that progesterone receptor mRNA is over-expressed in uterine leiomyoma compared to that in the adjacent normal myometrium. In the present study, we also provide evidence that progesterone is capable of increasing the expression of immunoreactive EGF proteins with a higher molecular mass relative to authentic EGF in leiomyoma cells, but that estradiol is not. Up-regulation by progesterone of the proliferating activity of leiomyoma cells and the expression of immunoreactive EGF proteins in leiomyoma cells is of great interest, as it is thought that EGF may be involved in the autocrine/paracrine regulation of leiomyoma growth. Nelson and associates[16] demonstrated in murine uterine tissues that the effect of estradiol may be mediated by EGF and that EGF is capable of replacing estradiol in the stimulation of female genital tract growth.

EGF is a 6-kDa polypeptide that is known to be generated by proteolytic processing of a larger molecular precursor, 133-kDa prepro-EGF[29,30]. EGF is shown to be present as prepro-EGF in the kidney and other tissues[31]. Taking these findings into account, the immunoreactive EGF proteins with higher molecular masses of 133 kDa and 71 kDa induced by progesterone treatment in cultured leiomyoma cells are postulated to be a prepro-EGF-like protein and an active species generated from the prepro-EGF protein, respectively. The presence of immunoreactive EGF protein and mRNA-encoding EGF in human myometrial cells and leiomyoma cells has previously been reported by Rossi and colleagues[18] using immunohistochemical techniques and by Yeh and associates[17] using the polymerase chain reaction (PCR). A potential role for EGF in the regulation of leiomyoma growth is also suggested on the basis of the observations of Lumsden and colleagues[32], who demonstrated that the shrinkage of uterine leiomyoma in conjunction with a reduction in estradiol levels in serum with GnRH agonist therapy was associated with a remarkable reduction in uterine EGF binding sites. In this connection, we have noticed in the present study that estradiol is capable of increasing the expression of EGF receptor in leiomyoma cells, but that progesterone is not. It is now likely that progesterone up-regulates the production of EGF-like proteins in leiomyoma cells, whereas estradiol up-regulates the expression of EGF receptor in leiomyoma cells. Progesterone and estradiol thus seem to participate in leiomyoma growth through the induction of EGF-like proteins and EGF receptor expression in leiomyoma cells, respectively. In support of this observation, we demonstrated that not only estradiol but also progesterone augmented the PCNA protein expression in cultured leiomyoma cells. The fact that progesterone up-regulates PCNA protein expression in cultured leiomyoma cells is in good agreement with the *in vivo* finding of a higher PCNA labeling index in leiomyoma tissues in the secretory, progesterone-dominated phase compared to that in the proliferative phase.

Bcl-2 protein expression in uterine myometria and leiomyomas throughout the menstrual cycle

Apoptosis was first described as a morphologic pattern of cell death characterized by cell shrinkage, membrane blebbing, and chromatin condensation culminating in cell fragmentation[33]. Despite the identification of genes necessary for apoptotic cell death, the essential biochemical events in apoptotic cell death remain largely unknown. Korsmeyer[20] reported that the *bcl-2* proto-oncogene was unique among cellular genes in its ability to block apoptotic cell death in multiple contexts. Overexpression of *bcl-2* in transgenic models leads to accumulation of cells due to evasion of normal cell death mechanisms[34]. Accordingly, *bcl-2* is thought to be a cell survival gene.

Immunohistochemical examinations of leiomyomas and normal myometrial tissues from the same individual uterus in the proliferative

phase of the menstrual cycle demonstrated that Bcl-2 protein was abundantly present in the cytoplasm of leiomyoma cells, but was scarcely present in normal myometrial smooth muscle cells. Comparison between immunostaining for Bcl-2 protein in leiomyoma tissues obtained in the proliferative phase (Figure 6a) and in the secretory phase (Figure 6b) showed that Bcl-2 protein expression in the leiomyoma cells in the secretory phase was much more abundant than that in the proliferative phase of the menstrual cycle. By contrast, there was no apparent difference in the intensity of immunostaining for Bcl-2 protein in normal myometrial smooth muscle cells between the proliferative phase and the secretory phase of the menstrual cycle.

Western blot analyses of protein extracts from leiomyoma and myometrial tissues revealed that 26-kDa Bcl-2 protein was abundantly present in leiomyoma tissue extracts, whereas in myometrial tissue extracts, Bcl-2 protein was undetectable (Figure 7).

Our present observation that Bcl-2 protein expression is predominant in leiomyoma cells compared to that in normal myometrial cells suggests the possibility that the greater abundance of Bcl-2 protein in leiomyoma cells may be responsible at least in part for the growth of leiomyoma by preventing apoptotic cell death[35]. In contrast, the scanty expression of Bcl-2 protein in normal myometrial cells raises the possibility that normal myometrial cells may be more susceptible to apoptotic cell death than leiomyoma cells. The increased expression of Bcl-2 protein in leiomyoma cells is likely to be

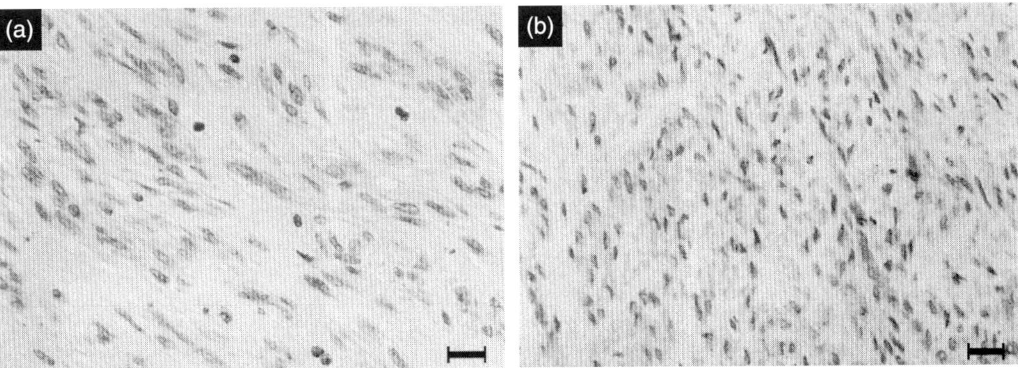

Figure 6 Immunohistochemical staining for Bcl-2 protein in leiomyoma tissues in the proliferative phase (a) and the secretory phase (b). The bars are 5 μm in length. Original magnification × 400

characteristic of leiomyomas and permits the growth of leiomyomas in the uterus. The enhanced growth of leiomyomas over normal myometria *in vivo* may, therefore, be attributed to the increased expression of Bcl-2 protein in leiomyoma cells relative to that in normal myometrial cells.

Sex steroidal regulation of Bcl-2 protein expression in leiomyoma cells

Effects of sex steroids on Bcl-2 protein expression in leiomyoma cells cultured *in vitro* have also been investigated. Western immunoblotting of proteins extracted from leiomyoma cells cultured for 72 h under serum-free conditions in the absence or presence of estradiol or progesterone showed that the cultured leiomyoma cells contained immunoreactive Bcl-2 protein with a molecular mass of approximately 26 kDa. The addition of progesterone (100 ng/ml) to the serum-free medium remarkably increased the expression of 26-kDa Bcl-2 protein in the cultured leiomyoma cells compared to that in control cultures (Figure 8). In contrast, the addition of estradiol (10 ng/ml) to the serum-free medium resulted in a somewhat lower expression of 26-kDa Bcl-2 protein in the cultured leiomyoma cells relative to that in control cultures (Figure 8). Unlike the cultured leiomyoma cells, neither treatment with progesterone nor treatment with estradiol affected the expression of Bcl-2 protein in cultured normal myometrial cells.

The fact that Bcl-2 protein expression in cultured leiomyoma cells was remarkably augmented by progesterone is consistent with our immunohistochemical observation of higher expression of Bcl-2 protein in leiomyomas in the secretory, progesterone-dominated phase compared to that in the proliferative phase. The molecular basis for progesterone action in the regulation of leiomyoma growth is not clear, but probably involves the progesterone-stimulated induction of Bcl-2 protein in leiomyoma cells. Since the Bcl-2 product has been shown to prolong cell survival by preventing apoptotic cell death, progesterone may act as a growth-promoting factor in regulating leiomyoma

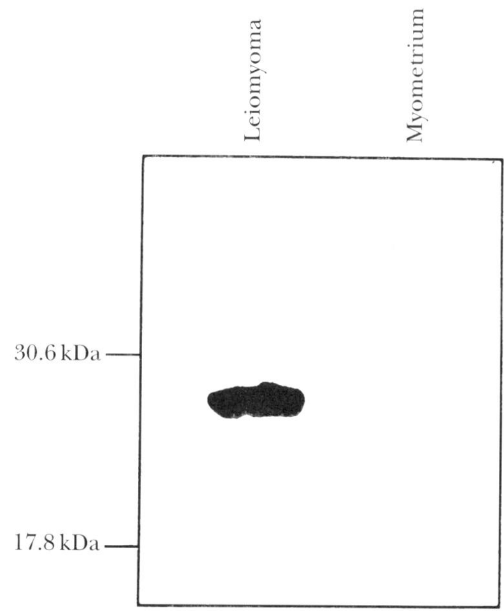

Figure 7 Western blot analysis of leiomyoma and myometrium tissue extracts with a monoclonal antibody to Bcl-2 protein. The 26-kDa Bcl-2 protein was abundantly present in leiomyoma tissue extracts, whereas in myometrial tissue extracts Bcl-2 protein was undetectable

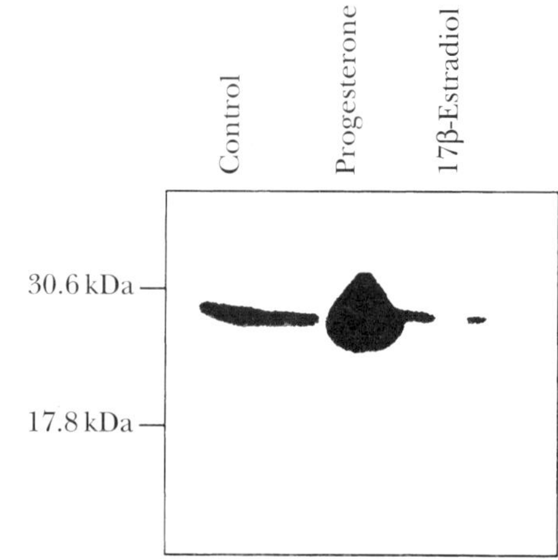

Figure 8 Effects of sex steroids on the expression of Bcl-2 protein in cultured leiomyoma cells as assessed by Western blot analysis. The addition of progesterone (100 ng/ml) remarkably increased the 26-kDa Bcl-2 protein expression in the cultured leiomyoma cells compared to that in control cultures, whereas the addition of estradiol (10 ng/ml) resulted in somewhat lower expression of the 26-kDa Bcl-2 protein

growth through the enhanced inhibition of apoptosis of leiomyoma cells. On the other hand, estradiol inhibited the induction of Bcl-2 protein in leiomyoma cells.

An inverse relationship between Bcl-2 expression and sex steroid hormones has been described in the endometrium. Up-regulation of Bcl-2 expression by estradiol and down-regulation by progesterone have been shown in the normal endometrium[36]. It must therefore be emphasized that the effects of sex steroid hormones on Bcl-2 protein expression vary among the different cell types even in the uterus. Indeed, in cultured normal myometrial cells, neither treatment with progesterone nor estradiol affected Bcl-2 protein expression. Furthermore, there was no apparent difference in the immunohistochemically-detected cellular levels of Bcl-2 protein in normal myometrial cells between the proliferative phase and the secretory phase of the menstrual cycle. This suggests that no cyclic changes in Bcl-2 protein expression exist in the normal myometrium throughout the menstrual cycle.

leiomyoma growth, it is conceivable that progesterone and estradiol act in combination to stimulate the proliferative potential of leiomyoma cells through the induction of EGF-like proteins and EGF receptor expression in human uterine leiomyoma. We have also demonstrated greater abundance of Bcl-2 protein in leiomyomas relative to the normal myometrium of the same individual uterus and that Bcl-2 protein expression in leiomyoma cells predominates in the secretory, progesterone-dominated phase of the menstrual cycle compared to that in the proliferative phase. Consistent with these findings, Bcl-2 protein expression in leiomyoma cells cultured *in vitro* under serum-free, phenol red-free conditions was up-regulated by progesterone, but down-regulated by estradiol (Figure 9). It therefore seems likely that progesterone may also participate in leiomyoma growth through the induction of Bcl-2 protein in leiomyoma cells. The abundant expression of Bcl-2 protein in leiomyoma may be one of the molecular bases for the enhanced growth of leiomyoma relative to that of normal myometrium in the uterus.

Conclusion

The growth of uterine myometria and leiomyomas has been known to be dependent on the presence of ovarian steroid hormones. The molecular mechanism underlying the sex steroidal regulation of myometria and leiomyoma growth, however, has not been defined. We have shown that progesterone up-regulates the PCNA protein expression in cultured leiomyoma cells. Consistently, the PCNA labeling index in leiomyoma tissues predominated in the secretory, progesterone-dominated phase of the menstrual cycle compared to that in the proliferative phase. Furthermore, we demonstrated that EGF-like protein expression in the cultured leiomyoma cells was up-regulated by progesterone, whereas EGF receptor expression in those cells was up-regulated by estradiol. As EGF is known to play a crucial role as a local factor in the autocrine/paracrine regulation of

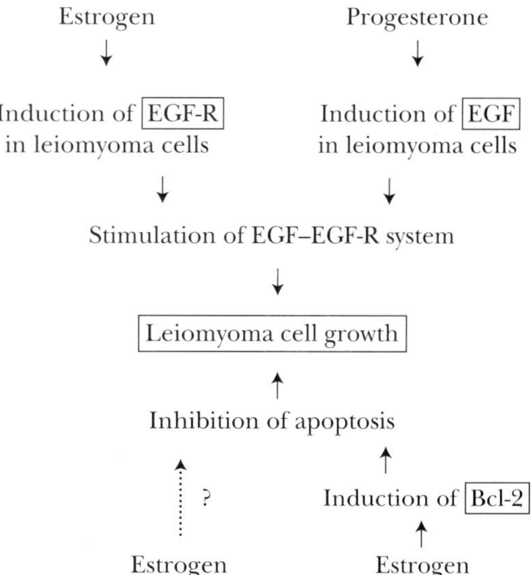

Figure 9 Schematic illustration of sex steroidal regulation of leiomyoma growth and apoptosis. EGF, epidermal growth factor; EGF-R, epidermal growth factor receptor

References

1. Wyllie AH, Kerr JFR, Currie AR. Cell death: the significance of apoptosis. *Int Rev Cytol* 1980;68:251–306

2. Marx J. Cell death studies yield cancer clues. *Science* 1993;259:760–2

3. Distelhorst CW. Glucocorticosteroids induce DNA fragmentation in human lymphoid leukemia cells. *Blood* 1988;72:1305–9

4. Sarraf CE, Bowen ID. Kinetic studies on a murine sarcoma: an analysis of apoptosis. *Br J Cancer* 1986;54; 989–98

5. Vollenhoven BJ, Lawrence AS, Healy DL. Uterine fibroids. *Br J Obstet Gynaecol* 1990;97:285–98

6. Buttram Jr VC, Reiter RC. Uterine leiomyoma: etiology, symptomatology and management. *Fertil Steril* 1981;36:433–47

7. Rein MS, Nowak RA. Biology of uterine myomas and myometrium *in vitro*. In Barbieri RL, ed. *Seminars in Reproductive Endocrinology*. New York: Thieme, 1992:310–19

8. Muran D, Gilleson M, Walters JH. Myomas of the uterus in pregnancy: ultrasonographic follow-up. *Am J Obstet Gynecol* 1980;138:16–19

9. West CP, Lumsden MA, Lawson S, *et al.* Shrinkage of uterine fibroids during therapy with goserelin (Zoladex): a luteinizing hormone-releasing hormone agonist administered as a monthly subcutaneous depot. *Fertil Steril* 1987;48:45–51

10. Huet-Hudson YM, Chakraborty C, Suzaki Y, *et al.* Estrogen regulates synthesis of epidermal growth factor in mouse uterine epithelial cells. *Mol Endocrinol* 1990;4:510–23

11. Murphy LJ, Ghahary A. Uterine insulin-like growth factor-1: regulation of expression and its role in estrogen-induced uterine proliferation. *Endocr Rev* 1990;11:443–53

12. Nelson KG, Takahashi T, Lee DC, *et al.* Transforming growth factor-α is a potential mediator of estrogen action in the mouse uterus. *Endocrinology* 1992;131:1657–64

13. Kurki P, Vanderlaan M, Dolbeare F, *et al.* Expression of proliferating cell nuclear antigen (PCNA)/cyclin during the cell cycle. *Exp Cell Res* 1986;166:209–19

14. Robbins BA, Vega DDL, Ogata K, *et al.* Immunohistochemical detection of proliferating cell nuclear antigen in solid human malignancies. *Arch Pathol Lab Med* 1987;111:841–5

15. Hofmann GE, Rao CV, Barrows GH, *et al.* Binding sites for epidermal growth factor in human uterine tissues and leiomyoma. *J Clin Endocrinol Metab* 1984;58:880–4

16. Nelson KG, Takahashi T, Bossert NL, *et al.* Epidermal growth factor replaces estrogen in the stimulation of female genital tract growth and differentiation. *Proc Natl Acad Sci USA* 1991;88:21–5

17. Yeh J, Rein M, Nowak R. Presence of messenger ribonucleic acid for epidermal growth factor (EGF) and EGF receptor demonstrable in monolayer cell cultures of myometria and leiomyoma. *Fertil Steril* 1991;56:997–1000

18. Rossi MJ, Chegini N, Masterson BJ. Presence of epidermal growth factor, platelet-derived growth factor, and their receptors in human myometrial tissue and smooth muscle cells: their action in smooth muscle cells *in vitro*. *Endocrinology* 1992;130:1716–27

19. Tsujimoto Y, Croce CM. Structure, transcripts, and protein products of Bcl-2, the gene involved in human follicular lymphoma. *Proc Natl Acad Sci USA* 1986;83:5214–18

20. Korsmeyer SJ. Bcl-2 initiates a new category of oncogenes: regulators of cell death. *Blood* 1992;80:879–86

21. Reed JC. Bcl-2 and the regulation of programmed cell death. *J Cell Biol* 1994;124:1–6

22. Kawaguchi K, Fujii S, Konishi I, *et al.* Mitotic activity in uterine leiomyomas during the menstrual cycle. *Am J Obstet Gynecol* 1989;160:637–41

23. Kawaguchi K, Fujii S, Konishi I, *et al.* Ultrastructural study of cultured smooth muscle cells from uterine leiomyoma and myometrium under the influence of sex steroids. *Gynecol Oncol* 1985;21:32–41

24. Murphy LJ, Ghahary A. Uterine insulin-like growth factor-1: regulation of expression and its role in estrogen-induced uterine proliferation. *Endocr Rev* 1990;11:443–53

25. Nichols AF, Sancar A. Purification of PCNA as a nucleotide excision repair protein. *Nucleic Acids Res* 1992;20:2441–6

26. Shimomura Y, Matsuo H, Samoto T, *et al.* Upregulation by progesterone of proliferating cell nuclear antigen and epidermal growth factor expression in human uterine leiomyoma. *J Clin Endocrinol Metab* 1998;89:2192–8

27. Eiletz J, Genz T, Pollow K. Sex steroid levels in serum, myometrium, and fibromyomata in correlation with cytoplasmic receptors and 17β-hydroxysteroid dehydrogenase activity in different age groups and phases of the menstrual cycle. *Arch Gynecol* 1980;229:13–20

28. Brandon DD, Bethea CL, Strawn EY, *et al.* Progesterone receptor messenger ribonucleic acid and protein are overexpressed in human uterine leiomyomas. *Am J Obstet Gynecol* 1993;169:78–85

29. Gray A, Dull J, Ullrich A. Nucleotide sequence of epidermal growth factor cDNA predicts a

128 000-molecular weight protein precursor. *Nature (London)* 1983;303:722–5

30. Scott J, Urdea M, Quiroga M, *et al.* Structure of a mouse submaxillary messenger RNA encoding epidermal growth factor and seven related proteins. *Science* 1983;221:236–40

31. Salido EC, Lakshmanan J, Shapiro LJ, *et al.* Expression of epidermal growth factor in the kidney and submandibular gland during mouse postnatal development. An immunocytochemical and *in situ* hybridization study. *Differentiation* 1990;45:38–43

32. Lumsden MA, West CP, Bramley T, *et al.* The binding of epidermal growth factor to the human uterus and leiomyomata in women rendered hypo-oestrogenic by continuous administration of an LHRH agonist. *Br J Obstet Gynaecol* 1988;95:1299–304

33. Kerr JER, Wylie AH, Currie AR. Apoptosis: a basic biological phenomenon with wide-ranging implications in tissue kinetics. *Br J Cancer* 1972; 26:239–57

34. Mcdonnell TJ, Deane N, Platt FM, *et al.* Bcl-2 immunoglobulin transgenic mice demonstrate extended B cell survival and follicular lymphoproliferation. *Cell* 1989;57:79–88

35. Matsuo M, Maruo T, Samoto T. Increased expression of Bcl-2 protein in human uterine leiomyoma and its up-regulation by progesterone. *J Clin Endocrinol Metab* 1997;82:293–9

36. Gowpel A, Sabourin JC, Martin A, *et al.* Bcl-2 expression in normal endometrium during the menstrual cycle. *Am J Pathol* 1994;144:1195–202

40

Unravelling the genetics of complex disorders of reproduction

J. F. Strauss, III

Substantial progress has been made in the identification of the molecular defects causing monogenic diseases that affect reproduction[1]. By and large, these disorders are relatively rare autosomal recessive or sex-chromosome-linked diseases that include mutations that inactivate gonadotropin β-subunit genes, the gonadotropin releasing hormone (GnRH) receptor, mutations that inactivate or activate gonadotropin receptors, mutations that inactivate steroidogenic enzymes and steroid hormone receptors[1]. In most cases, the mutant genes in question were identified by the clinical phenotype of the subjects, which pointed an incriminating finger at a specific candidate gene that was subsequently analyzed and shown to harbor a deleterious nucleic acid alteration. The challenge of the next decade is to elucidate the molecular genetics underlying the more common but complex disorders of reproduction, including polycystic ovary syndrome (PCOS), endometriosis, premature ovarian failure, pre-eclampsia and preterm birth. In each of these cases there exists evidence for familial clustering of these disorders, which makes it likely that there is a genetic component to the condition, although the modes of inheritance and penetrance are uncertain[2-7]. In contrast to the rare monogenic disorders mentioned above, the more common disorders are likely to be caused by several genetic variants, acting in concert or responding to environmental factors. Because the common disorders affect more than 2% of the population, the genetic differences that may be responsible for these disorders are not strictly speaking mutations, but rather polymorphisms; the distinction being that mutations are rare events and polymorphisms common variations in gene structure

that are present in 2% or more of the population. These polymorphisms form the basis of human diversity. Indeed, the human genome is estimated to contain some 200 000 single nucleotide polymorphisms within the coding regions of the estimated 80 000 genes. Repetitive DNA elements, di- or trinucleotide repeats, are also scattered throughout the human genome. These single base pair polymorphisms and the variable numbers of repetitive DNA elements may alter the level of expression of specific genes or the activities of the proteins that they encode, leading to phenotypic differences among individuals. With increasing knowledge of these polymorphisms, there is considerable interest in association studies that compare the prevalence of polymorphisms in candidate genes among affected and unaffected individuals. Association studies can be particularly useful in examining, in a preliminary fashion, genotype–environment interactions. The premise of such case–control studies is that, if an association is found, it is likely to be due to linkage disequilibrium, which is found only over small genetic map distances, implying close linkage between the marker examined and disease susceptibility. However, a significant association between a polymorphism and a phenotype in a case–control study should not be taken as proof of genetic linkage, since it is well known that heterogeneity in study populations can confound association studies and even suggest substantial association for unlinked loci. It is, however, a starting point for further exploration of the role of a candidate gene in a disease process.

Gene–environment interactions that result in disease can encompass exposure to environmental toxicants, infectious agents or changes in body physiology. These types of interactions have been suggested by the results of a number of association studies. For example, an association has been reported for the carriage of the null allele of the glutathione-*S*-transferase M1 (GSTM1) gene and endometriosis[5]. The GSTM1 gene encodes an enzyme involved in the phase 2 catabolism of xenobiotics. The homozygous state for the null allele in which individuals lack the GSTM1 enzyme could account for delayed clearance of xenobiotics that could influence endometrial tissue growth and invasion, predisposing individuals with this genotype to endometriosis upon exposure to these agents. A polymorphism in the promoter of the tumor necrosis factor-α gene, which confers increased transcriptional activity, has been associated with premature preterm rupture of the fetal membranes[6]. Carriers of this hyper-responsive allele may have a reproductive tract more responsive to low-grade infection (e.g. asymptomatic bacterial vaginosis), leading to increased production of tumor necrosis factor (TNF)-α, which in turn could activate matrix degrading enzymes, leading to premature fetal membrane rupture. Polymorphisms in the angiotensinogen gene[7], the angiotensin II type 1 receptor gene[8], a variant in the methylene-tetrahydrofolate reductase gene[9], leading to modest increases in plasma homocysteine concentrations, and the factor V Leiden mutation[10] have each been associated with pre-eclampsia or the severity of pre-eclampsia. Variants in these candidate genes could influence blood pressure, endothelial cell function and coagulation, respectively, in response to physiological changes associated with pregnancy, resulting in a predisposition to pre-eclampsia.

The identification of genetic loci that are truly linked to disorders that are likely to be caused by several genes is a more substantial challenge. This is especially true when there are no suitable animal models available (e.g. the mouse) to facilitate the search for the syntenic human loci. Unfortunately, this is the case for the more common disorders of human reproduction noted above. Family studies, such as the affected sib-pair analysis, which test for an excess of shared alleles among sibs in families in which more than one sib is affected, represent a

viable strategy for identification of disease susceptibility loci when little is known about the genetics of a disorder[11,12]. Genotyping families with affected sib pairs for 300–600 polymorphic markers with a high degree of heterozygosity separated by 10–20 cM can link disease susceptibility with specific genomic loci. These studies may require in the order of 300 affected sib pairs to achieve linkage. This represents no small task, since the phenotyping of family members must be rigorous and, in diseases such as endometriosis, requires extensive study with sophisticated methods (e.g. magnetic resonance imaging) or invasive techniques (e.g. laparoscopic surgery). This analysis is especially powerful when DNA from parents can be analyzed so that identity by descent of alleles (i.e. the transmission of alleles from parents to affected offspring) can be determined. A major advantage of the affected sib-pair analysis is that it requires no assumptions regarding frequency, penetrance or mode of inheritance of the disorder. In addition, the analysis has the ability to exclude loci as well as to link them to disease susceptibility. The transmission/disequilibrium test, originally developed to test for linkage when a marker near a candidate gene was found to be associated with a disease, is another tool for linking a complex disease with a genetic marker, even if there is no prior evidence of association[12]. At present there are several on-going family studies searching for genes linked to PCOS[2,13] and endometriosis[4].

The genome-wide screening methods usually fall short of identifying the specific genes involved. The disorder may be linked to a specific chromosome segment that may encompass several million base pairs. The next step is to further narrow the search in the region using educated guesses, in which genes already known to be in the chromosomal location of interest are examined for DNA sequence variations linked to disease susceptibility. A more laborious option is the systematic analysis of DNA in the linked region, which generally entails the sequence analysis of genomic DNA fragments and their assembly into contigs, overlapping DNA pieces, spanning the region of interest. Even with recent advances in manipulating genomic DNA, the human genome presents the daunting problem of being packed with large interruptions in most genes. These intervening sequences (introns) are interspersed among the exons, which contain the genetic information that encodes the amino acid sequence of proteins. Because introns can be quite large (kilobase pairs) and exons are generally small, averaging some 130 base pairs in size, much of the DNA sequence generated may be of little value to gene hunters. However, computer programs can usually pinpoint coding sequences in genomic DNA with accuracy based on the knowledge of characteristic boundary sequences surrounding exons and other motifs that are associated with genes.

The analysis of genomes of lower organisms has provided some efficient means of identifying genes in large fragments of the human genome. *Fugu ruprides*, the puffer fish, has a compact genome that is approximately one-eighth the size of the human genome[14]. The exons of puffer fish genes are separated by relatively small introns of about 100 base pairs. Because of the reasonably strong homology of genes between species, puffer fish homologs of human genes can be identified by screening puffer fish genomic DNA libraries with human genomic DNA fragments. The gene-rich puffer fish clones with their smaller introns can quickly yield potential candidates for further analysis of the human genome.

While the search for genes linked to susceptibility to common reproductive disorders such as PCOS and endometriosis represents a major enterprise engaging clinicians to recruit and phenotype families, and molecular geneticists to analyze genotypes and linkage, the rewards of these endeavors will be substantial in that the identification of genes linked to disease susceptibility will provide needed clues to the underlying pathophysiology of complicated disorders, effective means to identify subjects at risk so that the outcomes of therapeutic interventions can be clearly evaluated, and new therapeutic approaches.

References

1. Fauser BCJM, Hsueh AJW. Genetic basis of human reproductive endocrine disorders. *Hum Reprod* 1995;10:826–46
2. Franks S, Gharani N, Waterworth D, *et al*. The genetic basis of polycystic ovary syndrome. *Hum Reprod* 1997;12:2641–8
3. Legro RS, Driscoll D, Strauss JF III, Fox J, Dunaif A. Evidence for a genetic basis for hyperandrogenemia in polycystic ovary syndrome. *Proc Natl Acad Sci USA* 1998;95:14956–60
4. Kennedy S. Is there a genetic basis to endometriosis? *Semin Reprod Endocrinol* 1997;15:309–17
5. Baranova H, Bothorishvilli R, Canis M, *et al*. Glutathione *S*-transferase M1 gene polymorphism and susceptibility to endometriosis in a French population. *Mol Hum Reprod* 1997;3:775–80
6. Roberts AK, Monzon-Bordonaba F, Van Deerlin PG, *et al*. A polymorphism within the promoter of the tumor necrosis factor-α gene is associated with an increased risk of preterm premature rupture of the fetal membranes. *Am J Obstet Gynecol* 1999; in press
7. Morgan T, Craven C, Ward K. Human spiral artery–angiotensin system. *Hypertension* 1998;32:683–7
8. Morgan L, Crawshaw S, Baker PN, Brookfield JFY, Pipkin FB, Kalsheker, N. Distortion of maternal–fetal angiotensin II type 1 receptor allele transmission in pre-eclampsia. *J Med Genet* 1998;35:632–6
9. Sohda S, Arinami T, Hamada H, Yamada N, Hamaguchi H, Kubo T. Methelenetetrahydrofolate reductase polymorphism and pre-eclampsia. *J Med Genet* 1997;34:525–6
10. Dizon-Townson DS, Nelson LM, Easton K, Ward K. The factor V Leiden mutation may predispose women to severe pre-eclampsia. *Am J Obstet Gynecol* 1996;175:902–5

11. Weeks DE, Lathrop GM. Polygenic disease; methods for mapping complex disease traits. *Trends Genet* 1995;11:513 19
12. Spielman RS, Ewens WJ. The TDT and other family-based tests for linkage disequilibrium and association. *Am J Hum Genet* 1996;59:983–9
13. Urbanek M, Driscoll DA, Legro RS, Dunaif A, Strauss JF, Spielman RS. Genetic analysis of candidate genes for polycystic ovary syndrome (PCOS). *Am J Hum Genet* 1998;63:A312
14. Mileham P, Brown SDM. The pufferfish genome: small is beautiful? *BioEssays* 1994;16:153–4

Medical recommendations for the safe use of mifepristone

41

R. Sitruk-Ware

Introduction

Mifepristone is a synthetic steroid, with oral antiprogesterone and antiglucocorticoid activities. The molecule has been developed essentially for indications where the antiprogesterone activity was required, namely in the termination of early pregnancy. Under physiological conditions, progesterone helps to maintain the uterine cervix tightly closed. The antiprogesterone properties of mifepristone suppress this effect and result in the softening and opening of the cervical os, permitting a further surgical procedure for termination of pregnancy in the first trimester. Also, in the later stages of pregnancy, the antiprogesterone activity potentiates the activity of prostaglandin treatment, leading to an expulsion with reduced doses of prostaglandins.

The mifepristone molecule has several other potential indications due to its antiprogesterone and antiglucocorticoid properties[1]. Unfortunately, they have not been fully developed owing to the philosophical debate and controversies opposing further research on this compound. Nevertheless, since the early 1980s, researchers have developed the molecule for four indications with large development programs. Several pilot trials have also been started for various indications in large academic centers all over the world. When the controversies reached their peak level, forcing the manufacturers to stop their activities on this molecule, only the World Health Organization (WHO) and the Population Council still had access to the compound and could run further trials. Since 1997, a new company has been created in order to resume the manufacturing and development of this fascinating molecule.

For the time being the product is approved for four different indications in France, Sweden and the UK and a European application is pending. In the USA, the Food and Drug Administration delivered a preliminary approval in 1996 for the medical termination of early pregnancy, pending the manufacturing of the active principle. Unfortunately, the aggressive attitude of the pro-life movements in that country are discouraging the manufacturers and delaying the introduction of the compound. In China, another similar molecule is available and has been used by millions of women with a different regimen to that approved in other countries.

On the basis of more than 10 years of use, the efficacy and safety of mifepristone has been confirmed. Nevertheless, several conditions are in place to control the safe use of the product and should be maintained.

Information on efficacy and safety, first established by formal clinical research, has been verified by general use in over 400 000 cases. The recommended protocol for patient management, as detailed on the product labelling for each country of registration, endorses careful clinical assessment and close patient management. Generally the medical profession in those countries closely adheres to the recommendations. This close adherence to the patient management protocols has allowed for the safe and effective transfer of the treatment from clinical trials to routine medical use.

Overview of existing data

Medical alternative to surgical termination of early intrauterine pregnancy

In the original studies carried out between 1983 and 1987 and using mifepristone alone, the overall success rate of early pregnancy termination was not satisfactory, ranging from 63.3 to 89.4%[2]. Results obtained after repeated doses did not differ significantly from those observed after a single dose of 600 mg. Based on a comparison of consecutive trials conducted with a standard protocol with dosages of 200, 400, 600 and 800 mg, it appeared that lower doses of 200 or 400 mg gave lower success rates than the higher dose of 600 mg. Among the failures, the rate of ongoing pregnancies was the highest with the lower dose of 200 mg, particularly when pregnancies of more than 41 days' amenorrhea were included (26.7%), as compared with 600 mg (8.7%). Therefore, the dosage of 600 mg as a single dose was selected in further studies, but the overall success rate was still disappointing, ranging from 76.3 to 87.0%.

Bygdeman and Swahn[3] showed that the addition of a prostaglandin administered 36–48 h after mifepristone significantly improves the success rate. Prostaglandins enhance uterine contractions and antiprogestins increase endometrial prostaglandin concentrations by inhibiting prostaglandin dehydrogenase, the progesterone-dependent enzyme that metabolizes the active prostaglandins, PGE_2 and $PGF_{2\alpha}$. As a consequence, there is accumulation of these active prostaglandins[4,5]. Antiprogestins have also been shown to increase the myometrial response to exogenous prostaglandin[3]. Given the unsatisfactory results with mifepristone alone, the method was therefore modified by the sequential use of prostaglandins 36 to 48 h later. The success rate increased significantly with this combination, which is the current approved method of medical termination of pregnancy in France, Sweden and the UK.

The first prostaglandin used in combination with mifepristone was the PGE_2 analog sulprostone, which was administered by injection. However, because of the occurrence of a death from myocardial infarction in a 38-year-old smoker and cardiovascular side-effects in other subjects, this agent was withdrawn[2]. The prostaglandins currently used with mifepristone are the PGE_1 analogs, misoprostol (given by the oral or vaginal route) or the vaginal pessary gemeprost. To date, no untoward cardiovascular events have been reported when these two prostaglandins are used together with antiprogestins, after follow-up of more than 400 000 treatments.

The success rate has been recorded in several clinical trials with both types of prostaglandin. In the literature about 19 trials have been published including a total number of 26 348 patients exposed to the treatment. The main recent trials included a total of 5445 patients[6–9].

Table 1 summarizes the results of large trials using misoprostol as the prostaglandin analog administered 36–48 h after mifepristone[6–8]. In women with duration of gestation of less than 49 days, the success rate reaches 95.5%, when oral misoprostol is used. With that prostaglandin, the rate of successful pregnancy

Table 1 Termination of pregnancy (TOP): first-trimester efficacy results in pivotal clinical trials with mifepristone 600 mg single dose

Reference	Prostaglandin used	Length of pregnancy	Success rate (%)	Incomplete TOP (%)	Ongoing pregnancies (%)	Hemostatic curettage (%)
7	MIS 400 µg	≤ 49	95.3	2.8	1.5	0.3
6	MIS 400 µg	≤ 49	95.5	3.1	1.2	0.2
		≤ 63	92.9	3.9	2.3	0.9
8	MIS 400 µg	≤ 49	92.3	4.6	1	1.4
		≤ 63	85.5	6.2	3.9	2.6
*	GEM 1 mg	≤ 49	98.7	1.3	0	0
11	GEM 1 mg	≤ 63	94.8	4.5	0.3	0.4

*Data on file; MIS, misoprostol; GEM, gemeprost

Table 2 Failure rates in clinical trials using 600 mg mifepristone and prostaglandins for termination of pregnancy

Prostaglandin used	Length of pregnancy (days)	Incomplete abortion	Ongoing pregnancy	Hemostatic curettage
Misoprostol	≤ 49	2.8–4.6%	1–1.5%	0.3–1.4%
Misoprostol	≤ 63	3.9–6.2%	2.3–3.9%	0.9–2.6%
Gemeprost	≤ 63	4.5%	0.3%	0.4%

termination decreases after 49 days while with gemeprost the success rate is similar up to 63 days[6–11].

Table 2 indicates the failure rates according to the age of pregnancy and the type of prostaglandin used in various clinical trials[6–9]. It includes incomplete abortion, ongoing pregnancy, and hemostatic curettage. Incomplete abortion and missed abortion are differently reported by clinicians. This explains some differences between series. In addition to adoption of a surgical procedure on medical grounds, some vacuum aspirations are performed on request of the patients, who do not wish to wait for the full protocol completion. These are classified in any case as treatment failure[8].

The choice between misoprostol and gemeprost following administration of 600 mg mifepristone is largely based on local practice and specific country regulations. Vaginal misoprostol administration has been reported to give better results than the oral administration[10], but the product has not been developed in the appropriate pharmaceutical form for vaginal delivery. Gemeprost is more potent than misoprostol[11], and if it is used the window of application can be extended to duration of gestation of up to 63 days with excellent efficacy[9,11].

Misoprostol is convenient because it is given orally and can be stored at room temperature; it seems to be better tolerated, as the proportion of women requiring pain relief treatment is lower when compared to gemeprost. Clinical experience is very extensive, as it has been given at high doses for a long period of time in patients with gastrointestinal indications. Gemeprost is given vaginally. Suppositories must be stored at −15°C. The safety profile of the two compounds appears comparable and the same precautions apply for these two prosta-

glandin analogs. While no serious cardiovascular adverse events have been observed with these two compounds, use of this method is still not recommended in women over 35 years of age who are smokers (more than 10 cigarettes daily) and in women with cardiovascular disease or risk factors. As the outcomes of medical and surgical methods are quite similar in terms of safety and efficacy, the choice should be left to the patients themselves. Preference studies show that if given a choice, the majority of women opt for medical abortion[12–14].

The question of the optimal effective dosage of mifepristone was raised in 1993 following results coming from a WHO trial comparing three doses of mifepristone: 200, 400 and 600 mg followed by gemeprost 1 mg[15]. This study showed no statistically significant difference in the numbers of complete abortions; 93.8% in the 200 mg group and 94.3% in the 600 mg group. However, missed abortion was observed in three cases (0.8%) and one case (0.3%) in the 200 mg and 400 mg groups, respectively, while none were observed in the 600 mg group. An ongoing viable pregnancy was observed in only one case in the 600 mg group and in two cases in the 200 and 400 mg groups. The absence of loss of efficacy with low doses of mifepristone documented by this WHO trial encouraged other studies. McKinley and colleagues[16] found identical percentages of women (93.6%) who had a complete abortion in the two groups randomized either to mifepristone 200 mg or mifepristone 600 mg followed by misoprostol 600 μg in a single dose. However, the complete abortion rate was significantly higher in women with ≤ 49 days' amenorrhea compared to women with 50–63 days amenorrhea (97.5 versus 89.1%, respectively). When the subgroups were considered in women with ≤ 49 days' amenorrhea 59/61 who received 200 mg had a complete abortion (96.7%) and 57/58 who received 600 mg had complete success (98.3%). The difference was not statistically significant.

Other studies conducted with mifepristone 200 mg were non-comparative with another mifepristone dosage[11,17–22]. Moreover, the prostaglandin was not used according to the current recommendations of dose or route of administration. When combined with misoprostol given orally at 600 or 800 µg the percentage of ongoing pregnancies was 2.5 to 4%.

The ultimate goal of medical interruption of pregnancy is to obtain efficacy which is comparable with that of surgical procedures, with the added benefit of avoiding surgery, anesthesia, access to the theater, infections and related risks. An overall success rate of 95% is obtained with mifepristone 600 mg followed by misoprostol 400 µg orally up to 49 days of amenorrhea, or gemeprost 1 mg vaginally up to 63 days of amenorrhea. The development of mifepristone combined with a prostaglandin was based on the assumption that the lowest dose of prostaglandin analog should be selected for safety purposes. The large experience of mifepristone used according to approved recommendations confirmed the efficacy and safety profile of the 600 mg dosage. Given the safety data obtained over 10 years of post-marketing surveillance and more than 400 000 treatments with this dosage, it would be necessary to accumulate similar follow-up information with another regimen where the mifepristone would be lowered and the prostaglandin dose increased. This approach, although proposed by some authors on economic grounds is not substantiated by medical reasons. The prostaglandins are known to give side-effects, including painful uterine cramping, nausea, vomiting and diarrhea. It would not be advisable to increase the dose recommended at the moment without further assessment of safety and acceptability of these newly proposed regimens. Data from mifepristone 200 mg with gemeprost 1 mg are still limited to the results of one trial. Efficacy and safety results comparing mifepristone 200 mg with 600 mg followed by misoprostol 400 µg are still lacking.

After mifepristone and prostaglandin treatment the rate of women lost to follow-up (LFU) was 0.6 to 1.8% in clinical trials. The real incidence of LFU may be higher. Should a woman change her mind and not return to the clinic for the prostaglandin administration, the risk of failure and an ongoing pregnancy is higher with a 200 mg dose of mifepristone than with the higher dose of 600 mg, as described above[23]. This potential risk precludes any modification of the currently recommended dosage of 600 mg of mifepristone followed by a low dose of prostaglandin analog 36 to 48 h later, as an efficient and safe medical alternative to surgical termination of first-trimester pregnancy.

Softening and dilatation of the uterine cervix prior to surgical pregnancy termination

Antiprogestins have numerous other obstetric and gynecological applications. In addition to their ability to enhance myometrial contractility, antiprogestins also dilate and soften the uterine cervix. The available data indicate that antiprogestins do not act on the cervix by stimulating endogenous prostaglandin production[24]; rather, their action originates from inflammatory cells and chemotactic agents such as cytokines (e.g. interleukin-8 and interleukin-1)[25]. Indeed, it has been shown that progesterone inhibits and mifepristone stimulates interleukin-8 release in human choriodecidual cells *in vitro*[26]. Because of their action on the uterine cervix, antiprogestins are useful in the preoperative preparation of women for first-trimester vacuum aspiration. Mifepristone is usually administered 48 h prior to surgical abortion, is as effective as prostaglandins and has significantly fewer side-effects[27].

In a randomized double-blind, placebo-controlled dose-finding study[28], the effects of mifepristone at 50, 100, 200, 400 or 600 mg were evaluated at 24 and 48 h after administration. A total of 181 women were included (mean age 25.12 ± 0.39 years; mean gestational age 67.8 ± 0.75 days amenorrhea); 72 (40%) were nulliparous and 28% had had at least one previous termination of pregnancy.

Cervical dilatation increased over time ($p < 0.001$); maximal dilatation was observed at 48 h. There was a significant dose effect on dilatation of the cervix and the increase of cervical diameter was significantly different from placebo for each dose level from 100 mg (Dunnett's test, $p = 0.05$) at 48 h. As a function of parity, dilatation of the cervix was significantly increased in women with parity ≥ 1 at all times, but there was no significant difference in terms of increase in cervical dilatation. A significantly greater dilatation was observed at 48 h as a function of duration of amenorrhea ($p = 0.001$).

Decreased cervical resistance by mifepristone facilitates mechanical dilatation and shortens the duration of the surgical procedure. Indeed, a significant relation between dose of mifepristone and duration of surgical procedure was observed, the 600 mg group having a shorter duration by 4 min than the placebo group ($p = 0.003$)[28].

In several other studies[27,29–33], pretreatment with mifepristone caused significant dilatation of the cervix versus placebo. Also, cervical resistance was significantly reduced in all studies where mifepristone was administered at 200 or 600 mg, 24 to 48 h before aspiration, but not with a shorter interval of 12 h. A significant increase was seen in the percentage of women with easy dilatation as perceived by the surgeon[27,29–33].

In comparison with placebo, mifepristone has shown its efficacy in cervical dilatation and softening. Its cervical effects appear comparable with those of gemeprost and dilators. In comparison with dilators and prostaglandin analogs, mifepristone has the advantage of ease of administration (without need for monitoring or hospitalization before vacuum aspiration) and a superior safety profile (abdominal pain of moderate intensity, absence of hemodynamic risk). Moreover, mifepristone antagonizes the physiological effect of progesterone on the cervix and therefore appears more appropriate for this indication.

As far as side-effects are concerned, in the clinical trials no heavy bleeding was observed after mifepristone administration and before the surgical procedure. Peri- and postoperative blood loss was comparable with and without mifepristone preparation. The quantity of perioperative blood loss was not related to mifepristone dose or parity, but there was a significant increase in blood loss with duration of amenorrhea ($p < 0.001$).

Expulsion of products of conception occurred in 0.9% of cases before vacuum aspiration and required ultrasound examination to confirm the completeness of abortion. Although no case of heavy bleeding was recorded in the clinical trials, in post-marketing surveillance a few cases of heavy bleeding occurring after mifepristone and before surgery, and related to retained products after ovular expulsion, have been reported. In all cases the delay between mifepristone intake and the scheduled surgical procedure was longer than 48 h. These events led to the recommendation to limit to 36–48 h the interval between the treatment and the surgical procedure.

Preparation for the action of prostaglandin analogs in the termination of pregnancy for medical reasons (beyond the first trimester)

Termination of pregnancy for medical reasons in the second trimester can be performed either by surgical methods involving cervical dilatation and uterine evacuation, or by medical means using prostaglandins. However, surgical procedures expose patients to the risks of cervical damage and uterine perforation, which increase with duration of gestation. Prostaglandin-induced abortions are particularly unpleasant as the process lasts longer and is more painful than at earlier stages of gestation. The use of mifepristone has dramatically improved this procedure, in that it significantly reduces the time from first administration of prostaglandin to expulsion of the fetus, as well as reducing both prostaglandin and analgesic requirements.

Trials have been conducted in which mifepristone was used either in a placebo-controlled, randomized comparative manner, or in open studies[34–36]. The gestational ages of the women ranged between 12 and 21 weeks of amenorrhea. Primigravid patients and patients of mixed parity were included. The main efficacy criteria evaluated in these trials were as follows. Firstly, the interval between the initiation of prostaglandin treatment and fetal expulsion (induction-to-abortion interval) and the abortion rate within 12 h and 24 h were assessed. Also, efficacy was measured by recording the dose of prostaglandin used, and the need for adjuvant therapy or surgical procedure (in cases of incomplete expulsion or retained placenta), as well as the duration of hospital stay.

Pretreatment with mifepristone reduced the interval between prostaglandin administration and expulsion. Furthermore, the dose of prostaglandin required was reduced and the women experienced considerably less pain[34–36]. In most of the studies, the median induction-to-abortion time was about 7 h after pretreatment with mifepristone, and about 92 to 98% of women aborted within 24 h of starting the prostaglandin regimen. In a placebo-controlled study, the percentage of women expelling within 24 h was 91% in the mifepristone group versus 80% in the placebo group, receiving prostaglandin alone[34].

The dose of prostaglandin required to induce abortion with the use of mifepristone was reduced. In the study by Rodger and Baird[34], the median dose of gemeprost in the mifepristone group was 3 mg (range 1–10 mg), and 5 mg (range 2–10 mg) in the placebo group. Also, the duration of hospital stay was significantly reduced in the group of women treated with mifepristone versus placebo: 91% (mifepristone) vs. 72% (placebo) of women stayed two nights.

When compared to other methods such as the use of laminaria, the induction-to-abortion interval was significantly shorter after preparation with mifepristone[36].

In the interval between mifepristone administration and prostaglandin induction, vomiting, nausea and headache were the most commonly reported adverse events. During this period, a total of 7.3% of patients reported some vaginal bleeding and 28.5% of patients reported abdominal or pelvic pain. Following prosta-

glandin administration, vomiting, pelvic pain and nausea were the most frequently reported side-effects. At the follow-up visit 2–4 weeks post-termination, 19 patients (7.1%) reported vaginal bleeding or retained products.

In summary, in the context of therapeutic termination of pregnancy, mifepristone (600 mg dosage) has been shown to reduce the time between prostaglandin induction administered 36 to 48 h later and fetal expulsion. Consequently, the prostaglandin requirements are significantly reduced, as is the duration of stay in hospital. However, complications related to prostaglandins may occur and close monitoring is mandatory, especially in women with previous Cesarean section, due to the potential risk of uterine rupture.

Labor induction for expulsion of a dead fetus

Intrauterine fetal death during the second or third trimester exposes the mother to the risk of intrauterine sepsis and disseminated intravascular coagulation. These complications increase with prolongation of the induction–abortion interval. Different protocols for labor induction have been developed, using mainly prostaglandins. However, prostaglandins are known to induce side-effects, some of them serious (e.g. uterine rupture or hyperstimulation). Methods of cervical dilatation are therefore sought in order to reduce the dose of prostaglandin given and ensure safe expulsion of the dead fetus.

Two clinical studies comparing mifepristone with placebo confirmed the efficacy of mifepristone in termination of pregnancy after intrauterine death[37,38]. In both studies, significantly more patients expelled within 72 h after the first drug intake in the mifepristone group as compared to the placebo group. Bishop's scores after treatment were higher in the mifepristone group than in the placebo group. Cabrol and colleagues[37] recorded uterine contractions within 72 h of treatment intake in 47.2% of the patients in the placebo group and in 81% in the mifepristone group ($p < 0.002$). There was no significant variation in the mean systolic and diastolic blood pressures and in the mean heart rate during treatment, in either the placebo or the mifepristone groups. Painful uterine contractions were more frequent in the mifepristone group (40.5%) than in the placebo group (8.3%) ($p < 0.0006$). Uterine bleeding was reported as an adverse event in three cases but this bleeding was judged to be of mild or moderate intensity and did not require a hemostatic surgical procedure or a blood transfusion. No significant variations in the results of the hematological or biochemical examinations were observed after mifepristone or placebo. Cortisol and adrenocorticotropic hormone levels were significantly modified by mifepristone treatment[38]. This was secondary to the well-known antiglucocorticoid activity of mifepristone, with no clinical consequences.

These two placebo-controlled studies indicate that mifepristone can be useful in the management of intrauterine fetal death. The administration of 600 mg per day of mifepristone for 2 days provokes fetal expulsion within 72 h in 63% of cases. The observed changes in Bishop's scores confirm that mifepristone acts partly by inducing cervical ripening. Mifepristone is less rapidly effective than prostaglandins, but it is more physiological than prostaglandins as it antagonizes the progesterone effect on the cervix and can be a useful alternative in cases of contraindications to, or side-effects of, prostaglandins. The dose to be administered is 600 mg per day for 2 days. If fetal expulsion does not occur within 72 h after the first drug intake, other measures should be undertaken to provoke expulsion.

General safety issues and recommendations

For approved therapeutic indications, the use of mifepristone must follow the recommendations of the summary of product characteristics. In all instances this product should never be prescribed in the following situations: chronic adrenal failure; known allergy to mifepristone or to any component of the product; and severe asthma uncontrolled by corticosteroid therapy. Due to the antiglucocorticoid activity of mifepristone, the efficacy of long-term corticosteroid therapy may be decreased during the 3 to 4 days following mifepristone intake and therapy should be adjusted. As a precaution and in the absence of specific studies, mifepristone should not be used in patients with renal failure, liver failure and malnutrition.

Contraindications to the use of prostaglandin must be carefully excluded. According to the type of prostaglandin used, and due to the potent vasoconstrictive effect of some analogs, it is necessary to withdraw therapy from patients with a previous history of cardiovascular disease, especially of an ischemic nature.

The follow-up of patients is of the utmost importance. Firstly, it allows diagnosis of failure and ongoing pregnancy at an early stage, when surgery could complement the method. Secondly, should the woman still be bleeding at the follow-up visit, control of the β-human chorionic gonadotropin levels allows the diagnosis of an unnoticed ectopic pregnancy and appropriate therapy may be administered on time.

When used according to the recommendations, the product is well tolerated and no major issues are of concern. However, the main problems with the use of mifepristone in termination of pregnancy remain the event of heavy or prolonged bleedings and the issue of patients lost to follow-up and the risk of ongoing pregnancies.

Bleeding

All women included in the clinical trials experienced some bleeding as a result of the therapeutic process. Bleeding tended to increase from spotting–light before prostaglandin administration to light–moderate at 4 h post-prostaglandin. On average, 10% of women complained of excessive bleeding. Heavy bleeding needed hemostatic curettage in 0.3 to 1.4% (Table 2). Transfusion was needed in 0.25% of cases. Hemoglobin variations showed a small but significant decrease of 0.5 to 0.8 g/dl[6–8]. It is mandatory therefore to inform women about the risk of heavy bleeding and give them instructions to follow in case of emergency. Women living in areas where no medical facilities are available in the case of such events should not be included in the medical protocol for termination of pregnancy.

Ongoing pregnancies

There are several case reports of normal pregnancies and offspring when women have taken mifepristone alone or in combination with a prostaglandin, have not aborted and have elected to continue their pregnancies[39,40]. Medical termination of pregnancy efficacy is rated at 97% success but the overall risk of ongoing pregnancies according to the clinical studies varies between 0.3 and 1.4%. Between 1987 and 1998, 71 cases of ongoing pregnancies were recorded after medical termination, representing more than 10 years of surveillance[39]. Twenty-one cases used mifepristone alone and in 50 it was associated with a prostaglandin (misoprostol, $n = 22$; sulprostone, $n = 4$; gemeprost, $n = 10$; 14 cases with either a non-specific prostaglandin or unknown). Twenty-four normal babies were born but eight cases were reported with various defects identified at term or in the fetus. All but one of these abnormal cases used gemeprost, and no malformations were reported with mifepristone associated with misoprostol or sulprostone. However, it has been reported that misoprostol, when used alone and illegaly for pregnancy termination, may be associated with teratogenic effects[41,42]. In rabbits, occasional skull deformities occurred after exposure of the animals to mifepristone. Although these observations were not found in rats and mice, the rare anomalies seen in the rabbit were attributed to mechanical effects secondary to uterine contractions because of the decrease in progesterone activity[43]. Because of this, the manufacturer of mifepristone recommends firstly that the control visit takes place a mandatory 10–14 days after mifepristone intake, in order to control for the uterine vacuity, and secondly that in the case of failure of the method the pregnancy should be terminated by surgery.

Conditions of administration

The use of mifepristone for early medical termination of pregnancy has been part of a well-controlled protocol. The woman should receive the prostaglandin in a hospital or clinic setting, especially when gestation exceeds 49 days. However, it has recently been proposed that the present strict conditions of administration of the method should be relaxed, and the use of prostaglandins allowed at home, especially due to the good tolerability of misoprostol[44].

Although the results of a study conducted in the USA[44] concluded the feasibility of this change in the method, in less medically sophisticated environments, with reduced access to hospital facilities in case of emergency a hemorrhage could prove fatal. Although rare, hemorrhage requiring surgical intervention or transfusion can occur within the first few hours following administration of the prostaglandin, when the patient is under supervision in the hospital or clinic. Thus far these incidences have been managed quickly with good outcome and have not resulted in emergency readmission to hospital. Less controlled use may yield poorer and unacceptable outcomes.

Other potential indications

Mifepristone is under evaluation for labor induction. At this stage, no definite conclusion can be drawn concerning optimal dosage. In one placebo-controlled trial, 200 mg mifepristone caused onset of labor or favorable cervical conditions (Bishop score ≥ 6) in a higher percentage of women than in the placebo group[45]. More safety data are necessary, taking into consideration the observed higher rate of acute fetal distress under mifepristone than under placebo in some trials.

As emergency post-coital contraception, 600 mg mifepristone obtained comparable results to a high dose of estrogens and progestins[46–47]. Safety was satisfactory, with less nausea, vomiting or breast tenderness in the mifepristone group. In a recent study by the

WHO, lower doses of 10 and 50 mg showed similar efficacy in preventing pregnancy[48].

Early luteal contraception has been investigated (200 mg single dose, 2 days after the urinary luteinizing hormone surge on a monthly basis) but data are still limited[49]. Lower doses of 5 mg daily have been used in volunteers. The treatment resulted in a significant decrease in pregnancy rate without affecting the menstrual cycle or causing disturbing side-effects. However, the contraceptive effect needs to be improved[49,50]. Also, continuous administration of low doses of mifepristone associated with a progestin in the second part of the cycle proved effective in suppressing ovulation[5].

Information on the safety of mifepristone after repeated administration are provided by pilot studies in breast cancer[52,53], meningioma[54,55], endometriosis[56] and uterine leiomyomata[57], in which mifepristone was used according to indications at 50 to 200 mg daily for several months. Pilot phase 2 studies have been reported in advanced breast carcinoma. They were conducted either in patients who had failed with other therapy or in subjects who had received no previous medical therapy[52,53]. The results in these studies have been disappointing and no more than 18% complete or partial responses were recorded.

Antiprogestins have also been proposed in the treatment of tumors which contain steroid receptors, such as meningiomas. Antiprogestins inhibit growth of meningioma cells in culture and reduce the size of human meningiomas implanted into nude mice[13]. In pilot studies, 200 mg was given daily to patients with unresectable meningiomas[54,55]. In one study in which treatment was given for up to 62 months to a total of 28 patients, eight subjects demonstrated objective responses as shown by reduced tumor size on computed tomography or magnetic resonance scan and improvement in visual field examination[54]. A randomized double-blind placebo-controlled phase 3 trial is currently underway to confirm the activity of mifepristone in unresectable meningioma.

In clinical studies conducted in patients with endometriosis, with daily administration of mifepristone doses of 50 mg for 6 months, there was an improvement in pelvic pain and a decrease in the extent of disease as determined by laparoscopy[56].

Mifepristone has also been used in patients with leiomyomata. In a 3-month study of daily treatment with mifepristone in doses of 25 and 50 mg there was a significant decrease in leiomyoma volume[57].

Studies in animals have suggested that antiprogestins could be used for other tumors including gliomas and ovarian, prostate and endometrial cancers[2]. Mifepristone also binds to the glucocorticoid receptor and displays potent antiglucocorticoid properties applicable in Cushing's syndrome[1,2]. Higher doses of mifepristone are required to produce an antiglucocorticoid as compared to an antiprogestin effect[2]. High-dose continuous mifepristone administration (5–22 mg/kg/day) has been used to treat Cushing's syndrome due to ectopic adrenocorticotropic hormone (ACTH) secretion and adrenal carcinoma[58]. Mifepristone has been shown to normalize the Cushingoid phenotype, ameliorate depression, decrease hypertension, eliminate abnormal carbohydrate metabolism and correct glucocorticoid-induced gonadal and thyroid hormone suppression[58]. However, this drug cannot be used in Cushing's disease in which the hypothalamic–pituitary–adrenal axis is intact but regulated at a higher set point. Under these circumstances the mifepristone-induced increase in ACTH and cortisol secretion may overcome the glucocorticoid receptor blockade[2]. Mifepristone, however, could be used to prepare a patient for surgery. Moreover, it has few side-effects as compared to those observed with other agents used to treat these patients[2].

Conclusion

The discovery of mifepristone, the first antiprogesterone molecule, was a major breakthrough in reproductive medicine. Unfortunately, protests from pro-life groups have tried to intimidate researchers developing the many potential medical uses of this molecule. It is hard to understand why, in developed countries where abortion is legally accepted, the advantages offered by this medical alternative are denied to women. It is obvious that the molecule can bring to developing countries a tremendous improvement in abortive procedures, provided the therapy is used where surgical facilities exist but are over-stretched by the enormous demand. Besides the ethical debate on abortion in general, mifepristone has brought such important promise to the field of reproduction and research in general, that it is hard to believe its further development can now be stopped at the turn of the next millennium.

References

1. Baulieu EE. Contragestion and other clinical applications of RU 486, an antiprogesterone at the receptor. *Science* 1989;245:1351–7
2. Spitz IM, Bardin CW. Clinical pharmacology of RU 486 – an antiprogestin and antiglucocorticoid. *Contraception* 1993;48:403–44
3. Bygdeman M, Swahn ML. Progesterone receptor blockage. Effect on uterine contractility and early pregnancy. *Contraception* 1985;32:45–51
4. Cheng L, Kelly RW, Thong KJ *et al.* The effects of mifepristone (RU486) on prostaglandin dehydrogenase in decidual and chorionic tissue in early pregnancy. *Hum Reprod* 1993;8:705–9
5. Cheng L, Kelly RW, Thong KJ, *et al.* The effect of mifepristone (RU 486) on the immunohistochemical distribution of prostaglandin E and its metabolite in decidual and chorionic tissue in early pregnancy. *J Clin Endocrinol Metab* 1993;77:873–7
6. Peyron R, Aubeny E, Targosz V, *et al.* Early termination of pregnancy with mifepristone (RU 486) and the orally-active prostaglandin misoprostol. *N Engl J Med* 1993;328:1509–13
7. Aubeny E, Peyron R, Turpin CC, *et al.* Termination of early pregnancy (up to and after 63 days of amenorrhea) with mifepristone (RU 486) and increasing doses of misoprostol. *Int J Fertil* 1995;40:85–91
8. Spitz IM, Benton L, Bardin CW, *et al.* Early pregnancy termination with mifepristone and misoprostol in the United States. *N Engl J Med* 1998;338:1241–7
9. Urquhart DR, Templeton AA, Shimewi F, *et al.* The efficacy and tolerance of mifepristone and prostaglandin in termination of pregnancy of less than 63 days of gestation – U.K. multicenter study final results. *Contraception* 1997;55:1–5
10. El-Refaey H, Rajasekar D, Abdalla M, *et al.* Induction of abortion with mifepristone (RU 486) and oral or vaginal misoprostol. *N Engl J Med* 1995;332:983–7
11. Baird DT, Sukcharoen N, Thong KJ. Randomized trial of misoprostol and cervagem in combination with a reduced dose of mifepristone for induction of abortion. *Hum Reprod* 1995;10:1521–7
12. Bachelot A, Cludy L, Spira A. Conditions for choosing between drug-induced and surgical abortions. *Contraception* 1992;45:547–59
13. Henshaw RC, Naji SA, Russell IT, *et al.* Comparison of medical abortion with surgical vacuum aspiration: women's preferences and acceptability of treatment. *Br Med J* 1993;307:714–17
14. Howie FL, Henshaw RC, Naji SA, *et al.* Medical abortion or vacuum aspiration? Two-year follow-up of a patient preference trial. *Br J Obstet Gynaecol* 1997;104:829–33
15. Van Look PFA, the WHO. Taskforce on postovulatory methods of fertility regulation. Termination of pregnancy with reduced doses of mifepristone. *Br Med J* 1993;307:532–7
16. McKinley C, Thong KJ, Baird DT. The effect of dose of mifepristone and gestation on the efficacy of medical abortion with mifepristone and misoprostol. *Hum Reprod* 1993;8(9):1502–5
17. El Refaey H, Templeton A. Early abortion induction by a combination of mifepristone and oral misoprostol: a comparison between two dose regimens of misoprostol and their effect on blood pressure. *Br J Obstet Gynaecol* 1994;101:792–6
18. Penney GC, McKessock L, Rispin R, *et al.* An effective, low-cost regimen for early medical abortion. *Br J Fam Plann* 1995;21:5–6
19. Thong KJ, Baird DT. Induction of abortion with mifepristone and misoprostol in early pregnancy. *Br J Obstet Gynaecol* 1992;99:1004–7
20. Weeks AD, Stewart P. The use of low-dose mifepristone and vaginal misoprostol for first-trimester termination of pregnancy. *Br J Fam Plann* 1995;21:85–6
21. Prasad RNV, Choolani M. Termination of early human pregnancy with either 50 mg or 200 mg

single oral dose of mifepristone in combination with either 0.5 mg or 1 mg vaginal gemeprost. *Aust NZ J Obstet Gynaecol* 1996;36(1):20–3

22. Ashok PW, Penney GC, Flett GMM, *et al.* An effective regimen for early medical abortion: a report of 2000 consecutive cases. *Hum Reprod* 1988; 13(10):2962–5

23. Ulmann A, Barnard J. Termination of pregnancy with mifepristone. *Br Med J* 1993;307:684

24. Radestad A, Bygdeman M. Are prostaglandins mediators of mifepristone (RU 486)-induced cervical softening in early pregnancy? *J Lipid Mediators* 1993;6:503–7

25. Chwalisz K, Stockemann K, Fuhrmann U, *et al.* Mechanism of action of antiprogestins in the pregnant uterus. *Ann NY Acad Sci* 1995;761: 202–23

26. Kelly RW, Leask R, Calder AA. Choriodecidual production of interleukin-8 and the mechanism of parturition. *Lancet* 1992;339:776–7

27. Henshaw RC, Templeton AA. Pre-operative cervical preparation before first-trimester vacuum aspiration: a randomized controlled comparison between gemeprost and mifepristone (RU 486). *Br J Obstet Gynaecol* 1991;98:1025–30

28. Lefebvre Y, Proulx L, Elie R, *et al.* The effects of RU-38486 on cervical ripening. *Am J Obstet Gynecol* 1990;162:61–5

29. Cohn M, Stewart P. Pretreatment of the primigravid uterine cervix with mifepristone 30 h prior to termination of pregnancy: a double-blind study. *Br J Obstet Gynaecol* 1991;98:778–82

30. Rädestad A, Christensen NJ, Stromberg L. Induced cervical ripening with mifepristone in first-trimester abortion. *Contraception* 1988;38: 301–12

31. Urquhart DR, Templeton AA. Mifepristone (RU 486) for cervical priming prior to surgically-induced abortion in the late first trimester. *Contraception* 1990;42:191–9

32. World Health Organization. The use of mifepristone (RU 486) for cervical preparation in first-trimester pregnancy termination by vacuum aspiration. *Br J Obstet Gynaecol* 1990;97:260–6

33. Gupta JK, Johnson N. Should we use prostaglandins, tents or progesterone antagonists for cervical ripening before first-trimester abortion? *Contraception* 1992;46:489–97

34. Rodger MW, Baird DT. Pretreatment with mifepristone (RU 486) reduces interval between prostaglandin administration and expulsion in second-trimester abortion. *Br J Obstet Gynaecol* 1990;97:41–5

35. UK Multicenter Study Group. Oral mifepristone 600 mg and vaginal gemeprost for mid-trimester induction of abortion. *Contraception* 1997;56: 361–6

36. Ho PC, Tsang SSK, Ma HK. Reducing the induction-to-abortion interval in termination of second-trimester pregnancies: a comparison of mifepristone with laminaria tent. *Br J Obstet Gynaecol* 1995;102:648–51

37. Cabrol D, Dubois C, Cronje H, *et al.* Induction of labor with mifepristone (RU 486) in intrauterine fetal death. *Am J Obstet Gynecol* 1990;163:540–2

38. Padayachi T, Moodley J, Norman RJ, *et al.* Termination of pregnancy with mifepristone after intrauterine death. Clinical and hormonal effects. *S Afr Med J* 1989;75:540–2

39. Sitruk-Ware R, Davey A, Sakiz E. Fetal malformation and failed medical termination of pregnancy. *Lancet* 1998;352:323

40. Pons J-C, Imbert M-C, Elefant E, *et al.* Development after exposure to mifepristone in early pregnancy. *Lancet* 1991;338:763

41. Fonseca W, Alencar AJC, Mota FSB, *et al.* Misoprostol and congenital malformations. *Lancet* 1991;338:56

42. Gonzalez CH, Vargas FR, Perez ABA, *et al.* Limb deficiency with or without Mbius sequence in seven Brazilian children associated with misoprostol use in the first trimester of pregnancy. *Am J Med Genet* 1993;47:59–64

43. Jost A. Animal reproduction. New data on the hormonal requirement of the pregnant rabbit: partial pregnancies and fetal anomalies resulting from treatment with a hormonal antagonist, given at a sub-abortive dosage. *CR Acad Sci Paris* 1986;303(111):281–4

44. Schaff EA, Stadalius LS, Eisinger SH, *et al.* Vaginal misoprostol administered at home after mifepristone (RU486) for abortion. *J Fam Pract* 1997;44:353–60

45. Frydman R, Lelaidier C, Baton-Saint-Mleux C, *et al.* Labor induction in women at term with mifepristone (RU486): a double-blind, randomized, placebo-controlled study. *Obstet Gynecol* 1992;80:972–5

46. Glasier A, Thong KJ, Dewar M, *et al.* Mifepristone (RU 486) compared with high-dose estrogen and progestogen for emergency postcoital contraception. *N Engl J Med* 1992;327:1041–4

47. Webb AMC, Russell J, Elstein M. Comparison of Yuzpe regimen, danazol, and mifepristone (RU 486) in oral postcoital contraception. *Br Med J* 1992;305:927–31

48. Piaggio G, Von Hertzen H, Grimes D, Van Look P. Task Force on Postovulatory Methods of Fertility Regulation. Comparison of three single doses of mifepristone as emergency contraception: a randomized trial. *Lancet* 1999;353:697–702

49. Gemzell-Danielsson K, Swahn M-L, Svalander P, *et al.* Early luteal phase treatment with mifepristone (RU 486) for fertility regulation. *Hum Reprod* 1993;8:870–3

50. Marions L, Gemzell-Danielsson K, Swahn ML, *et al.* Contraceptive efficacy of low doses of mifepristone. *Fertil Steril* 1998;70:813–16

51. Croxatto HB, Salvatierra AM, Croxatto HD, *et al.* Effects of continuous treatment with low-dose mifepristone throughout one menstrual cycle. *Hum Reprod* 1993;8:201–7

52. Romieu G, Maudelonde T, Ulmann A, *et al.* The antiprogestin RU 486 in advanced breast cancer: preliminary clinical trial. *Bull Cancer* 1987;74: 455–61

53. Perrault D, Eisenhauer EA, Pritchard Kl, *et al.* Phase II study of the progesterone antagonist mifepristone in patients with untreated metastatic breast carcinoma: a National Cancer Institute of Canada Clinical Trials Group Study. *J Clin Oncol* 1996;14:2709–12

54. Grunberg SM, Weiss MH, Spitz IM, *et al.* Treatment of unresectable meningiomas with the antiprogesterone agent mifepristone. *J Neurosurg* 1991;74:861–6

55. Lamberts SWJ, Fanghe HLJ, Avezaat CJJ, *et al.* Mifepristone (RU 486) treatment of meningiomas. *J Neurol Neurosurg Psychiatr* 1992;55: 486–90

56. Kettel LM, Murphy AA, Morales AJ, *et al.* Preliminary report on the treatment of endometriosis with low-dose mifepristone (RU 486). *Am J Obstet Gynecol* 1998;178:1151–6

57. Murphy AA, Morales AJ, Kettel LM, *et al.* Regression of uterine leiomyomata to the antiprogesterone RU 486: dose–response effect. *Fertil Steril* 1995;64:187–90

58. Nieman LK, Chrousos GP, Kellner C, *et al.* Successful treatment of Cushing's syndrome with the glucocorticoid antagonist RU 486. *J Clin Endocrinol Metab* 1985;61:536–40

Abortion induction with misoprostol 42

A. Faúndes

Introduction

Misoprostol is a synthetic analog of prostaglandin E_1. It has important differences from other prostaglandin analogs: it is stable at room temperature, is active by the oral and vaginal route, has fewer gastrointestinal effects, and has a much lower cost than other prostaglandins. Marketed under the commercial name of Cytotec, misoprostol has been licensed for the treatment of peptic ulcers in many countries.

The effectiveness of misoprostol for abortion induction was first tested as a complement to the administration of mifepristone[1]. In the same study the administration of oral misoprostol alone was rather inefficient in inducing abortion. After that, several other authors found that orally administered misoprostol was as effective as other prostaglandins, when used as a complement to mifepristone for the induction of early abortion, with a sucess rate of 90 to 95%[2,3].

The first study showing the effectiveness of vaginal administration of the drug was carried out in Mozambique by Bugalho and colleagues[4]. Based in the hypothesis that the mechanism of action of prostaglandins is through the induction of changes in the cervix, these authors decided to apply the tablets in the vagina, where they dissolve rapidly in the presence of minimal moisture. The study set out to evaluate the capacity of misoprostol to induce second- trimester abortion and found a 91% effectiveness with an initial dose ranging from 200 to 800 μg, followed by 200 μg every 12 h, always by the vaginal route. The authors concluded that 200 μg every 12 h was enough to induce second- trimester abortion, and that the dose should be repeated only if the cervix was not dilated and uterine contractility had not been established. Vacuum aspiration of the uterine cavity was carried out in all women, in order to prevent hemorrhage. Consequently, the authors did not have information on the proportion of abortions that were complete. Other authors confirmed the effectiveness of vaginal misoprostol for the induction of second-trimester abortion, using dosages of 200 to 400 μg, with intervals as short as every 3 h[5,6].

Another approach was tried by Creinin and Darney[7], who found that the administration of vaginal misoprostol was significantly more efficient in inducing first-trimester abortion when administered 4 days after receiving methotrexate at a dose of 50 mg/m^2 intramuscularly. Creinin found that such a regimen was not as effective when used after 56 days of amenorrhea[8], while it has 80% to 100% effectiveness in earlier pregnancies[9]. He used intramuscular or oral methotrexate, followed by 800 μg misoprostol 3 or 7 days later[10].

Another combination, successfully tested more recently, is the administration of 800 μg of vaginal misoprostol twice with a 24-h interval, after 4 days of treatment with 20 mg oral tamoxifen per day. A success rate of 92% in the termination of early pregnancy of 56 days or less was obtained with this regimen[11].

The use of misoprostol alone for the induction of first-trimester abortion is less effective than later in pregnancy, with a success rate of between 40 and 65%[12–14], using either one single dose of 800 μg, or 200 to 400 μg every 4 to 12 h, for a maximum of 48 h of treatment. Bugalho and colleagues[14] found that the higher the dose and the longer the duration of use, the greater the success rate of vaginal misoprostol alone for termination of early pregnancy. Abortion was obtained in 67% of women receiving 400 μg every 12 h and in 45% of those who used 200 μg of misoprostol at the same intervals. On the other hand, the success rate with 400 µg was just over 40% at 12 h, 50% at 24 h, 58% at 36 h and 67% at 48 h of treatment. Based on that observation the authors conclude 'that better results may be achieved by further increasing each dose, the frequency of administration, the duration of treatment or a combination of the three'[14]. Accordingly, Carbonell and associates[15] increased the dose to 800 µg and doubled the duration of treatment to 4 days, although they increased the interval to every 48 h. They reported a sucess rate of 93%.

What is not very clear in the analysis of the different studies is which proportion of the abortions can be classified as complete. The problem is that the definition of complete abortion varies from one author to another, and while some are willing to wait for up to 3 or 4 weeks, with the women tolerating moderate bleeding, others aspirate the uterine contents if there is any suspicion of remaining embryonic tissue. On the other hand, all authors coincide in concluding that even in the cases of failure to induce abortion, misoprostol administration promotes softening and dilatation of the cervix, which facilitates the surgical evacuation of the uterus by vacuum aspiration[16].

From a review of available literature, including reports on the use of vaginal misoprostol for the induction of labor, it is clear that there is a direct association between duration of pregnancy and sensitivity of the cervix and uterus to misoprostol. While the effective dose in early pregnancy appears to be no less than 800 µg, repeated several times, 200 µg appears to be sufficient in the second trimester, 100 µg is sufficient for the induction of labor at around 30 weeks, at least in the presence of fetal death[17], and only 50 to 25 µg are required for induction of labor at term[18–22].

The process of learning which is the appropriate interval between individual doses has been rather slow. Intervals ranging from every 3 to every 48 h can be found in the literature. Little attention has been given to one study of the plasma levels of misoprostol after oral and vaginal administration[23]. It shows rather stable levels that remain high for a longer period after vaginal administration, while a higher concentration, but with a much shorter half-life, is obtained with the oral administration. This study showed that the plasma levels remain close to the nadir up to 4 h after vaginal administration, suggesting that any interval shorter than 6 to 8 h would cause a summation of doses. The attending physician who prescribes misoprostol should be well aware of the presence of residual levels when the drug is given at short intervals. While this may not have very significant effects in the termination of early pregnancy, it may be disastrous at later gestational ages, up to the point of causing rupture of the uterus and maternal death.

It is also important to be aware of the secondary effects observed during the use of vaginal misoprostol. Although they are fewer than with oral administration and are negligible with the 25 µg dose used for labor induction, they are significant when doses of 400 or 800 µg are administered. Nausea is present in about 20% of subjects, vomit and fatigue in about 10% and diarrhea in 6 to 7%. However, the most common side-effect is low abdominal pain (70–75%), which is probably unavoidable and has to be treated with appropriate sedation, according to the severity of the symptom.

The availability of misoprostol in Brazil

The use of misoprostol for termination of early pregnancy was first reported in Fortaleza, the capital of the state of Ceará, situated in the northeast of Brazil. A survey of maternity records showed that misoprostol was mentioned in 12% of the induced abortion cases treated in 1988. By 1990, this proportion had increased to 70%[24]. In Goiânia, the capital of the state of Goiás, there was a three-fold increase in sales of misoprostol from 1987 to 1989, and sales remained at about the same level until 1991[25].

The rapid diffusion of the use of misoprostrol as an abortifacient in Brazil can be better understood considering that, for many years, women with delayed menses consulted staff in pharmacies, where they were given a drug that would make them bleed. A variety of different drugs have been used for this purpose. The information for patients in the commercially marketed product containing misoprostol includes a warning that it should not be used by pregnant women as it may provoke an abortion. This was good news for the pharmacy clerks, interested in selling, who thus obtained a more effective remedy for 'delayed menses' than those prescribed until then.

Not only pharmacy clerks, but the media and women themselves, were all responsible for disseminating information about the drug. A study carried out in Rio de Janeiro showed that most women who had used misoprostol (84%) had learnt about the drug from friends, relatives or colleagues and a small proportion (10%) directly from the pharmacist[26]. As news of the use of misoprostol to induce abortion entered the public domain, and considering that abortion is basically illegal in Brazil, the Ministry of Health decided, in 1991, to modify the regulations under which the drug could be marketed, in an attempt to restrict its use as an abortifacient. Under the new regulations, misoprostol may only be sold in drugstores, which retain a copy of the doctor's prescription for official use. Some states established even more severe restrictions. In Ceará, Cytotec was totally banned, and in Rio de Janeiro and Minas Gerais its use was limited to hospitals[27]. In São Paulo, the drug could be sold for gastrointestinal purposes only, with access limited to a few registered drugstores. Gynecological use in hospitals required authorization from the Ministry of Health. The analysis of sales shows a 50% decrease in the number of units sold in São Paulo between 1991 and 1996. The same data show that in a single month of 1996, 1186 units were sold in the state of São Paulo, while 3578 were sold in the much smaller state of Pernambuco, where less restrictive regulations were in place.

The government efforts to limit use of misoprostol were only partially successful. Studies carried out in Fortaleza, Goiânia and Recife between 1992 and 1996 showed that between 40 and 78% of women hospitalized with complications of induced abortion had used misoprostol[25,28,29]. The pharmacies continued to be the main source of supply. Misoprostol was available without prescription in 26% of 194 pharmacies visited by investigators in a study carried out in Recife in 1996.

The restrictions in the marketing of the drug resulted in a substantial increase in its cost. Nearly half of the women in the Recife study reported paying between US $30 and 40 for four tablets; at least five times the six dollars reported by women in 1991 in Rio de Janeiro[26].

The doses of misoprostol reported by women studied in Rio de Janeiro in 1991, when misoprostol was freely sold in flasks of 28 tablets of 200 µg each, varied from 200 to 16 800 µg (1–64 tablets); 65% took the drug by mouth, 29% used both oral and intravaginal routes of administration and 6% the vaginal route only[26]. It was obvious that women and pharmacy clerks had no idea which was the appropriate dose or route of administration[30].

The restrictions to the sale of misoprostol resulted in the creation of a black market and in an increase in the price. This had the positive effect of reducing the amount of drug used for abortion induction and, consequently, the risk of overdose was also reduced. This was shown by studies carried out after 1991, which showed that most women had induced abortion with doses of four tablets, administered simultaneously by mouth and intravaginally (90%, 75% and 78% in Fortaleza, Goiânia and Recife, respectively).

The concept that the vaginal route of administration is more efficient for abortion induction than the oral route was also slowly learnt by the Brazilian population, as shown by the increasing proportion of women who used misoprostol vaginally, in combination or not with oral administration, in the most recent studies[25].

A very important finding of studies carried out from 1995 on, is the lower complication rate among misoprostol users than among users of other methods. Hospital-based studies carried out in Goiânia and Recife showed a much lower rate of complication than in the Rio de Janeiro study of 1991, which may be related to the lower dose being used. In addition, these two studies confirmed that the rate of post-abortion infection and of severe infection (tubo-ovarian abscess and sepsis) was much lower than after any other form of clandestinely induced abortion[25,29]. The rate of infection reported by the most recent studies in Fortaleza and Recife was also considerably lower (9% and 15%, respectively) than that observed in 1991 in Rio de Janeiro, possibly reflecting women's improved understanding of the method as well as health professionals' improved management of misoprostol patients[28,31].

It has also been argued that although the complications following misoprostol use may be less severe, the widespread use of the drug may have given rise to a substantial increase in the numbers of women who decide to abort, reflected in the total number of hospital admissions for abortion complications[32]. The lack of reliable baseline data makes it difficult to evaluate whether such an increase occurred in the country in general. Nevertheless, a study conducted in the city of Goiânia, for the period 1987 to 1991, found no association between increased misoprostol sales and hospital admissions for complications of abortion[25].

The use of misoprostol is decreasing as the legislation becomes more restrictive. At the same time, a proportionate increase in the use of herbal teas and catheter insertion has been observed. The available data strongly suggest that misoprostol may have replaced some of the more dangerous abortion methods in the late 1980s and early 1990s, but the restrictions to the sale of the drug led to a return to the old abortion methods and, consequently, to an increase in the rate of severe complications in recent years. Although the available data are very limited, some recent studies give reason to be worried. A three-fold increase in maternal deaths resulting from abortion complications was observed in the city of Campinas, between 1991 and 1996[33]. As the numbers are small and the data are limited to one city, these results are not conclusive, but they indicate the need to be alert to a possible new burst of severe abortion complications, which had substantially decreased during the years misoprostol was widely available[29].

References

1. Wong KS, Ngai CSW, Chan KS, *et al.* Termination of second-trimester pregnancy with gemeprost and misoprostol: a randomized double-blind placebo-controlled trial. *Contraception* 1996;54:23–5
2. Thong KJ, Baird DT. Induction of abortion with mifepristone and misoprostol in early pregnancy. *Br J Obstet Gynaecol* 1992;99:1004–7
3. Guo-wei S, Li-Ju W, Qing-Xian S, *et al.* Termination of early pregnancy by two regimens of mifepristone with PG05 – a multicentre randomized clinical trial in China. *Contraception* 1994;50: 501–10
4. Bugalho A, Bique C, Almeida L, Faúndes A. The effectiveness of intravaginal misoprostol (Cytotec) in inducing abortion after 11 weeks of pregnancy. *Stud Fam Plann* 1993;24(5):319–23
5. Jain JK, Mishell DR Jr. A comparison of intravaginal misoprostol with prostaglandin E_2 for termination of second-trimester pregnancy. *N Engl J Med* 1994;331(5):290–3
6. Wong KS, Ngai CSW, Wong AYK, *et al.* Vaginal misoprostol compared with vaginal gemeprost in termination of second-trimester pregnancy. *Contraception* 1998;58:207–10
7. Creinin MD, Darney PD. Methotrexate and misoprostol for early abortion. *Contraception* 1993; 48(4):339–48
8. Creinin MD. Methotrexate and misoprostol for abortion at 57–63 days' gestation. *Contraception* 1994;50(6):511–15
9. Crenin MD, Vittinghoff E. Methotrexate and misoprostol vs. misoprostol alone for early abortion. *J Am Med Assoc* 1994;272:1190–5
10. Creinin MD. Oral methotrexate and vaginal misoprostol for early abortion. *Contraception* 1996;54:15–18
11. Mishell DR Jr, Jain JK, Byrne JD, Lacarra MDC. A medical method of early pregnancy termination using tamoxifen and misoprostol. *Contraception* 1998;58:1–6

12. Creinin MD, Park M. Acceptability of medical abortion with methotrexate and misoprostol. *Contraception* 1995;52:41–4

13. Koopersmith TB, Mishell DR Jr. The use of misoprostol for termination of early pregnancy. *Contraception* 1996;53(4):238–42

14. Bugalho A, Faúndes A, Jamisse L, *et al.* Evaluation of the efficacy of vaginal misoprostol to induce first-trimester abortion. *Contraception* 1996;53:243–6

15. Carbonell JLL, Varela L, Velazco A, Fernandez C. The use of misoprostol for termination of early pregnancy. *Contraception* 1997;55:165–8

16. Bokstrom H, Atterfelt M, Alexandersson M, *et al.* Preparative cervical softening before first-trimester legal abortion by mifepristone and misoprostol. *Contraception* 1998;58:157–63

17. Bugalho A, Bique C, Machungo F, Faúndes A. Induction of labor with intravaginal misoprostol in intrauterine fetal death. *Am J Obstet Gynecol* 1994;171(2):538–41

18. Bugalho A, Bique C, Machungo F, Faúndes A. Low-dose vaginal misoprostol for induction of labor with a live fetus. *Int J Gynecol Obstet* 1995;49:149–155

19. Wing DA, Jones MM, Rahall A, *et al.* A comparison of misoprostol and prostaglandin E_2 gel for preinduction cervical ripening and labor induction. *Am J Obstet Gynecol*, 1995;172(6):1804–10

20. Wing DA, Rahall A, Jones MM, *et al.* Misoprostol: an effective agent for cervical and labor induction. *Am J Obstet Gynecol* 1995;172(6):1811–16

21. Wing DA, Ortiz-Omphroy G, Paul RH. A comparison of intermittent vaginal administration of misoprostol with continuous dinoprostone for cervical ripening and labor induction. *Am J Obstet Gynecol* 1997;177(3):612–18

22. Farah LA, Sanchez-Ramos L, Rosa C, *et al.* Randomized trial of two doses of the prostaglandin E_1 analog misoprostol for labor induction. *Am J Obstet Gynecol* 1997;177(2):364–71

23. Zieman M, Fong SK, Benowitz NL, *et al.* Absorption kinetics of misoprostol with oral or vaginal administration. *Obstet Gynecol* 1997;90(1):88–92

24. Barros JAC. A medicalização da mulher no Brasil. In Wolffers I, Hardon A, Janssen J, eds. *O Marketing da Fertilidade.* São Paulo: Editora HUCITEC, 1991

25. Viggiano MGC, Faúndes A, Borges AL, *et al.* Disponibilidade de misoprostol e complicações de aborto provocado em Goiânia. *J Bras Ginec* 1996;106(3):55–61

26. Costa SH, Vessey PV. Misoprostol and illegal abortion in Rio de Janeiro, Brazil. *Lancet* 1993;341:1258–61

27. Sociedade Brasileira de Vigilância de Medicamentos, Instituto de Defesa do Consumidor (IDEC). (Approved by Comissão Técnica de Assessoramento em Assuntos de Medicamentos e Correlatos) *Technical Report on Misoprostol,* 1997

28. Fonseca W, Misago C, Corréia LL, *et al.* Determinantes do aborto provocado entre mulheres admitidas em hospitais em localidade da região Nordeste do Brasil. *Rev Saúde Pública* 1996;30(1):13–18

29. Faúndes A, Santos LC, Carvalho M, Gras C. Post-abortion complications after interruption of pregnancy with misoprostol. *Adv Contracept* 1996;12:1–9

30. Barbosa RM, Arilha M. The Brazilian experience with Cytotec. *Stud Fam Plann* 1993;24(4):236–40

31. Molina A. Acesso ao misoprostol para interrupcao da gravidez indesejada do Grande Recife. Presented at the *XII Jornada Pernambucana de Ginecologia e Obstetrícia,* Recife, March 1997

32. Coelho HLL, Teixeira AC, Santos AP, *et al.* Misoprostol and illegal abortion in Fortaleza, Brazil. *Lancet* 1993;341:1261–3

33. Parpinelli MA, Faúndes A, Surita FGC, Pereira BG, Cecatti JG. Mortalidade materna na cidade de Campinas, no período 1992 a 1994. *J Bras Ginec Obstet* 1999;in press

Studies of gossypol in the treatment of cancer

M. M. Reidenberg

Introduction

While most of the interest in gossypol in the past has been for its antifertility effect[1-5], there has been ongoing research into its potential as an antineoplastic drug.

In 1974, gossypol was entered into the US National Cancer Institute primary screening program. Its activity did not meet the criteria for further consideration at that time. The effect of gossypol in uncoupling oxidative phosphorylation of tumor cells was observed *ex vivo* in Ehrlich ascites tumor cells in 1983[6]. Gossypol was shown to be cytocidal to murine erythroleukemia cells in tissue culture in 1984[7]. Also in 1984, gossypol was given systemically to mice with implanted Ehrlich ascites tumors and found to prolong the life of the treated mice compared to controls[8]. Thus, by 1984, gossypol had been shown to be cytocidal to mouse cancer cells, and had prolonged the life of a murine model cancer. The proposed mechanism of action was related to energy metabolism, probably uncoupling oxidative phosphorylation or even inhibition of respiration.

During the 1980s, there was also interest in testing gossypol in many cancer cell lines for evidence of selective toxicity in cancer. Tuszynski and Cossu[9] tested gossypol in eight cancer cell lines and one normal fibroblast line. They found that most of the cancer cells (melanoma and colon carcinoma lines) were more sensitive to gossypol than the fibroblast line, demonstrating selective toxicity for the cancer. They also tried to evaluate the mechanism of action and found that the sensitive cell lines had mainly cathodic forms of lactic dehydrogenase (LDH) while the resistant cell lines had high levels of anodic LDH[9]. This research therefore supported the hypothesis that an effect on energy metabolism was the mechanism of action of gossypol.

In vivo testing of gossypol treatment of tumor-bearing mice revealed a prolonged survival of treated mice with a mouse breast adenocarcinoma but no prolongation of life of mice with two forms of mouse leukemia[10]. Other studies in the 1980s found human carcinoma cell lines more sensitive to gossypol than bone marrow stem cells, with sensitivity among the carcinoma lines correlating with the level of cathodic LDH in these cell lines[11]. A study of 14 human cell lines *in vitro* did not find selectivity for the cancer lines compared to fibroblasts or stimulated lymphocytes but did find the (−)enantiomer of gossypol to be several times more potent an antiproliferative drug than the (+)enantiomer[12]. Other early work on mechanism found that gossypol caused cell cycle arrest[13], inhibited DNA polymerase[14], inhibited topoisomerase II[15] and increased microviscosity of intracellular membranes[16].

Additional studies of tumor cell lines in tissue culture have revealed activity against human adrenocortical carcinoma[16], human gliomas[17], human breast cancers[18-19], human melanomas[20] and human prostate cancer cell lines[21]. Some of these studies also attempted to identify the mechanism of the cytotoxic effect. A study of five glioma cell lines[17] found that the sensitivity of the line correlated with the fraction of LDH that was cathodic. Two studies of the same human breast cancer cell lines (MCF-7 and MCF-7$_{Adr}$) found that sensitivity to gossypol was present in cells that expressed multidrug resistance[18,22].

A different mechanistic approach was taken by Benz and colleagues[23]. They found that gossypol, especially the (−)enantiomer, injured tumor endothelial cells reducing tumor blood flow in rats with implanted pancreatic tumors. It also increased the phosphorylated 27-kDa heat shock protein of cultured endothelial cells. They postulated an oxyradical injury of endothelial cells similar to the injury of ischemia–reperfusion[23].

A study of prostate cancer cells found that gossypol stimulated the expression of transforming growth factor-β[21]. Studies of both prostate and breast cancer cell lines found an arrest of cells in the G_0/G_1 phase, with failure of cells to advance to S phase[19,21]. One study of MCF-7 cells also found that gossypol inhibited the expression of cyclin D_1 and the retinoblastoma gene protein (Rb)[19].

Clinical trials

In addition to *in vitro* work, the study of human adrenocortical carcinoma cells has included implanting them in nude mice. The gossypol-treated mice had a lower tumor prevalence and a lower mortality at 12 weeks (8.3% vs. 41.6%)[16]. Based on this result, a clinical trial at the National Institutes of Health and the New York Hospital–Cornell Medical Center was carried out. Twenty-one patients were entered into the study. Nineteen had tumor progression while on mitotane and two had refused it. Eighteen patients completed at least 6 weeks of therapy at doses ranging from 30–70 mg/day of racemic gossypol acetic acid. Three had partial responses; one lasted 8 months, one 4 months, and one 1 year. The plasma gossypol concentrations in the three responders were similar to those in the non-responders. Side-effects were frequent but tolerable (xerostomia, transient transaminase elevation, dry skin, fatigue). No patient developed hypokalemia while on gossypol. Four patients developed paralytic ileus after 3 months of 40 mg/day or more. The paralytic ileus resolved in 1–2 weeks after stopping the gossypol[24].

The study of glioma cells lines has also included an *in vivo* experiment. Nude mice received implants of the BRW cell line from a patient with a primitive neuroectodermal tumor. Gossypol treatment inhibited tumor growth by 50% after 4 weeks of treatment compared to untreated controls[17]. Based on these results a clinical trial was carried out. Gossypol was given at a dose of 20 mg/day to 26 patients with recurrent glioblastomas or anaplastic astrocytomas. Of 22 evaluable patients, two had partial responses, four had stable disease, and 16 progressed. The partial responses lasted 8 and 71 weeks. Plasma gossypol levels were similar in the responders and non-responders. Eight patients developed hypokalemia. All were receiving dexamethasone in addition to the gossypol. Potassium supplementation corrected the problem[25,26].

With the data on breast cancer cell lines described above, we thought a breast cancer trial was warranted. To date, 14 women with metastatic breast cancer whose tumors were resistant to at least two chemotherapy regimens have been entered into the study. The doses given have ranged from 30–50 mg/day. Treatment was stopped for disease progression, toxicity, or lack of response after 8 weeks. The mean age of the patients was 52 (range 36–72), the mean number of organ system sites of metastases was three (1–5), and the mean number of prior chemotherapy regimens was three (2–6). The mean plasma gossypol concentration in seven patients was 311 ng/ml (range 214–465 ng/ml) after 4 weeks of therapy of 30 or 40 mg/day. Immunohistochemistry of serial biopsies of metastatic soft tissue lesions taken before and during gossypol treatment in four patients showed an increase in nuclear Rb and nuclear cyclin D_1 expression in three patients. In one patient, nuclear Rb increased and no cyclin D_1 was detected in either of the biopsies. Gossypol caused grade I–II fatigue, nausea, emesis, diarrhea and dysgeusia (altered taste sensation) in some patients. Two of three patients receiving 50 mg/day had dose-limiting skin toxicity. There were four evaluable patients receiving 30 mg/day, five receiving 40 mg/day, and one receiving 50 mg/day. One patient on 40 mg/day had a minor response. Two patients on 30 mg/day had decreased serum marker (BR2729)[27]. This study is being continued.

A preliminary study of 31 patients with a variety of advanced cancers was carried out by Stein and colleagues[28]. The doses of gossypol ranged from 30–180 mg per week (equivalent to 4–26 mg/day) for a median duration of 4 weeks. Some additional patients then received higher doses. Among 20 evaluable patients there were no episodes of tumor regression. Three patients had stable disease for 16, 19 and 23 weeks[28].

Current work to identify mechanism of action

The work outlined above suggests that gossypol may be promising as a new antineoplastic drug. Yet its mechanism of action is not clear. For these reasons, we have initiated an attempt, using molecular biological techniques, to determine the mechanism of cytotoxic action of gossypol. The controlled random homozygous knockout technique of Li and Cohen[29] is being used.

Mouse endothelial cells were infected with a retroviral gene search vector containing a regulated antisense promoter. Activation of the promoter produces antisense RNA to block transcripts from the adjacent gene (homozygous knockout). Cells resistant to gossypol indicate the knocked-out gene is involved in gossypol-induced cell death. Culture of wild-type cells for 2 days produces confluence, while with $8\mu M$ gossypol only a few cells are in the culture with 25% survival of those using fluorescent activated cell sorter analysis. Cells from a clone with active reverse transcriptase (T5g31) are near confluence after 2 days in $8\mu M$ gossypol with 89% survival while cells from this clone but with the reverse transcriptase inactivated (T5g31-cre) have a moderate number of adherent cells after 2 days in $8\mu M$ gossypol and 84% survival. Culture in $10\mu M$ gossypol for 2 days does not change the growth of T5g31 cells with 80% survival but further reduces the growth of T5g31-cre cells with 65% survival. Culture in $20\text{-}\mu M$ gossypol kills all cells. We conclude that at low concentrations, gossypol kills cells through a pathway dependent on a specific gene(s) yet to be identified[30]. This may account for the selectivity of the antifertility and antineoplastic effects of gossypol. Identification of this gene may be the first step leading to definitive knowledge about the mechanism of the selective cytotoxic action of gossypol. This knowledge may enable the design of a drug based on this mechanism that will be better than gossypol as an antineoplastic or antifertility drug.

References

1. Adams R, Geissman TA, Edwards JD. Gossypol, a pigment of cottonseed. *Chem Rev* 1960;60:555–74
2. National Co-ordinating Group on Male Anti-fertility Agents. Gossypol – a new antifertility agent for males. *Chin Med J* 1978;4:417–28
3. Qian SZ, Wang ZG. Gossypol: a potential anti-fertility agent for males. *Ann Rev Pharmacol Toxicol* 1984;24:329–60
4. Segal S, ed. *Gossypol: a Potential Contraceptive for Men*. New York, London: Plenum Press, 1985
5. Wu D. An overview of the clinical pharmacology and therapeutic potential of gossypol as a male contraceptive agent and in gynaecological disease. *Drugs* 1989;38:333–41
6. Floridi A, D'Atri S, Menichini R, *et al*. The effect of the association of gossypol and lonidamine on the energy metabolism of Ehrlich ascites tumor cells. *Exp Mol Pathol* 1983;38:322–35
7. Haspel HC, Ren YF, Watanabe KA, *et al*. Cytocidal effect of gossypol on cultured murine erythroleukemia cells is prevented by serum protein. *J Pharmacol Exp Ther* 1984;229:218–25
8. Tso WW. Gossypol inhibits Ehrlich ascites tumor cell proliferation. *Cancer Lett* 1984;24:257–61

9. Tuszynski GP, Cossu G. Differential cytotoxic effect of gossypol on human melanoma, colon carcinoma, and other tissue culture cell lines. *Cancer Res* 1984;44:768–71

10. Rao PN, Wang YC, Lotzova E, *et al.* Antitumor effects of gossypol on murine tumors. *Cancer Chemother Pharmacol* 1985;15:20–5

11. Benz C, Keniry M, Goldberg H. Selective toxicity of gossypol against epithelial tumors and its detection by magnetic resonance spectroscopy. *Contraception* 1988;37:221–8

12. Band V, Hoffer AP, Band H, *et al.* Antiproliferative effect of gossypol and its optical isomers on human reproductive cancer cell lines. *Gynecol Oncol* 1989;32:273–7

13. Wang YC, Rao PN. Effect of gossypol on DNA synthesis and cell cycle progression of mammalian cells *in vitro*. *Cancer Res* 1984;44:35–8

14. Rosenberg LJ, Adlakha RC, Desai DM, *et al.* Inhibition of DNA polymerase-α by gossypol. *Biochim Biophys Acta* 1986;866:258–67

15. Adlakha RC, Ashorn CL, Chan D, *et al.* Modulation of 4′-(9-acridinylamino) methanesulfon-*m*-anisidide-induced, topoisomerase II-mediated DNA cleavage by gossypol. *Cancer Res* 1989;49:2052–8

16. Wu Y-W, Chik CL, Knazek RA. An *in vitro* and *in vivo* study of antitumor effects of gossypol on human SW-13 adrenocortical carcinoma. *Cancer Res* 1989;49:3754–8

17. Coyle T, Levante S, Shetler M, *et al.* *In vitro* and *in vivo* cytotoxicity of gossypol against central nervous system tumor cell lines. *J Neurol Oncol* 1994;19:25–35

18. Gilbert NE, O'Reilly JE, Chang CJG, *et al.* Antiproliferative activity of gossypol and gossypolone on human breast cancer cells. *Life Sci* 1995;57:61–7

19. Ligueros M, Jeoung D, Tang B, *et al.* Gossypol inhibition of mitosis, cyclin D1 and Rb protein in human mammary cancer cells and cyclin-D1-transfected human fibrosarcoma cells. *Br J Cancer* 1997;76:21–8

20. Blackstaffe L, Shelley MD, Fish RG. Cytotoxicity of gossypol enantiomers and its quinone metabolite gossypolone in melanoma cell lines. *Melanoma Res* 1997;7:364–72

21. Shidaifat F, Canatan H, Kulp SK, *et al.* Inhibition of human prostate cancer cell growth by gossypol is associated with stimulation of transforming growth factor-β. *Cancer Lett* 1996;107:37–44

22. Jaroszewski JW, Kaplan O, Cohen JS. Action of gossypol and rhodamine 123 on wild-type and multidrug-resistant MCF-7 human breast cancer cells: 31P nuclear magnetic resonance and toxicity studies. *Cancer Res* 1990;50:6936–43

23. Benz CC, Iyer SB, Asgari HS, *et al.* Gossypol effects on endothelial cells and tumor blood flow. *Life Sci* 1991;49:PL67–72

24. Flack MR, Pyle RG, Mullen NM, *et al.* Oral gossypol in the treatment of metastatic adrenal cancer. *J Clin Endocrinol Metab* 1992;76:1019–24

25. Bushunow P, Reidenberg MM, Wasenko J, *et al.* Gossypol treatment of recurrent adult malignant gliomas. Naunyn-Schmiedeberg's *Arch Pharmacol* 1998;358(Suppl. 2):R533

26. Bushunow P, Reidenberg MM, Wasenko J, *et al.* Gossypol treatment of recurrent adult malignant gliomas. *J Neurol Oncol* 1999; in press

27. Seidman AD, Rosen P, Ligueros M, *et al.* Gossypol in advanced breast cancer. *J Invest Med* 1998;3:213A

28. Stein RC, Joseph AEA, Matlin SA, *et al.* A preliminary clinical study of gossypol in advanced human cancer. *Cancer Chemother Pharmacol* 1992;30:480–2

29. Li L, Cohen S. Tsg101: a novel tumor susceptibility gene isolated by controlled homozygous functional knockout of allelic loci in mammalian cells. *Cell* 1996;88:143–54

30. Qiu J, Reidenberg MM, Levin LR, *et al.* The search for gene(s) conferring sensitivity to cell killing by gossypol. *Fed Proc* 1999; in press

Index